Diagnosis and Treatment of Diseases of the Facial Skeleton, Oral Cavity, and Paranasal Sinuses

Diagnosis and Treatment of Diseases of the Facial Skeleton, Oral Cavity, and Paranasal Sinuses

Guest Editors

Kamil Nelke
Maciej Dobrzyński
Marceli Łukaszewski

MDPI

Basel • Beijing • Wuhan • Barcelona • Belgrade • Novi Sad • Cluj • Manchester

Guest Editors
Kamil Nelke
Maxillo-Facial Surgery Ward
EMC Hospital
Wrocław
Poland

Maciej Dobrzyński
Department of Pediatric
Dentistry and
Preclinical Dentistry
Wroclaw Medical University
Wroclaw
Poland

Marceli Łukaszewski
Department of Anesthesiology
and Intensive Care
Sokołowski Hospital
Wałbrzych
Poland

Editorial Office
MDPI AG
Grosspeteranlage 5
4052 Basel, Switzerland

This is a reprint of the Special Issue, published open access by the journal *Medicina* (ISSN 1648-9144), freely accessible at: https://www.mdpi.com/journal/medicina/special_issues/X7YMBI2F41.

For citation purposes, cite each article independently as indicated on the article page online and as indicated below:

Lastname, A.A.; Lastname, B.B. Article Title. *Journal Name* **Year**, *Volume Number*, Page Range.

ISBN 978-3-7258-6520-8 (Hbk)
ISBN 978-3-7258-6521-5 (PDF)
https://doi.org/10.3390/books978-3-7258-6521-5

Contents

Kamil Nelke, Maciej Dobrzyński and Marceli Łukaszewski
Editorial for the Special Issue "Diagnosis and Treatment of Diseases of the Facial Skeleton, Oral Cavity, and Paranasal Sinuses"
Reprinted from: *Medicina* **2025**, *61*, 2191, https://doi.org/10.3390/medicina61122191 1

Rahma Gamal Mostafa, Mohammad Ibrahim Hashim, Ahmed Abdulwahab Bawahab, Razan Abed A. Baloush, Mohammed S. Abdelwahed, Abdulkarim Hasan, et al.
Immunohistochemical Expression of Glucose Transporter-1 in Oral Epithelial Dysplasia and Different Grades of Oral Squamous Cell Carcinoma
Reprinted from: *Medicina* **2025**, *61*, 557, https://doi.org/10.3390/medicina61040557 5

Nurul Inaas Mahamad Apandi, Siew Wui Chan and Yen Fa Toh
Differential Expression of Mucin in Salivary Gland Tumours
Reprinted from: *Medicina* **2024**, *60*, 920, https://doi.org/10.3390/medicina60060920 15

Mohamed Abdulla, Osama Refaat, Mohamed Alahmer, Ayman Yehia, Hesham Abdelsalam, Khaled Abdelaal and Mohamed Shams Eldin
Prelacrimal Recess Approach in Unilateral Maxillary Sinus Lesions: What Is the Impact and Efficacy?
Reprinted from: *Medicina* **2024**, *60*, 222, https://doi.org/10.3390/medicina60020222 26

Rafał Pokrowiecki, Barbora Šufliarsky and Maciej Jagielak
Esthetic Surgery of the Chin in Cis- and Transgender Patients—Application of T-Genioplasty vs. Single-Piece Segment Lateralization
Reprinted from: *Medicina* **2024**, *60*, 139, https://doi.org/10.3390/medicina60010139 38

Rafał Pokrowiecki, Barbora Šufliarsky and Maciej Jagielak
Feminization Surgery of the Upper Face as the Crucial Factor in Gender Confirmation—Pearls and Pitfalls
Reprinted from: *Medicina* **2024**, *60*, 120, https://doi.org/10.3390/medicina60010120 54

Monika Morawska-Kochman, Ziemowit Miłosz Malecha, Krzysztof Zub, Jakub Kielar, Krzysztof Dudek, Kamil Nelke and Tomasz Zatonski
Physical Conditions Prevailing in the Nasal and Maxillary Sinus Cavities Based on Numerical Simulation
Reprinted from: *Medicina* **2023**, *59*, 1094, https://doi.org/10.3390/medicina59061094 68

Kazuya Yoshida
Long-Standing Temporomandibular Joint Dislocation: A Comprehensive Review and Proposal of a Treatment Algorithm
Reprinted from: *Medicina* **2025**, *61*, 1505, https://doi.org/10.3390/medicina61091505 80

Cristian Mârțu, Ștefan Dragoș Tîrnovanu, Ioana Mârțu, Dan Ferariu, Dan Mârțu, Alexandra Jităreanu and Luminița Rădulescu
Alveolar Rhabdomyosarcoma of Nasopharynx and Paranasal Sinuses in Children Diagnosis and Treatment—Review of the Literature and Case Report
Reprinted from: *Medicina* **2025**, *61*, 80, https://doi.org/10.3390/medicina61010080 97

Zofia Resler, Monika Morawska-Kochman, Katarzyna Resler and Tomasz Zatoński
Fibrous Dysplasia of the Ethmoid Bone Diagnosed in a 10-Year-Old Patient
Reprinted from: *Medicina* **2025**, *61*, 45, https://doi.org/10.3390/medicina61010045 116

Won-Bae Park, Jina Shin, Seungil Shin and Ji-Youn Hong
A Clinical Approach for the Removal of a Large Antral Pseudocyst with Simultaneous Maxillary Sinus Augmentation: A Case Series
Reprinted from: *Medicina* **2024**, *60*, 838, https://doi.org/10.3390/medicina60050838 . . . . **123**

Kamil Nelke, Maciej Janeczek, Edyta Pasicka, Krzysztof Żak, Marceli Łukaszewski, Radosław Jadach and Maciej Dobrzyński
The Temporary Mental Nerve Paresthesia as an Outcome of Dentigerous Cyst Removal during Preparation for Dental Implant Placement: A Case Report
Reprinted from: *Medicina* **2023**, *59*, 711, https://doi.org/10.3390/medicina59040711 . . . . **134**

medicina

MDPI

Editorial

Editorial for the Special Issue "Diagnosis and Treatment of Diseases of the Facial Skeleton, Oral Cavity, and Paranasal Sinuses"

Kamil Nelke [1,2,*], Maciej Dobrzyński [3] and Marceli Łukaszewski [4]

1 Maxillo-Facial Surgery Ward, EMC Hospital, Pilczycka 144, 54-144 Wroclaw, Poland
2 Academy of Applied Sciences, Health Department, Academy of Silesius in Wałbrzych, Zamkowa 4, 58-300 Wałbrzych, Poland
3 Department of Pediatric Dentistry and Preclinical Dentistry, Wroclaw Medical University, Krakowska 26, 50-425 Wroclaw, Poland
4 Department of Anaesthesiology and Intensive Care, Sokołowski Hospital, Sokołowskiego 4, 58-309 Wałbrzych, Poland
* Correspondence: kamil.nelke@gmail.com

The scope of diseases and lesions that might be present and found in the facial skeleton, oral cavity, and paranasal sinus is very broad and wide-reaching. Each might have various etiological factors and a stage of local growth and development. When evaluating each patient's local status, a good radiological evaluation, followed by patient anamnesis, accurate differential diagnostics, and adequate preparation for surgery, impact on the final results. Current trends in maxillo-facial surgery not only include the usage of patient individual solutions, virtual planning, and 3D-designed hardware, but also implementations in patient-selected surgical cases to improve patient outcomes and prognosis. Because some lesions tend to be more or less common in the facial skeleton area, the possible treatment methods and algorithms can differ greatly based on case, surgeon, and many other individual factors [1,2]. An intraoral approach is more common than an intranasal approach alone; however, a combination of intraoral approach with an endoscope is also used more commonly by maxillofacial surgeons [3–5]. CBCT planning makes approaching the sinus floor safer [3]. Possible local nerve paresis can be treated with good outcomes using pharmacological agents, especially vitamin B with or without alpha-lipoic acid oral intake, as suggested by some researchers [4].

At present, many jawbone and adjacent tissue lesions can be evaluated and diagnosed with CBCT (cone-beam computed tomography). The role of this imaging method is helpful in estimating the presence of some odontogenic or non-odontogenic lesions, as it carefully evaluates bone structure within tooth-bearing structures. The usage of AI (artificial intelligence) for pattern evaluation in CBCT is the next step. Studies like that of Al-Haj Husain and others confirm that CBCT focuses on not only jawbone structures and conditions, but also sinuses and their patency or spread of inflammation within [6]. Appropriate diagnosis helps identify the pattern of certain sinus lesions, as well as their boundaries and possible anatomical variations in future operable areas [6–8]. The study by Morawska-Kochman et al. indicates that airflow in the sinuses and nasal cavity might experience disturbances stemming from both anatomical and post-operative factors [9].

Studies, like those by Mclean et al. and Omami and Yeoh, summarize the occurrence and possible patterns and characteristics of various typical jaw cysts and tumors that can be found during radiological and clinical patient evaluation [10,11]. It is worth noting that the radiolucent, radiopaque, or mixed appearance of each bone lesion could be characteristic of some tumor of odontogenic, non-odontogenic, or other bone lesion abnormalities. The authors in this Special Issue emphasize the role of individual case-related studies and planning the scope of each surgery based on 3D models. Sometimes, CBCT can be useful, detecting incidental tumors or lesions that are not found under normal circumstances. The usage of CT and CBCT is important for assessing disturbances in nasal airflow and smell sensation and distinguishing between an odontogenic-like lesion and fibrous dysplasia, as presented in Resler et al.'s case report [12].

On the other hand, the scope of maxillary sinus radiological imaging and all paranasal sinus diseases and their conditions might have different possible etiological factors, including odontogenic and non-odontogenic sources, where odontogenic sinusitis (ODS) plays a role in the majority of related cases [13,14]. A recent review by Craig (2022) indicates that collaboration between general dentists, laryngologists, and maxillofacial surgeons could benefit the treatment and patient outcomes when all aspects of ODS are treated equally using a team-based approach [14]. Perhaps future improvements might include a combination of simultaneous FESS-CBCT (functional endoscopic sinus surgery–cone beam computed tomography) navigation for not only ODS but also minimally invasive sinus surgery. All diagnostic approaches should also take into consideration that the area of the maxillary alveolar process and maxillary sinuses can be not only occupied by bone anomalies like fibrous dysplasia, ossifying fibromas, cemento-ossifying lesions, but also more aggressive lesions like squamous cell carcinoma or rhabdomyosarcoma, as demonstrated in the studies by Resler et al. and Mârțu et al. [12,15]. As elucidated in the following sections, each lesion requires sufficient diagnoses and tumor sampling to establish the most accurate approach for each patient.

Currently, all lesions and diseases of the jaw bones, sinuses, and surrounding tissues can be treated using many different approaches. Some important aspects include studying the expression of certain markers to determine patients' outcomes and the necessity and scope of each surgery. Mostafa et al. investigate the expression of glucose transporter-1 in oral epithelial dysplasia, while Mahamad Apandi et al. examine the expression of mucin; the results of these studies may help both histopathologists and surgeons understand how certain lesions are diagnosed, progress in time, and what treatment is more suitable in those cases [16,17].

The three-dimensional proportions and relations between the lower, middle, and upper areas of the face and skull also influence decision-making. In the most common dento-alveolar skeletal malocclusion cases, which can be treated with great overall success with different orthognathic surgery steps, it is also worth remembering that the scope of CBCT and 3D planning can affect any other different surgeries that include feminization and masculinization procedures, with goals that are mostly related to facial beauty and esthetics [18,19]. Both surgical scopes depend on individual 3D planning protocols, surgical guides, 3D models, and individual PEEK or other implants; however, Beyer et al. conclude that precise surgical guides promote better, more accurate, and predictable results with less unstable long-term results [19]. Individually designed and manufactured 3D-printed models may take less time when new dental materials include 3D-bone-like meshes, which are now quite commonly used to evaluate and plan cis- and trans-patients' surgeries, establishing the scope of surgery by improving patients' outcomes, satisfaction levels, and quality of life. Recent studies by Pokrowiecki et al. highlighted a possible new methodology for the following surgeries [20,21].

Each pathology can be treated with many possible methods and approaches; however, some interesting cases can open new possibilities and treatment modalities or present a novel or atypical scope of the disease. Paranasal sinus pathologies are not only related to cysts, tumors, or lesions; the scope of possible teeth-related and odontogenic origins should also be considered. Some more aggressive lesions might include oral cancer spreading towards the sinuses, the occurrence of small and major salivary gland tumors, or the presence of sarcomas, vascular tumors, neurogenic tumors, and other conditions that can be found in the facial skeleton area [22,23]. Some approaches, including neuronavigation and computed tomography, should be used simultaneously in the virtual reality environment to minimize the risk of any real in vivo surgery. In each surgery, care should be taken to reduce damage, luxation, trauma, or temporo-mandibular joint overload. A recent review by Yoshida highlights the important aspect of TMJ dislocation [24]. On the other hand, any joint or mandibular asymmetries, problems with occlusion, TMJ acoustic symptoms, and possible related malocclusion should always be differentiated from unilateral condylar hyperplasia (UCH) [25].

In conclusion, a majority of surgical procedures in the facial skeleton area can influence patients' quality of life; improve bite, chewing, and function; and enhance esthetics and overall patient confidence. Improvements in healthcare and new technologies, specifically diagnostic approaches used in different jawbone and facial skeleton surgeries, are promising for the future of more specialized maxillofacial surgery.

We believe that these eleven contributions improve our current understanding of certain fields, i.e., oral, jawbone, maxillary sinus, and related facial skeleton diseases, and have the potential to stimulate further research.

Author Contributions: Writing—original draft preparation, K.N.; writing—review and editing, K.N., M.D. and M.Ł. All authors have read and agreed to the published version of the manuscript.

Funding: This work was financed by a subsidy from Wrocław University of Environmental and Life Sciences.

Conflicts of Interest: The authors declare no conflicts of interest.

References

1. Chen, H.S.; Hsiao, S.Y.; Lee, K.T. Analysis of Facial Skeletal Morphology: Nasal Bone, Maxilla, and Mandible. *BioMed Res. Int.* **2021**, *2021*, 5599949. [CrossRef] [PubMed] [PubMed Central]
2. Foster, B.L.; Ramnitz, M.S.; Gafni, R.I.; Burke, A.B.; Boyce, A.M.; Lee, J.S.; Wright, J.T.; Akintoye, S.O.; Somerman, M.J.; Collins, M.T. Rare bone diseases and their dental, oral, and craniofacial manifestations. *J. Dent. Res.* **2014**, *93*, 7S–19S. [CrossRef] [PubMed] [PubMed Central]
3. Park, W.-B.; Shin, J.; Shin, S.; Hong, J.-Y. A Clinical Approach for the Removal of a Large Antral Pseudocyst with Simultaneous Maxillary Sinus Augmentation: A Case Series. *Medicina* **2024**, *60*, 838. [CrossRef]
4. Nelke, K.; Janeczek, M.; Pasicka, E.; Żak, K.; Łukaszewski, M.; Jadach, R.; Dobrzyński, M. The Temporary Mental Nerve Paresthesia as an Outcome of Dentigerous Cyst Removal during Preparation for Dental Implant Placement: A Case Report. *Medicina* **2023**, *59*, 711. [CrossRef]
5. Abdulla, M.; Refaat, O.; Alahmer, M.; Yehia, A.; Abdelsalam, H.; Abdelaal, K.; Shams Eldin, M. Prelacrimal Recess Approach in Unilateral Maxillary Sinus Lesions: What Is the Impact and Efficacy? *Medicina* **2024**, *60*, 222. [CrossRef]
6. Al-Haj Husain, A.; Döbelin, Q.; Giacomelli-Hiestand, B.; Wiedemeier, D.B.; Stadlinger, B.; Valdec, S. Diagnostic Accuracy of Cystic Lesions Using a Pre-Programmed Low-Dose and Standard-Dose Dental Cone-Beam Computed Tomography Protocol: An Ex Vivo Comparison Study. *Sensors* **2021**, *21*, 7402. [CrossRef] [PubMed] [PubMed Central]
7. Nelke, K.; Diakowska, D.; Morawska-Kochman, M.; Janeczek, M.; Pasicka, E.; Łukaszewski, M.; Żak, K.; Nienartowicz, J.; Dobrzyński, M. The CBCT Retrospective Study on Underwood Septa and Their Related Factors in Maxillary Sinuses-A Proposal of Classification. *J. Pers. Med.* **2023**, *13*, 1258. [CrossRef] [PubMed] [PubMed Central]
8. Mistretta, F.; Magnini, A.; Cinci, L.; Zanobini, P.; Pisano, M.; Barcali, E.; Bocchi, L.; Nardi, C. A systematic review and meta-analysis on the concept of bone quality in dento-maxillofacial Cone Beam Computed Tomography. *Radiol. Med.* **2025**, *130*, 1193–1206. [CrossRef] [PubMed]
9. Morawska-Kochman, M.; Malecha, Z.M.; Zub, K.; Kielar, J.; Dudek, K.; Nelke, K.; Zatonski, T. Physical Conditions Prevailing in the Nasal and Maxillary Sinus Cavities Based on Numerical Simulation. *Medicina* **2023**, *59*, 1094. [CrossRef] [PubMed]
10. McLean, A.C.; Vargas, P.A. Cystic Lesions of the Jaws: The Top 10 Differential Diagnoses to Ponder. *Head Neck Pathol.* **2023**, *17*, 85–98. [CrossRef] [PubMed] [PubMed Central]

11. Omami, G.; Yeoh, M. Cysts and Benign Odontogenic Tumors of the Jaws. *Dent. Clin.* **2024**, *68*, 277–295. [CrossRef] [PubMed]
12. Resler, Z.; Morawska-Kochman, M.; Resler, K.; Zatoński, T. Fibrous Dysplasia of the Ethmoid Bone Diagnosed in a 10-Year-Old Patient. *Medicina* **2025**, *61*, 45. [CrossRef]
13. Allevi, F.; Fadda, G.L.; Rosso, C.; Martino, F.; Pipolo, C.; Cavallo, G.; Felisati, G.; Saibene, A.M. Diagnostic Criteria for Odontogenic Sinusitis: A Systematic Review. *Am. J. Rhinol. Allergy* **2021**, *35*, 713–721. [CrossRef] [PubMed]
14. Craig, J.R. Odontogenic sinusitis: A state-of-the-art review. *World J. Otorhinolaryngol. Head Neck Surg.* **2022**, *8*, 8–15. [CrossRef] [PubMed] [PubMed Central]
15. Mârțu, C.; Tîrnovanu, Ș.D.; Mârțu, I.; Ferariu, D.; Mârțu, D.; Jităreanu, A.; Rădulescu, L. Alveolar Rhabdomyosarcoma of Nasopharynx and Paranasal Sinuses in Children Diagnosis and Treatment—Review of the Literature and Case Report. *Medicina* **2025**, *61*, 80. [CrossRef] [PubMed]
16. Mostafa, R.G.; Hashim, M.I.; Bawahab, A.A.; Baloush, R.A.A.; Abdelwahed, M.S.; Hasan, A.; Ismail, K.A.; Abd-Elhameed, N.R.; Embaby, A.; Sharfeldeen, A.E.R.M. Immunohistochemical Expression of Glucose Transporter-1 in Oral Epithelial Dysplasia and Different Grades of Oral Squamous Cell Carcinoma. *Medicina* **2025**, *61*, 557. [CrossRef] [PubMed]
17. Mahamad Apandi, N.I.; Chan, S.W.; Toh, Y.F. Differential Expression of Mucin in Salivary Gland Tumours. *Medicina* **2024**, *60*, 920. [CrossRef] [PubMed]
18. Callen, A.L.; Badiee, R.K.; Phelps, A.; Potigailo, V.; Wang, E.; Lee, S.; Talbott, J.; Glastonbury, C.; Pomerantz, J.H.; Narvid, J. Facial Feminization Surgery: Key CT Findings for Preoperative Planning and Postoperative Evaluation. *Am. J. Roentgenol.* **2021**, *217*, 709–717. [CrossRef] [PubMed]
19. Beyer, M.; Abazi, S.; Tourbier, C.; Burde, A.; Vinayahalingam, S.; Ileșan, R.R.; Thieringer, F.M. Innovations in gender affirmation: AI-enhanced surgical guides for mandibular facial feminization surgery. *Clin. Oral Investig.* **2025**, *29*, 390. [CrossRef] [PubMed] [PubMed Central]
20. Pokrowiecki, R.; Šufliarsky, B.; Jagielak, M. Esthetic Surgery of the Chin in Cis- and Transgender Patients—Application of T-Genioplasty vs. Single-Piece Segment Lateralization. *Medicina* **2024**, *60*, 139. [CrossRef] [PubMed]
21. Pokrowiecki, R.; Šufliarsky, B.; Jagielak, M. Feminization Surgery of the Upper Face as the Crucial Factor in Gender Confirmation—Pearls and Pitfalls. *Medicina* **2024**, *60*, 120. [CrossRef] [PubMed]
22. Kessler, A.T.; Bhatt, A.A. Review of the Major and Minor Salivary Glands, Part 2: Neoplasms and Tumor-like Lesions. *J. Clin. Imaging Sci.* **2018**, *8*, 48. [CrossRef] [PubMed] [PubMed Central]
23. Young, A.; Okuyemi, O.T. Malignant Salivary Gland Tumors. In *StatPearls*; StatPearls Publishing: Treasure Island, FL, USA, 2023. Available online: https://pubmed.ncbi.nlm.nih.gov/33079504/ (accessed on 22 November 2025). [PubMed]
24. Yoshida, K. Long-Standing Temporomandibular Joint Dislocation: A Comprehensive Review and Proposal of a Treatment Algorithm. *Medicina* **2025**, *61*, 1505. [CrossRef]
25. Nelke, K.H.; Pawlak, W.; Morawska-Kochman, M.; Łuczak, K. Ten years of observations and demographics of hemimandibular hyperplasia and elongation. *J. Cranio-Maxillofac. Surg.* **2018**, *46*, 979–986. [CrossRef] [PubMed]

medicina

MDPI

Article

Immunohistochemical Expression of Glucose Transporter-1 in Oral Epithelial Dysplasia and Different Grades of Oral Squamous Cell Carcinoma

Rahma Gamal Mostafa [1], Mohammad Ibrahim Hashim [1], Ahmed Abdulwahab Bawahab [2], Razan Abed A. Baloush [2], Mohammed S. Abdelwahed [2,3], Abdulkarim Hasan [3,*], Khadiga A. Ismail [4], Nageh Rady Abd-Elhameed [5], Ahmed Embaby [6,7] and Abd El Rahman M. Sharfeldeen [1,8]

1 Department of Oral and Maxillofacial Pathology, Faculty of Dentistry, Assiut University, Assiut 71524, Egypt
2 Department of Basic Medical Sciences, College of Medicine, University of Jeddah, Jeddah 23218, Saudi Arabia
3 Department of Pathology, Faculty of Medicine, Al-Azhar University, Cairo 11561, Egypt
4 Department of Clinical Laboratory Sciences, College of Applied Medical Sciences, Taif University, Taif 21944, Saudi Arabia
5 Department of Pathology, Faculty of Medicine, Al-Azhar University, Assiut 71524, Egypt
6 Department of Surgical Oncology, Faculty of Medicine, Al-Azhar University, Cairo 11561, Egypt
7 Department of General Surgery, Lister Hospital, Stevenage SG1 4AB, UK
8 Department of Oral Pathology, College of Dentistry, City University Ajman, Ajman P.O. Box 18484, United Arab Emirates
* Correspondence: a.abdel@cu.ac.ae or abdulkarim.hasan@azhar.edu.eg

Abstract: *Background and Objectives*: Glucose Transporter-1 (GLUT1) is the key target gene for hypoxia-inducible factor (HIF), which helps cells uptake glucose during cell division, malignant transformation, and nutrient depletion. Cancer hypoxia is a well-known condition caused by an oxygen imbalance in the cancer microenvironment. During chronic hypoxia, certain cancer cells can survive and adapt. These cellular alterations can make cancer more aggressive, causing invasion and metastasis. The study investigated the presence of GLUT1 in oral epithelial dysplasia (OED) and various histopathological grades of oral squamous cell carcinoma (OSCC) to assess the significance of GLUT1 as a prognostic indicator. *Material and Methods*: A total of 40 samples of tissue blocks, including 5 cases of normal oral mucosa, 5 cases of epithelial dysplasia, and 30 cases of OSCC with 10 cases each of well-differentiated, moderately differentiated, and poorly differentiated OSCCs, these cases were diagnosed using the Hematoxylin and Eosin (H&E) staining technique. GLUT1 expression was assessed using immunohistochemical staining, which involved evaluating the location of the stain and the percentage of staining. *Results*: The mean area percent was highest in poorly differentiated cases (47.37) and lowest in well-differentiated cases (13.42). In poorly differentiated cases, diffuse expression was observed in almost all malignant cells, exhibiting membrane, cytoplasmic and nuclear staining. A significant difference ($p < 0.001$) between all groups in regard to immunostaining was detected. *Conclusions:* GLUT1 expression increased from oral epithelial dysplasia to oral squamous cell carcinoma histological grades. GLUT1 in actively dividing cells may reflect the tumor's aggressiveness and treatment response. Hypoxia increases this marker's expression, indicating division and proliferation.

Keywords: oral epithelial dysplasia; glucose transporter-1; prognostic marker; oral squamous cell carcinoma

 https://doi.org/10.3390/medicina61040557

1. Introduction

Oral cancer is a widespread global health problem characterized by substantial rates of illness and death. Despite the existence of preventive strategies, this cancer continues to be highly prevalent, highlighting the necessity for enhanced diagnostic and prognostic techniques [1].

More than 90% of OSCCs are the most prevalent and deadly malignant tumors in the head and neck area. Approximately 380,000 new cases are anticipated annually, making it one of the most common tumors globally. This tumor accounts for 2% of all cancer cases and will rank eighteenth in 2020 [2].

Oral potentially malignant disorders (OPMDs) frequently occur before the development of neoplastic tumors [3]. These lesions, including leukoplakia, oral lichen planus, and oral lichenoid lesions, are part of this group [4]. Previously, conditions such as OED, proliferative verrucous leukoplakia, submucous fibrosis, and HPV-associated dysplasic lesions were categorized as OPMDs [5].

The majority of instances of OSCC are detected in advanced stages. That may be attributed to the patient's lack of awareness, as most cases are asymptomatic in the early stages. There is a requirement to create novel immunohistochemistry markers for the early detection of OSCC patients to commence therapy and enhance the survival rate of this severe disease [6,7].

Glucose transporters are membrane proteins transporting hexoses like glucose and fructose through plasma membranes. Glucose Transporter-1 (GLUT1) is the main target gene for hypoxia-inducible factor (HIF), enabling glucose entry into cells during settings with heightened metabolic demands, such as cell division, malignant transformation, and nutrient insufficiency [8].

GLUT1 is a glycoprotein located in the cell membrane. Its primary function is to transfer glucose into cells without sodium ions. Research has shown changes in the expression of GLUT1 in several lesions that can potentially become cancerous or are already cancerous [9].

Cancer hypoxia is a widely recognized occurrence that arises from an inequity between the availability and utilization of oxygen within the microenvironment of the cancer. During prolonged periods of low oxygen levels, specific cancer cells can survive and undergo adaptations in response to hypoxia. These cellular changes can contribute to a more aggressive cancer phenotype, leading to invasion and metastasis [10].

GLUT1 may play an essential role in carcinogenesis. High GLUT1 expression has been reported in head and neck squamous cell carcinoma [11]. GLUT-1 expression in various head and neck tumors has shown different correlations with factors such as progression and prognosis [12]. This study investigated the presence of GLUT11 in oral epithelial dysplasia and various histological grades of OSCC to assess the significance of GLUT1 as a prognostic indicator.

2. Material and Methods

After the study received ethical approval from the Faculty of Dental Medicine ethics committee, Al-Azhar University in Assiut, Egypt, we collected forty formalin-fixed, paraffin-embedded tissue specimens from our institution's pathology archives in Assiut, Egypt. Related clinical and demographic data were retrieved from medical files.

The specimens were initially preserved in a 10% buffered formalin solution for 24 h following the extraction of third molars. Group I comprised five normal oral mucosa (NOM) samples, serving as controls, which were collected from the gingival and vestibular mucosa. Group II included five cases, as defined by the OED. Group III consisted of thirty cases of

OSCC, which were further classified into ten cases each of well-differentiated, moderately differentiated, and poorly differentiated OSCC.

The histopathological diagnosis and grading were reviewed by at least two pathologists (on-site or remote examination) to confirm the included cases. Exclusion criteria included non-Egyptian patients and cases with missing data or insufficient material in the cell block.

2.1. Immunohistochemical Study

Paraffin-embedded tissue specimens were cut into 4 μm thick sections and subjected to immunohistochemistry using the streptavidin biotin-peroxidase method. The primary antibody used was the rabbit monoclonal antibody GLUT1 EP141.

The sections were deparaffinized by immersion in xylene twice for five minutes each, followed by rehydration using a graded ethanol series (100%, 95%, and 70%). The slides were then washed in phosphate-buffered saline (PBS) to facilitate antigen recovery. Antigenic sites were revealed using heat-induced antigen retrieval with citrate buffer (pH 6.0) or Tris-EDTA buffer (pH 9.0), typically by heating at 95 °C for 15–20 min in a microwave or water bath. Following a 20 min cooling period at room temperature, the slides were washed with PBS to remove buffer residues.

To mitigate background staining, endogenous peroxidase activity was inhibited with a peroxidase-blocking solution for 10 min, followed by washing with PBS. A blocking buffer containing 5% bovine serum albumin (BSA) or normal serum was applied for 30 min to prevent nonspecific binding. The primary antibody, anti-GLUT1, was then applied at an optimum dilution (typically 1:100–1:500) and incubated overnight at 4 °C or for 1–2 h at room temperature. After incubation, the slides were washed three times with PBS, each lasting five minutes.

A secondary antibody conjugated to HRP or alkaline phosphatase, corresponding to the host species of the primary antibody, was applied and incubated for 30 min at room temperature. The slides were then washed three more times in PBS before the addition of a chromogenic substrate, such as 3,3′-diaminobenzidine (DAB) for HRP-based detection, producing a brown stain. The reaction was monitored under a microscope and terminated by washing the slides with distilled water.

For contrast, sections were counterstained with hematoxylin for 30 to 60 s, then rinsed in running tap water. The slides were subsequently dehydrated using a graded ethanol series, cleared with xylene, and mounted with a permanent medium for visualization. Under microscopic examination, positive GLUT1 expression appeared as brown membrane staining in cells, while negative regions remained unstained except for the counterstain. Internal positive controls, including red blood cells, exhibited GLUT1 positivity to ensure staining reproducibility. This refined procedure ensured precise and consistent detection of GLUT1 expression across different tissues, facilitating research and diagnostic applications, such as tumor characterization and metabolic investigations.

Microscopic images were captured using a SOPTOP EX20 biological microscope (Ningbo Sunny Instruments Co., China, Yuyao), an HD camera (model No. XCAM1080PHB) (manufactured by ToupTek Photonics, Hangzhou, China), and Image View software at $\times$100 and $\times$200 magnification.

Immunohistochemical stained sections were examined using high power fields (X200) by light microscope, and the positive reaction's most homogenous areas were evaluated. The image analyzer computer system applying Imagej 1.53e software (USA) was used for automated measurement of area percent of Glut-1 positivity. It was performed in a standard frame area of 5.04×10^6 μm^2.

2.2. Statistical Methods

The results were evaluated through statistical analysis using the SPSS software (version 24). The Shapiro–Wilk test of normality was employed to assess the normality assumption for all continuous variables. The One-way analysis of variance (ANOVA) test was used to determine the presence of a statistically significant difference among the groups under investigation. Subsequently, the Tukey–Kramer Post hoc test was conducted to further examine the statistically significant findings. Statistical significance was determined by considering *p*-values less than or equal to 0.05.

3. Results

3.1. Immunohistochemical Findings of GLUT-1

The greatest mean area percent was recorded in poorly differentiated cases (47.37), whereas the lowest value was recorded in well-differentiated cases (13.42). One-way analysis of variance (ANOVA) test revealed that the difference between all groups was statistically significant ($p < 0.001$) with Cohen's d effect size = 10.4 and 95% CI [7.3176, 13.4266]. Tukey's post hoc showed that all groups were significantly different from each other (when comparing every two groups) (Table 1, Figure 1).

Table 1. Difference in mean GLUT1 area between different groups using ANOVA statistical test.

Groups	Mean GLUT1 Area%					
	Mean	SD	Min	Max	F-Value	*p*-Value
OED	17.13	3.02	14.209	20.239	348.026	<0.0001 *
WDSCC	13.42	3.309	10	17.208		
MDSCC	38.78	3.692	35.887	42.939		
PDSCC	47.37	2.392	43.913	50.552		

* significant at $p < 0.05$.

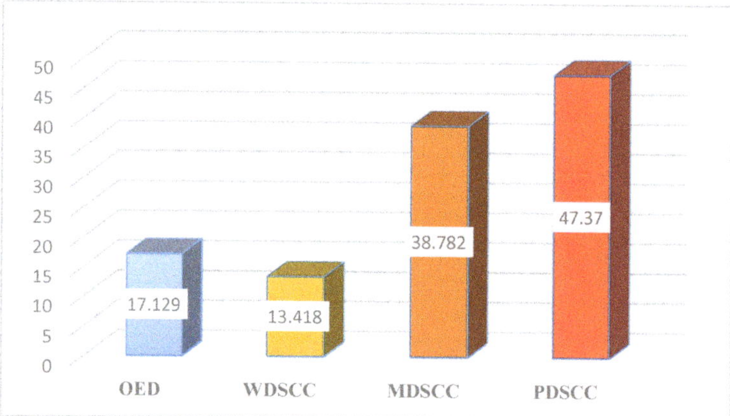

Figure 1. Mean area percentage of GLUT1 among groups.

These results suggest a potential role of differentiation status in influencing the observed parameter, warranting further investigation into the underlying biological mechanisms.

Tukey's post hoc test means sharing the same superscript letter is not significantly different.

3.2. Evaluation of GLUT-1 Immunostaining

In oral epithelial dysplasia cases, GLUT1 immunostaining was more intense in the basal and suprabasal layers of the epithelium, with a gradual reduction in reactivity observed in the most superficial layers. This staining pattern suggests an increased metabolic demand in proliferative regions, consistent with cellular adaptation to hypoxia. Notably, GLUT1 expression was predominantly localized at the tumor periphery, where cells are likely experiencing a higher proliferative rate, while significantly weaker staining was observed in the central regions of the tumor areas, possibly due to reduced metabolic activity or necrotic changes (Figure 2).

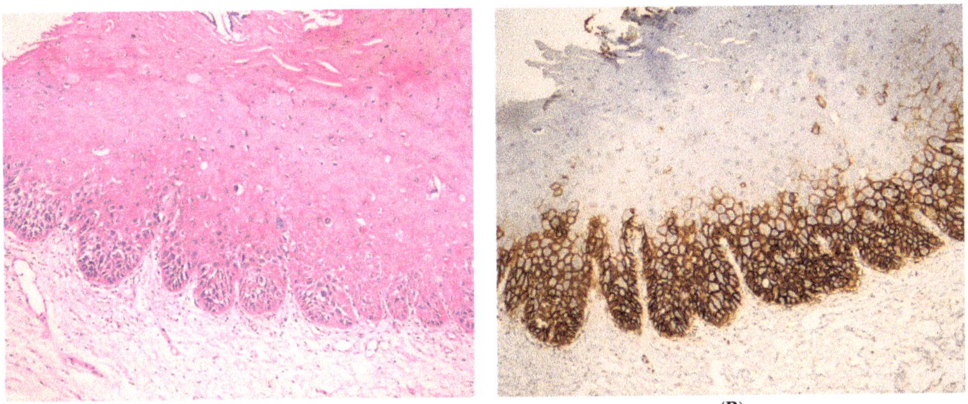

(A) (B)

Figure 2. (**A**) Photomicrograph showing oral epithelial dysplasia (H&E, ×100). (**B**) Photomicrograph showing moderate expression of GLUT1, which extends to the mid-spinous layers in oral epithelial dysplasia (IHC, ×100).

GLUT1-positive expression was identified in all cases of oral squamous cell carcinoma (OSCC), indicating its ubiquitous presence across different grades of malignancy. A detailed comparison of GLUT1 immunoexpression in relation to tumor grade revealed a progressive shift in staining distribution. As the grade of OSCC increased, the expression pattern changed from being predominantly localized in peripheral cells of tumor islands to a more diffuse pattern, encompassing both peripheral and central tumor cells. This shift may reflect altered tumor microenvironment conditions, such as increased glucose demand and hypoxia-driven metabolic adaptation in more aggressive tumors.

In well-differentiated OSCC cases, immunostaining was most pronounced in cells at the periphery of tumor cell nests, while keratin pearls exhibited negative expression. The observed membranous localization of GLUT1 suggests its functional role in glucose transport at the tumor-stroma interface, where active proliferation occurs (Figure 3). In moderately differentiated OSCC cases, the immunostaining pattern was more heterogeneous, with patchy expression detected in the central tumor cells, indicating a more diffuse metabolic adaptation. Interestingly, positive GLUT1 immunoreactivity was also noted in the endothelial lining of blood capillaries, suggesting a potential role in tumor-associated angiogenesis (Figure 4). These findings underscore the dynamic nature of GLUT1 expression in OSCC progression and its potential relevance as a biomarker for tumor metabolism and aggressiveness.

In poorly differentiated cases, diffuse expression was observed in almost all malignant cells, exhibiting membrane, cytoplasmic and nuclear staining (Figure 5).

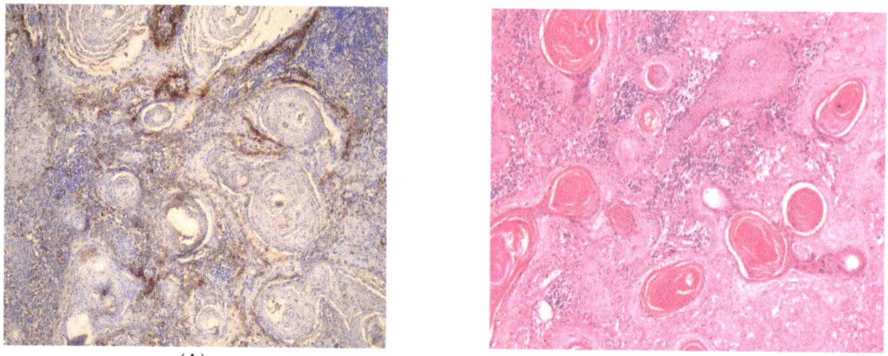

(A) (B)

Figure 3. (**A**) Photomicrograph showing well-differentiated OSCC (H&E, ×100). (**B**) Photomicrograph showing mild expression of GLUT1 in well-differentiated OSCC showing peripheral tumor cells showing membranous expression of GLUT1 (IHC, ×100).

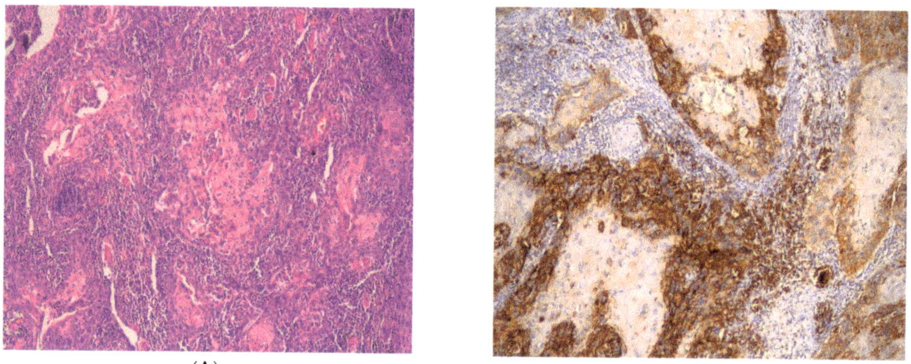

(A) (B)

Figure 4. (**A**) Photomicrograph showing moderately differentiated OSCC (H&E, ×100) (**B**) Photomicrograph showing moderate expression of GLUT1 in tumor islands of moderately differentiated OSCC showing intense GLUT1 expression in peripheral cells of tumor island (IHC, ×100).

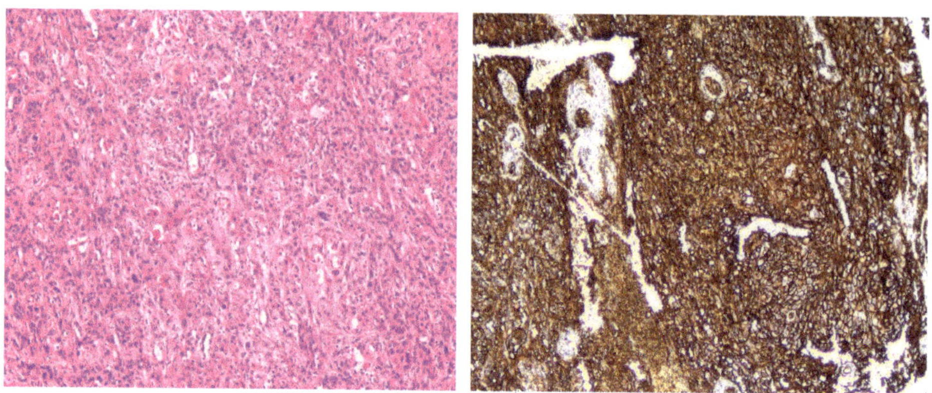

(A) (B)

Figure 5. (**A**) Photomicrograph showing poorly differentiated OSCC (H&E, ×100). (**B**) Photomicrograph shows intense expression of GLUT1 in peripheral and central cells of tumor island in poorly differentiated OSCC with membranous and cytoplasmic staining (IHC, ×100).

4. Discussion

Progress in surgical procedures, radiation, and chemotherapy has enhanced organ preservation and the overall quality of life while reducing morbidity. Nevertheless, further comprehension of the molecular pathways that govern the progression from normal epithelium to pre-malignancy to invasive oral cancer is imperative to enhance the long-term survival rates of affected patients [13].

Oral squamous cell carcinoma (OSCC) is a prevalent malignancy often linked to poor prognosis. OSCCs demonstrate the Warburg effect, relying heavily on an increased glucose supply to sustain tumor growth and metabolism. In various cancers, glucose transporters (GLUTs) are overexpressed, playing a crucial role in tumor progression. Their excessive production has been associated with treatment resistance, adverse clinical outcomes, and reduced overall survival rates [14].

Aerobic glycolysis, often referred to as the Warburg effect, produces significantly less adenosine triphosphate (ATP) per glucose molecule compared to mitochondrial oxidative phosphorylation (OXPHOS). However, the rate of glucose metabolism via aerobic glycolysis is markedly higher, allowing cells to rapidly generate lactate from glucose at a rate 10 to 100 times faster than the complete oxidation of glucose through OXPHOS [15]. This metabolic shift enables proliferating cells to sustain their energetic and biosynthetic demands despite their lower ATP.

For a cell—whether normal or altered—to actively proliferate, it must duplicate its DNA content along with essential cellular components such as membranes, proteins, and organelles. This process requires an increased intake of nutrients, particularly glucose, which not only fuels ATP production but also provides metabolic intermediates essential for biosynthesis. Additionally, amino acids play a crucial role as building blocks for protein synthesis, supporting the structural and functional needs of dividing cells.

Importantly, proliferating cells can reroute carbons from glycolysis at the pyruvate or lactate stage into anabolic pathways, such as lipid and nucleotide synthesis, rather than fully oxidizing them in the mitochondria. This metabolic flexibility allows cells to balance energy production with the synthesis of macromolecules necessary for growth and division, reinforcing the role of aerobic glycolysis in supporting rapid proliferation [16,17].

To keep growing and proliferating, tumor cells must ingest an overabundance of glucose. GLUT1 is an energy-free glucose transporter. Although low levels of GLUT1 expression are found in normal tissues and benign lesions, high levels of expression are frequently associated with carcinogenesis and can suggest a bad prognosis or recurrence [16].

The current study was conducted to examine the expression of GLUT1 in oral epithelial dysplasia and various histological grades of OSCC to assess its efficacy as a prognostic marker.

In the current study, poorly differentiated OSCC cases had the highest mean area percentage (47.37), while well-differentiated OSCC cases had the lowest value (13.42).

The current work investigated the expression of GLUT1 in oral epithelial dysplasia. GLUT1 expression was observed in the basal and suprabasal layers of the epithelium, but it was reduced in the most superficial layers. GLUT1 expression was observed mainly in the periphery of the tumor. These findings aligned with the study by Ehtisham et al. [8] and Patlolla et al., in 2020 [14].

The elevated expression of GLUT1 in oral epithelial dysplasia than in well-differentiated OSCC in present research is similar to that found in the study of Pereira et al. [16]; this overexpression is observed in conditions when cells require glucose as an energy source, such as during ischemia or hypoxia. These conditions might arise due to inadequate oxygen supply caused by poor blood movement [18,19].

We examined the distribution of GLUT1 immunostaining across invading islands in OSCC grades. In WDOSCC, GLUT1 expression was most noticeable on the tumor islands' periphery and nonexistent in central keratin pearls. These findings agree with Patlolla et al. [14], who explained that greater glycogen buildup in keratin pearls is inversely associated with GLUT1 expression, indicating that mature and differentiated cells in keratinized areas do not express GLUT1. Glycogen is related to squamous epithelium cellular maturation but vanishes during neoplastic transformation as differentiation occurs. An antistromal staining pattern in PDOSCC areas lacking squamous development and keratinization may be produced by hypoxia-driven GLUT1 activation.

In the current study, the intracellular localization of GLUT1 expression showed a major transition from being primarily located in the cell membrane to being located in the cytoplasm and eventually to a combination of both membrane and cytoplasmic positives. The results of this investigation were consistent with the research conducted by Airley et al. [20], which investigated the relationship between the presence of GLUT1 in tumors and the duration and severity of hypoxia in various regions. Their proposal suggests that the presence of GLUT1 close to the Golgi apparatus results in the simultaneous production of this protein in both the cell membrane and the cytoplasm.

Recent research targeting GLUT1 has demonstrated the potential to improve prognosis and increase survival rates. However, additional studies using larger sample sizes are necessary to determine the clinical relevance of GLUT1 as a prognostic marker for evaluating the risk and prognosis of OSCC [21].

GLUT-1 expression did not show a significant correlation with factors such as gender, age, alcohol consumption, or regional recurrence. However, it was prejudiced by proliferation rate, oxygen availability, malignant transformation, tumor progression, histological grading, clinical staging, lymph node involvement, tobacco use, and distant metastasis [22]. In their analysis, Yu M et al. reported that GLUT-1 overexpression was linked to increased aggressiveness and invasive potential of the lesion [23].

The use of ImageJ software for quantitative measurement of GLUT1 expression offers significant advantages over traditional semi-quantitative scoring methods. Unlike subjective visual assessment, which is prone to interobserver variability, ImageJ provides objective and reproducible quantification of immunohistochemical staining by analyzing pixel intensity and area percentage. This automated approach can reduce human bias and enhance evaluation accuracy in histological examination and immunohistochemical assessment [24].

Despite the strengths of this study on Egyptian patients, certain limitations should be acknowledged. First, the sample size was relatively small, which may limit the generalizability of our findings to a broader population. Larger, multi-center studies are needed to validate these results. Second, the study design was retrospective, which prevents the establishment of a definitive causal relationship between the observed variables. A longitudinal study would provide more robust evidence regarding the temporal sequence of these associations in addition to future studies incorporating functional validation through in vitro assays or exploring co-expression patterns with additional hypoxia-related markers to further elucidate GLUT1's role in OSCC progression. Future studies could also explore whether GLUT1 expression varies significantly between different intraoral subsites to provide additional insights into tumor behavior and prognosis. Lastly, while we use immunohistochemistry to assess Glut1, this approach has inherent limitations, including potential variability in interpretation and technical constraints, complementary genetic testing could provide additional insights.

5. Conclusions

The level of GLUT1 expression was elevated from oral epithelial dysplasia to various histological grades of OSCC. The presence of GLUT1 in actively dividing cells could indicate the tumor's aggressiveness and susceptibility to different treatment approaches. More expression of this marker indicates more division and proliferation under hypoxic conditions.

Author Contributions: Study design: R.G.M., M.I.H., A.H., R.A.A.B., K.A.I., N.R.A.-E., A.E. and A.E.R.M.S. Methodology: R.G.M., M.I.H., A.H., A.A.B., R.A.A.B., K.A.I., N.R.A.-E., M.S.A., A.E. and A.E.R.M.S. Data analysis: R.G.M., M.I.H., A.E. and A.E.R.M.S. Writing—review and editing. R.G.M., M.I.H., A.H., A.A.B., R.A.A.B., K.A.I., N.R.A.-E., M.S.A., A.E. and A.E.R.M.S. Collection of data, writing—original drafts: R.G.M., M.I.H., A.H., A.A.B., R.A.A.B., K.A.I., M.S.A., M.S.A., A.E. and A.E.R.M.S. All authors have read and agreed to the published version of the manuscript.

Funding: This research was funded by Taif University, Saudia Arabia, Project No. (TU-DSPP-2024-81).

Institutional Review Board Statement: Ethical approval was obtained from the Ethics committee of the Faculty of Dental Medicine, Al-Azhar University, Assuit Branch, Egypt. The code number is AUAREC20240005-10. Date: 7 May 2024.

Informed Consent Statement: Waived due to the nature of the study as a retrospective analysis from the archived data and paraffin blocks.

Data Availability Statement: All data generated or analyzed in this study are included in this published article. The data are available on request.

Acknowledgments: The authors would like to thank Taif University Project No. (TU-DSPP-2024-81).

Conflicts of Interest: The authors declare no conflicts of interest.

References

1. Zdrojewski, J.; Nowak, M.; Nijakowski, K.; Jankowski, J.; Scribante, A.; Gallo, S.; Pascadopoli, M.; Surdacka, A. Potential Immunohistochemical Biomarkers for Grading Oral Dysplasia: A Literature Review. *Biomedicines* **2024**, *12*, 3. [CrossRef] [PubMed]
2. Sung, H.; Ferlay, J.; Siegel, R.L.; Laversanne, M.; Soerjomataram, I.; Jemal, A.; Bray, F. Global Cancer Statistics 2020: GLOBOCAN Estimates of Incidence and Mortality Worldwide for 36 Cancers in 185 Countries. *CA Cancer J. Clin.* **2021**, *71*, 209–249. [CrossRef] [PubMed]
3. Gupta, N.; Gupta, R.; Acharya, A.K.; Patthi, B.; Goud, V.; Reddy, S.; Garg, A.; Singla, A. Changing Trends in oral cancer—A global scenario. *Nepal J. Epidemiol.* **2016**, *6*, 613–619. [CrossRef]
4. Sriram, S.; Hasan, S.; Alqarni, A.; Alam, T.; Kaleem, S.M.; Aziz, S.; Durrani, H.K.; Ajmal, M.; Dawasaz, A.A.; Saeed, S. Efficacy of Platelet-Rich Plasma Therapy in Oral Lichen Planus: A Systematic Review. *Medicina* **2023**, *59*, 746. [CrossRef] [PubMed]
5. Muller, S.; Tilakaratne, W.M. Update from the 5th Edition of the World Health Organization Classification of Head and Neck Tumors: Tumours of the Oral Cavity and Mobile Tongue. *Head Neck Pathol.* **2022**, *16*, 54–62. [CrossRef]
6. Salama, D.E.; Hasan, A.; Balbola, G.A.; Taha, A.M.; Abdel-Samia, H.M.; Taha, A.K.; Radwan, G.S.; Rifat, R.; Abdel-Maqsoud, M.F.; Samman, A.; et al. Immunohistochemical comparison of CD44 and hypoxia inducible Factor-1 alpha (HIF-1α) in Oral squamous cell carcinoma and Oral epithelial dysplasia: A comparative study. *J. Med. Chem. Sci.* **2024**, *7*, 9–23.
7. Fayed TM, M.E.; Abd Algaleel, M.A.; El Azony, H.A. Pattern of Recurrence of Oral Cavity Squamous Cell Carcinoma; A clinicopathological study. *Al-Azhar Int. Med. J.* **2024**, *5*, 33. [CrossRef]
8. Ehtisham, M.; Gupta, S.; Khan, S. Expression of Glut-1 in Oral Epithelial Dysplasia and OSCC: An Immunohistochemical Study. *Int. J. Contemp. Med. Res.* **2020**, *7*, 15–19.
9. Augustin, R. The protein family of glucose transport facilitators: It's not only about glucose after all. *IUBMB Life* **2010**, *62*, 315–333. [CrossRef]
10. Poon, E.; Harris, A.L.; Ashcroft, M. Targeting the hypoxia-inducible factor (HIF) pathway in cancer. *Expert Rev. Mol. Med.* **2009**, *11*, e26. [CrossRef]
11. Kumar, D. Regulation of glycolysis in head and neck squamous cell carcinoma. *Postdoc J. J. Postdr. Res. Postdr. Aff.* **2017**, *5*, 14–28. [CrossRef] [PubMed]

12. Yang, H.; Zhong, J.-T.; Zhou, S.-H.; Han, H.-M. Roles of GLUT-1 and HK-II expression in the biological behavior of head and neck cancer. *Oncotarget* **2019**, *10*, 3066–3083. [CrossRef]
13. Nakazato, K.; Mogushi, K.; Kayamori, K.; Tsuchiya, M.; Takahashi, K.-I.; Sumino, J.; Michi, Y.; Yoda, T.; Uzawa, N. Glucose metabolism changes during the development and progression of oral tongue squamous cell carcinomas. *Oncol. Lett.* **2019**, *18*, 1372–1380. [CrossRef] [PubMed]
14. Patlolla, P.; Shyam, N.D.V.N.; Kumar, G.K.; Narayen, V.; Konda, P.; Mudududla, P. Evaluation of glucose transporter-1 expression in oral epithelial dysplasia and oral squamous cell carcinoma: An immunohistochemical study. *J. Oral Maxillofac. Pathol. JOMFP* **2020**, *24*, 578. [CrossRef] [PubMed]
15. Liberti, M.V.; Locasale, J.W. The Warburg Effect: How Does it Benefit Cancer Cells? *Trends Biochem. Sci.* **2016**, *41*, 211. [CrossRef]
16. Pereira, K.M.A.; Chaves, F.N.; Viana, T.S.A.; Carvalho, F.S.R.; Costa, F.W.G.; Alves, A.P.N.N.; Sousa, F.B. Oxygen metabolism in oral cancer: HIF and GLUTs (Review). *Oncol. Lett.* **2013**, *6*, 311–316. [CrossRef]
17. Singh, D.; Arora, R.; Kaur, P.; Singh, B.; Mannan, R.; Arora, S. Overexpression of hypoxia-inducible factor and metabolic pathways: Possible targets of cancer. *Cell Biosci.* **2017**, *7*, 62. [CrossRef]
18. Pereira, K.M.A.; Feitosa, S.G.; Lima, A.T.T.; Luna, E.C.M.; Cavalcante, R.B.; Lima, K.C.D.; Chaves, F.N.; Costa, F.W.G. Immunohistochemical Evaluation of Glucose Transporter Type 1 in Epithelial Dysplasia and Oral Squamous Cell Carcinoma. *Asian Pac. J. Cancer Prev.* **2016**, *17*, 147–151. [CrossRef]
19. Reisser, C.; Eichhorn, K.; Herold-Mende, C.; Born, A.I.; Bannasch, P. Expression of facilitative glucose transport proteins during development of squamous cell carcinomas of the head and neck. *Int. J. Cancer* **1999**, *80*, 194–198. [CrossRef]
20. Airley, R.; Loncaster, J.; Davidson, S.; Bromley, M.; Roberts, S.; Patterson, A.; Hunter, R.; Stratford, I.; West, C. Glucose transporter glut-1 expression correlates with tumor hypoxia and predicts metastasis-free survival in advanced carcinoma of the cervix. *Clin. Cancer Res. Off. J. Am. Assoc. Cancer Res.* **2001**, *7*, 928–934.
21. Haneef, A.N.M.; Gopalakrishnan, S.; Jayaseelan, V.P.; Ramamurthi, R.; Muniapillai, S. GLUT1 Expression in Oral Squamous Cell Carcinoma and Its Significance. *Middle East J. Cancer* **2024**, *15*, 189–198.
22. Attur, S.K.; Patel, A.; Attur, K.M. Study of expression of GLUT-1 in oral potentially malignant disorders and oral squamous cell carcinoma: An immuno-histochemical analysis. *J. Oral Maxillofac. Pathol.* **2024**, *28*, 70–76. [CrossRef] [PubMed]
23. Yu, M.; Yongzhi, H.; Chen, S.; Luo, X.; Lin, Y.; Zhou, Y.; Jin, H.; Hou, B.; Deng, Y.; Tu, L.; et al. The Prognostic value of GLUT-1 in cancers:A systematic review and meta-analysis. *Oncotarget* **2017**, *8*, 43356–43367. [CrossRef] [PubMed]
24. Bankhead, P.; Loughrey, M.B.; Fernández, J.A.; Dombrowski, Y.; McArt, D.G.; Dunne, P.D.; McQuaid, S.; Gray, R.T.; Murray, L.J.; Coleman, H.G.; et al. QuPath: Open source software for digital pathology image analysis. *Sci. Rep.* **2017**, *7*, 16878. [CrossRef]

medicina

MDPI

Article

Differential Expression of Mucin in Salivary Gland Tumours

Nurul Inaas Mahamad Apandi [1,*], Siew Wui Chan [2] and Yen Fa Toh [3]

1 Fakulti Pergigian, Universiti Kebangsaan Malaysia, Kuala Lumpur 50300, Malaysia
2 Fakulti Pergigian, Universiti Malaya, Kuala Lumpur 50603, Malaysia; swuichan@um.edu.my
3 Jabatan Patologi, Pusat Perubatan Universiti Malaya, Kuala Lumpur 50603, Malaysia; yenfa@um.edu.my
* Correspondence: nurulinaas@ukm.edu.my

Abstract: *Background and Objectives*: Mucin has been implicated via various mechanisms in the development and growth of tumour cells. However, mucin expression studies in salivary gland tumours are limited, especially with samples from minor salivary glands. This study aims to investigate and compare mucin expression in benign and malignant salivary gland tumours of minor and major salivary gland origins. *Materials and Methods*: Special stains were used to stain neutral mucin (Periodic acid Schiff), sialomucin (Alcian Blue) and sulfomucin (Aldehyde Fuschin) within tissues from six normal salivary glands and 73 salivary gland tumours including 31 pleomorphic adenomas, 27 mucoepidermoid carcinomas, and 15 adenoid cystic carcinomas. A semi-quantitative approach was used to evaluate mucin expression within ductal lumens. Sialomucin was the most expressed mucin in all salivary gland tumours, regardless of origin. *Results*: A significant difference was observed in the mucin expression between benign and malignant salivary gland tumours, as pleomorphic adenoma showed three times significantly higher expression of sialomucin compared to mucoepidermoid carcinoma and adenoid cystic carcinoma ($p = 0.028$). Pleomorphic adenomas of major glands showed 42 times significantly higher expression of sialomucin compared to those of minor glands ($p = 0.000$). *Conclusions*: Sialomucin content in pleomorphic adenomas of major glands was vastly increased compared to that in minor glands. Differential sialomucin expression in benign and malignant salivary gland tumours suggests a role in diagnosing of borderline salivary gland tumours.

Keywords: pleomorphic adenoma; mucoepidermoid carcinoma; Alcian blue; sialomucin; sulfomucin

1. Introduction

Salivary gland neoplasms are relatively infrequent, accounting for 2–6.5% of head and neck tumours, with approximately 75% benign [1]. Secretory mucin has been postulated to play a significant role in disease development [2,3], as mucin differs in quality and quantity under normal and neoplastic conditions [3]. Mucin can be differentiated into epithelial mucin and connective tissue mucin. Epithelial cell components secrete neutral and acidic mucins, with acidic mucin further classified into sialomucin and sulfomucin. On the other hand, connective tissue mucin contains more acidic mucosubstances including, chondroitin sulphates, keratin sulphates, hyaluronic acid and dermatan sulphates [3].

Development and growth of tumour cells have been linked to the dysregulation of mucin protein core expression. Through this selection process, enzyme-modified tumour cells are presumed to express novel mucin forms, enhancing their survival. Mucin may influence the biological properties of tumour cells in several ways. Unlike epithelial cells, mucin could confer protection and serve as a barrier to tumour cells. This allows the tumour cells to be sheltered from toxic compounds, rendering them resistant towards acids, chemotherapeutic agents and cytotoxic compounds [4].

The mucin layer could capture biologically active molecules such as growth factors and cytokines that may promote tumour growth, offering an indirect influence over the regulation and interaction of the immune system, inflammatory response and stromal cell interaction with tumour cells. Differentiation and proliferation of tumour cells are governed by cell surface mucin via morphogenetic signal transduction and ligand-receptor interaction. Overexpression of mucin leads to signalling interaction via the mitogen-activated protein kinase (MAPK) pathway [5], which can be triggered in response to external growth factors. Mucin has also been associated with tumour metastasis by its involvement in a molecular process that regulates anti-adhesion and adhesion effects [6]. The modulation of leukocyte activity is possible, as high levels of soluble mucin form a barrier that nullifies the effects of leucocytes on tumour cells. The presence of these mucins within the blood and lymphatics would also obstruct the antigen-presenting mechanism against tumour cells [4].

Mucin can be stained with different single stains and a combination of stains, thus enabling them to be classified. Both epithelial and connective tissue mucins can be stained for identification. Stains available for mucin include Periodic Acid Shiff (PAS), Alcian blue (AB), Mucicarmine (MC), High Iron Diamine (HID), Aldehyde Fuchsin (AF), Hale Colloidal Iron and Toluidine blue staining. Epithelial neutral mucin can be stained with PAS, while epithelial acidic mucin can be stained with PAS, MC and AB. For the distinction between the two types of acidic mucin, sialomucin can be stained with PAS, MC, AB (pH 2.5) and hale colloidal iron, while sulfomucin can be stained with AB (pH 0.5), AF and HID. Connective tissue mucin can be highlighted with AB and Hale colloidal iron [7]. A summary is shown in Figure 1. Hence, in this study, we will use a combination of PAS, AB and AF stains to achieve better contrast. A PAS/AB stain will be used to identify neutral and acidic mucin, while AB/AF will be used for identification of acidic mucin. AB at pH 2.5 is specific to highlight the presence of sialomucin, while AF is specific for traces of sulfomucin.

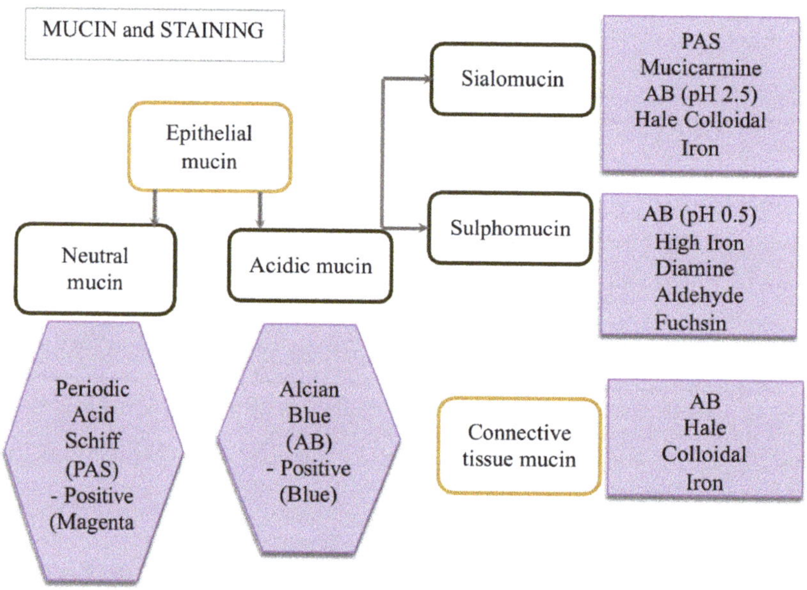

Figure 1. Diagrammatic representation of mucins and their corresponding stains, modified from various sources.

In salivary gland tumours, it has been shown that sialomucin was predominant within benign tumours and in combination with sulfomucin in the malignant types. This is shown in PA, whereby, there is a predominance of sialomucin and neutral mucin [3]. Meanwhile, higher traces of sialomucin and sulfomucin were found in MEC of salivary glands compared to MEC of the oesophagus [8]. AdCC also showed more sialomucin presence and neutral mucin in focal areas [9]. Another study demonstrated that periodic acid Schiff diastase (PAS-D) positive granules were helped differentiate various salivary gland neoplasms [10].

Mucin expression studies in salivary gland tumours are few and far between, with existing studies limited by sample size or restricted to a few types of salivary gland tumours due to the generally rare incidence of these tumours. No study explores salivary gland origin as a possible confounding factor for mucin expressions within the same type of salivary gland tumours. This study investigated mucin expression in benign and malignant salivary gland tumours of minor and major salivary gland origins to explore the potential of mucin histochemistry as an indicator of clinical behaviour in salivary gland tumours.

2. Material and Methods

2.1. Tissue Sample

Sample size calculation was done using G*Power software, version 3.1.9.4 for this study. Based on the effect size of 0.25 and power of 0.86, the estimated sample size was 32 for each group. Unfortunately, 5 PA cases, 9 MEC cases and 7 AdCC cases from minor salivary glands had to be replaced because the initial selected blocks were eaten by rats. After staining, 1 MEC case from a minor salivary gland had to be discarded due to insufficient tumour tissue. Two more cases (1 PA and 1 AdCC) from the major salivary gland were rejected as the wrong tissue blocks were provided. At the final count, the sample collection was at 79. The sample consisted of 6 control group tissues, from normal salivary gland tissues, of which, 3 were from submandibular glands (major salivary gland), 3 were from normal labial mucosa region (minor salivary gland) and 73 were histologically diagnosed salivary gland neoplasms which included 31 cases of pleomorphic adenoma (PA), 27 cases of mucoepidermoid carcinoma (MEC) and 15 cases of adenoid cystic carcinoma (AdCC) from 1995 to 2019. PAs consisted of 15 cases from major glands and 16 from minor glands. For MEC, 12 were from major glands and gradings are as follows; 6 low grade, 2 intermediate grade and 4 high grade, while 15 were from minor glands and all were low grade except 1, which was intermediate grade. For AdCC, 3 were from major glands while 12 were from minor glands, and all of cribriform patterns except those for 1 minor gland displayed a solid arrangement, as shown in Table 1. Major glands utilized for the majority of the samples were from the Parotid gland and Submandibular glands, while minor glands utilized the majority were from the palatal and retromolar region. The corresponding formalin-fixed paraffin-embedded tissue blocks were sourced from the archives of the Oral Pathology Research and Diagnostic Laboratory, Department of Oral and Maxillofacial Clinical Science, Faculty of Dentistry, University of Malaya (UM) and Anatomical Pathology Division of Department of Pathology, University Malaya Medical Centre (UMMC). Control group tissues composed of normal salivary tissue from intraoral mucoceles and normal submandibular glands obtained from surgical specimens with neck dissections. This study was approved by the Medical Ethics Committee, Faculty of Dentistry, UM [DF OS1911/0044(P)] and the Medical Research Ethics Committee, UMMC (20200622-8793).

Table 1. Distribution of cases included in study.

Salivary Gland Tumour	Minor Glands	Major Glands
PA	16	15
MEC	15 (14 low-grade, 1 intermediate-grade)	12 (6 low-grade, 2 intermediate-grade and 4 high-grade)
AdCC	12 (All tubular and cribriform pattern)	3 (2 tubular and cribriform pattern, 1 solid pattern)

PA: Pleomorphic adenoma; MEC: Mucoepidermoid carcinoma; AdCC: Adenoid cystic carcinoma.

2.2. Histochemistry

Histochemical re-staining was done on 4–5 µm-thick sections cut by a microtome and mounted on glass slides. Histological staining was performed with Harris Haematoxylin and Eosin. Harris Haematoxylin and Eosin were used as they provide crisp clear nuclear detail. The combination of Alcian Blue-Periodic Acid Schiff (AB-PAS) staining was performed according to Mowry [11] while a combination of Alcian Blue-Aldehyde Fuschin (AB-AF) staining was performed according to Spicer and Mayer [12]. PAS-stained magenta for neutral mucin, AB-stained blue for sialomucin (acidic mucin) and AF-stained purple for sulfomucin (acidic mucin). Staining reagents or kits were procured from Premier Diagnostics Sdn Bhd, Malaysia (Alcian blue (pH 2.5) 100 test/kit, Hamburg, Germany; Gomori's paraldehyde fuschins, 1 kit (100 tests); Hematoxylin) and Labchem Sdn Bhd, Malaysia (Sigma Aldrich Schiffs Fuschin, sulfite reagent, Bayswater, Australia) suitable for detection of glycoproteins, 500 mL; Periodic acid for analysis, Merck, Rahway, NJ, USA).

2.3. Semi-Quantitative Analysis

The localizations of AB, PAS, and AF were examined under a virtual microscope (Olympus 534630, Hamburg, Germany) and the images were captured by using a digital microscope (Olympus BX51, Hamburg, Germany) at a high resolution of 4080 × 3072 pixels. Tumour tissue from biopsied specimens was entirely utilized while tissue from surgical specimens, a few different sections, were evaluated before selecting a final suitable representative section. Distribution of the stains within the tumour microenvironment was assessed, with the findings recorded as (+) indicating the presence of stain and (−) indicating the absence of stain. A semi-quantitative approach was used to further evaluate the expression of mucin within the ductal lumens. This approach was considered due to the categorical data nature of the percentage of surface areas highlighted by the special stains. For each sample, the entire surface area of the tumour microenvironment was examined under 20× to 100× magnifications using Toupview software (Version: V3.4_20230223) to assess the percentage of stains within lumens of ductal structures. Intra-examiner and inter-examiner calibrations involving three examiners were conducted and verified to minimise discrepancies. To avoid the possibility of inaccurate scoring, areas of intense inflammation and necrosis were excluded. The extent of scoring was categorized as follows: 0, less than 25% of surface area positivity; 1, 25–50% of surface area positivity; 2, 50–75% of surface area positivity and 3, more than 75% of surface area positivity. The scoring was further classified into two as follows: less than 50% of surface area positivity and more than 50% of surface area positivity.

2.4. Statistical Analysis

Result analysis was performed using IBM Statistical Package for Social Sciences (SPSS) version 26 obtained from SPSS Inc., Chicago, IL, USA. Comparative analysis was performed using Chi-square test and Fisher's exact where applicable, for mucin expression (AB, PAS and AF) in relation to minor or major salivary gland tumours and benign or malignant salivary gland tumours. Post-hoc analysis was done using Binary logistic regression. For all the statistical analyses, p Value < 0.05 indicates statistical significance.

3. Results

3.1. Sample Details

The salivary gland tumours involved patients ranging from 15 to 81 years of age. Benign tumours like PA occurred significantly more often in younger patients while malignant tumours often affected the elderly. Details on the presentations of salivary gland tumours are summarized in Table 2.

Table 2. Clinical presentations of salivary gland tumours in this study.

		PA (n = 31)		MEC (n = 27)		AdCC (n = 15)	
		Minor	Major	Minor	Major	Minor	Major
Age * n(%)	<47	14 (45)	9 (29)	7 (26)	2 (7)	2 (13)	1 (7)
	>47	2 (6)	6 (19)	8 (30)	10 (37)	10 (67)	2 (13)
Gender n(%)	F	12 (39)	11 (35)	4 (15)	11 (41)	8 (53)	1 (7)
	M	4 (13)	4 (13)	4 (15)	8 (30)	4 (27)	2 (13)
Ethnicity n(%)	Chinese	9 (29)	8 (26)	7 (26)	6 (22)	6 (40)	2 (13)
	Malay	4 (13)	4 (13)	6 (22)	5 (19)	6 (40)	1 (7)
	Indian	3 (10)	3 (10)	2 (7)	1 (4)	-	-
Intraoral sites n(%)	Palate	11 (35)	-	7 (26)	-	2 (13)	-
	Non-palate	5 (16)	-	8 (30)	-	10 (67)	-
Extraoral sites n(%)	Parotid	-	9 (29)	-	11 (41)	-	2 (13)
	Non-parotid	-	6 (19)	-	1 (4)	-	1 (7)

* Median age of 47 years was used as cut-off point for age binary measurement. PA: Pleomorphic adenoma; MEC: Mucoepidermoid carcinoma; AdCC: Adenoid cystic carcinoma.

3.2. Mucin Expression in Salivary Gland Tumours

Variable amounts of all three types of mucins were present in PA, MEC and AdCC (Figures 2 and 3). Generally, all the salivary gland tumours, regardless of origin, showed greater dominance of AB-positive mucin (sialomucin). A significant difference between the expression of AB within PA of minor and major salivary glands was also shown (Table 3). Expression of AB within PA of major salivary glands was 42 times higher compared to PA of minor glands.

Table 3. Comparison of mucin expression between minor and major salivary gland tumours.

Stain	AB, n(%)		p Value	AF, n(%)		p Value	PAS, n(%)		p Value
	Low	High		Low	High		Low	High	
PA									
Minor n = 16	13 (81)	3 (19)	^{c*} 0.000	8 (53)	7 (47)	^{c} 0.484	9 (75)	3 (25)	^{f} 0.242
Major n = 15	2 (13)	13 (87)		8 (67)	4 (33)		1 (33)	2 (67)	
MEC									
Minor n = 15	15 (94)	1 (6)	^{f} 1.000	15 (100)	-	$^{\alpha}$ -	12 (100)	-	$^{\alpha}$ -
Major n = 12	15 (100)	-		12 (100)	-		3 (100)	-	
AdCC									
Minor n = 12	15 (94)	1 (6)	^{f} 1.000	12 (80)	3 (20)	^{c} 0.756	12 (100)	-	$^{\alpha}$ -
Major n = 3	15 (100)	-		9 (75)	3 (25)		3 (100)	-	

Significant level p = 0.05, ^{c}: Pearson Chi-square; ^{f}, Fisher's Exact test; low, <50%; high, ≥50; $^{\alpha}$ p-values were not computed as figures did not meet statistical test requirements; ^{c*} Binary logistic regression showed higher AB expression within major PA compared to minor PA by 42, folds (p = 0.000); PA, Pleomorphic adenoma; MEC, Mucoepidermoid carcinoma; AdCC, Adenoid cystic, carcinoma; AB, Alcian blue; AF, Aldehyde Fuschin; PAS, Periodic acid–Schiff.

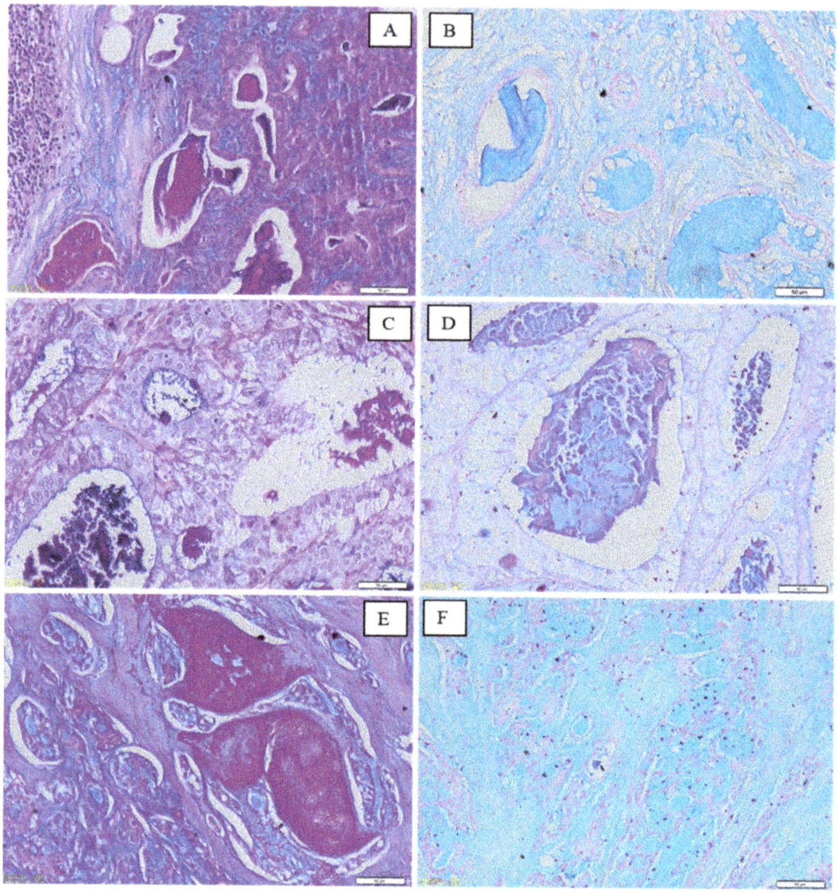

Figure 2. Photomicrograph shows staining in samples from minor salivary gland tumours: PA (**A**,**B**), MEC (**C**,**D**) and AdCC (**E**,**F**). (**A**) Luminal areas showing PAS-positivity with AB-PAS staining. (**B**) Predominance of AB staining within the lumens with AB-AF staining. (**C**) AB and PAS presence within lumen with AB-PAS staining. (**D**) Dominance of AB with traces of AF within lumens with AB-AF staining. (**E**) Dominance of AB with traces of PAS within the pseudocystic spaces with AB-PAS staining. (**F**) Dominance of AB within the pseudocystic spaces with AB-AF staining. [Magnification ×200].

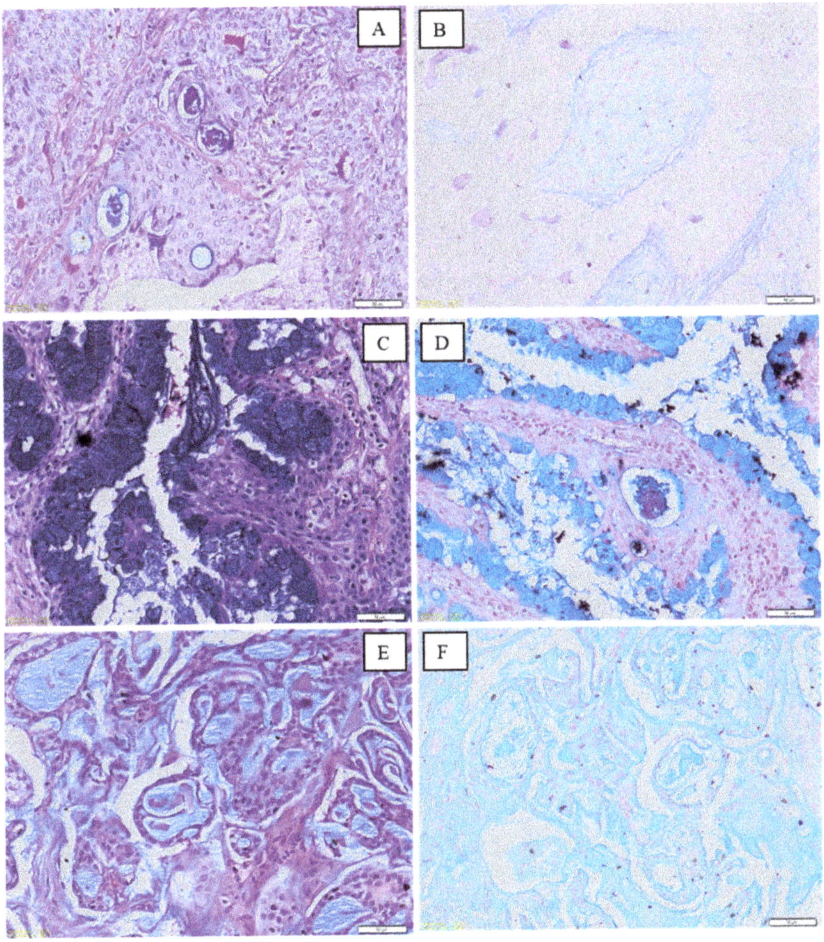

Figure 3. Photomicrograph shows staining in samples from major salivary gland tumours; PA (**A**,**B**), MEC (**C**,**D**) and AdCC (**E**,**F**). (**A**) Presence of both AB and PAS within luminal areas with AB-PAS staining. (**B**) Presence of AB and AF within luminal areas with AB-AF staining. (**C**) Mucous cells show AB-positivity with traces of luminal PAS-positivity with AB-PAS staining. (**D**) Dominance of AB and traces of AF within luminal areas with AB-AF staining (**E**) Dominance of AB within pseudocystic spaces with AB-PAS staining. (**F**) Dominance of AB within pseudocystic spaces in AB-AF staining. [Magnification ×200].

Benign salivary gland tumours demonstrated three times more expression of AB compared to malignant salivary gland tumours (Table 4).

Table 4. Comparison of mucin expression between benign and malignant salivary gland tumours.

Stain	Benign $n = 31$		Malignant $n = 42$		p Value [c]
	Low	High	Low	High	
AB, n(%)	12 (39)	19 (61)	29 (69)	13 (31)	0.016 *
AF, n(%)	31 (100)	-	41 (98)	1 (2)	0.387
PAS, n(%)	28 (90)	3 (10)	38 (90)	4 (10)	0.982

Significant level: $p = 0.05$, [c]: Pearson Chi-square test, Low: <50%, High: ≥50%, Benign—PA, Malignant—MEC & AdCC, * Binary logistic regression showed higher expressions of AB within benign tumours than malignant, tumours by 3 folds ($p = 0.028$); PA: Pleomorphic adenoma; MEC: Mucoepidermoid carcinoma; AdCC: Adenoid cystic carcinoma; AB: Alcian blue; AF: Aldehyde Fuschin; PAS: Periodic Acid-Schiff.

4. Discussion

Mucin is a complex molecule rich in protein and polysaccharide components, generally divided into epithelial and connective tissue mucin [3]. However, this study focused on neutral and acidic mucins secreted by epithelial cell components, considering only PA is a mixed tumour. Neutral mucins comprise hexosamines and hexose units without a free acidic group but with increased amounts of uncharged monosaccharides. Meanwhile, acidic mucin is further divided into sialomucin or sulfomucin based on the presence of terminal sialic acid or sulphate groups on the oligosaccharide chain respectively [13].

Salivary gland secretions are dependent on the composition and types of acini; serous, mucous or mixed. Generally, parotid glands are composed of mainly serous acini, sublingual glands of mainly mucous acini, and submandibular glands and minor glands of mixed acini [2,14]. A descriptive study found that mucin content in mucous cells was composed of sulfomucin and sialomucins, while serous acini contained other highly sulfated substances that were AB-positive but may not have been mucins [3]. The authors also noted that mucous acini in submandibular glands demonstrated varied heterogeneity; similarly, this is reflected in our findings [3]. In another study, neutral mucin was predominant, with little acidic mucin within parotid glands [13]. These staining variations reiterate the complexity and heterogeneous nature of salivary glands and their tumours, though it seems that mucous acini tend to produce acidic mucin, especially sialomucin.

Salivary gland tumours were shown to be sialomucin-dominant within benign tumours and demonstrated a sialomucin–sulfomucin combination within malignant tumours [3], but all our samples showed greater sialomucin expression, regardless of origin (Table 5). A possible explanation for the ubiquitous sialomucin content could be derived from the role of human mucin gene, MUC4, also known as a sialomucin complex, which shares similar ascitic sialoglycoprotein subunit and receptor domains. MUC4 expression was elevated throughout the epithelial thickness in normal or dysplastic mucosa close to the invasive tumour, indicating a cellular protective function of the mucin in reaction to the tumour and its predisposing environmental factors [15]. Sialomucin or its associated cells may possess similar protective functions.

Table 5. Summary of high mucin expression (>50%) in luminal spaces.

	Minor Glands	Major Glands
Normal	>Sialomucin (100%)	* Mixed neutral and acidic mucin (100%)
PA	>Sialomucin (19%)	>Sialomucin (86%)
MEC	>Sialomucin (47%) and neutral mucin (20%)	>Sialomucin (33%) and neutral mucin (25%)
AdCC	>Sialomucin (34%)	>Sialomucin (67%)

* Submandibular gland; PA, pleomorphic adenoma; MEC, mucoepidermoid carcinoma; AdCC, adenoid cystic carcinoma.

The exceptionally high sialomucin content in major PA compared to minor PA cannot be attributed to the original acini composition of the glands, since minor glands arguably contain more mucous acini. We could only speculate that maybe PA in major glands consisted of abundant luminal structures in comparison to minor glands. Previously, Naag et al. (2010) found elevated neutral and sialomucin content within PA of major salivary glands [3]. The sialomucin and neutral mucin combination in MEC of either origin also differs from other studies that reported a mixture of sialomucin and sulfomucin in MEC [3]. Relatively higher sialomucin content was a consistent finding but sulfomucin was barely detected in MEC in this study. The disparate sulfomucin detection patterns could be due to the use of different staining kits. In contrast to our findings, Lam et al. (1993) noted that oesophageal MEC had higher sialomucin content compared to MEC of the salivary gland, which had higher sulfomucin and sialomucin content, and histogenetic origin of the mucin-producing components was suggested as a possible explanation [8]. Comparing findings of AdCC from either origin was not feasible due to the imbalanced cases but the elevated sialomucin content within pseudocystic spaces in AdCC coincided with previous studies [16]. Other studies involving AdCC reported dominant sialomucin with focal areas of faint neutral mucin [3,8] or the presence of both sulfomucin and sialomucin [17]. To the best of our knowledge, no similar research was done specifically on minor salivary glands. Comparing mucin expression between minor and major salivary glands would ensure that mucin profiling done on salivary gland tumours is not undermined by their origin. However, we acknowledge that our findings would probably apply best to salivary glands of similar variants, as cystic or tubular variants theoretically express more mucin.

Greater sialomucin expression in benign salivary gland tumours compared to the malignant ones suggests a possible role of sialomucin or sialomucin-producing cells in the malignant progression of salivary gland neoplasms, correlating well with many of the reported roles of mucin in growth and development of tumour cells. Mucin is known for its wide-ranging influence over tumour cells via control of the local environment, regulation of differentiation and cell proliferation, tumour suppression, invasion, metastases and regulation of inflammation and immune response [2]. This finding is also consistent with the reported observations in many tumours that acidic mucin content was elevated as tumorigenesis progressed [18,19].

Mucin expression has also been linked to the histological tumour grade and prognosis of MEC [20]. MUC1 was expressed in high-grade MEC and associated with poor prognosis and shorter disease-free survival intervals, while MUC4 was highly expressed in low-grade MEC with a better prognosis and longer disease-free survivals. Our findings suggest that AB staining may be useful in distinguishing benign salivary gland tumours from malignant ones, like the use of AB (pH 2.5) in differentiating benign prostate hyperplasia and well-differentiated prostate adenocarcinoma [21]. Mucin studies in salivary gland tumours were found to be extremely lacking for further comparisons as most researchers tend to gravitate towards more precise immunohistochemical studies. Existing mucin studies mainly concentrated on gastrointestinal tumours, where grading is based on the postulated theory that there would be sulfomucin predominance in malignancy and increased neutral mucin expression with progressive differentiation of gastrointestinal tumours [22–24]. In addition to neutral mucin promotion, sulfomucin demotion during progressive tumour differentiation was also reported in later studies [18,19]. Although insignificant, a greater extent of neutral mucin content among MEC was seen compared to PA in our study. Unfortunately, the concept of differentiation is not applicable to these tumours. Then again, the results were also varied and inconsistent even amongst gastrointestinal mucin studies. Gad (1982) reported that well-differentiated carcinomas expressed more sialomucin compared to sulfomucin [19], while another study showed a marked increase of sialomucin content in more extensive tumours [22].

Salivary mucin secretion may also be affected by underlying obstructive disease, which is commonly seen in submandibular glands [25]. Submandibular duct papillae are often involved due to the ductal course; that is, against gravity, in addition to its long and curved anatomical structure [26]. Although, in our samples, there was no history of obstructive disorder; however, it can be evaluated further, especially for the two samples of PA from the submandibular gland in our study.

We acknowledge that this study had some limitations. Firstly, although the sample size was larger than it was in previous studies, there was an unequal distribution within each type of salivary gland tumour, especially for AdCC. Secondly, the varied histological features of each type of salivary gland tumour could influence the amount of mucinous content highlighted by the special stains. This problem was particularly prominent when a minute or an absence of mucinous composition was noted within solid tumour variants. This study could be improved by selecting salivary gland tumours of the same variants. We also had issues with the Aldehyde Fuschin kit stain because the reagents given as counterstains for nuclei were red while AF was violet and these colours were of similar intensity, thus making interpretation a laborious procedure. Lastly, histochemistry is only limited to portraying the presence of mucosubstances and does not allow the depiction of the refined element of these mucosubstances. Therefore, future studies need to be carried out to further explore the complex nature of salivary gland tumours.

5. Conclusions

In conclusion, sialomucin was the most expressed mucin in all salivary gland tumours irrespective of origin, inferring that alcian blue is the best special stain to visualize mucin components during microscopic examination. Significantly higher sialomucin expression in benign salivary gland tumours compared to malignant tumours suggests a possible role in the diagnosis of borderline salivary gland tumours. Perhaps further insight could be derived by investigating the role of sialomucin or sialomucin-producing cells in the malignant evolution of salivary gland tumours, with the use of PA and carcinoma ex-PA samples. Sialomucin expression within PA of major glands was excessively elevated in comparison to minor glands, while mucin expressions in MEC and AdCC were not significantly affected by their origin. Hence, caution is advised in samplings of PA for future research of a similar nature.

Author Contributions: Conceptualization N.I.M.A. and S.W.C.; methodology, N.I.M.A., S.W.C. and Y.F.T.; validation S.W.C. and Y.F.T.; formal analysis, N.I.M.A.; investigation, N.I.M.A.; resources, S.W.C. and Y.F.T.; data curation, N.I.M.A.; writing—original draft preparation, N.I.M.A.; writing—review and editing, S.W.C.; visualization, Y.F.T.; supervision, S.W.C. and Y.F.T.; project administration, S.W.C.; funding acquisition, S.W.C. All authors have read and agreed to the published version of the manuscript.

Funding: This research was financed by Research University Grant, Faculty of Dentistry, University of Malaya (GPF008E-2019).

Institutional Review Board Statement: The study was conducted in accordance with the Declaration of Helsinki, and approved by the Medical Ethics Committee, Faculty of Dentistry, University of Malaya (DF OS1911/0044(P)) and the Medical Research Ethics Committee, University Malaya Medical Centre (20200622-8793) on 31 December 2019.

Informed Consent Statement: Not applicable.

Data Availability Statement: The original contributions presented in the study are included in the article, further inquiries can be directed to the corresponding author.

Acknowledgments: The author conveys gratitude to the consultants and technical laboratory staff for their endless guidance and assistance.

Conflicts of Interest: The authors declare that there are no conflicts of interest regarding the publication of this paper.

References

1. Bobati, S.S.; Patil, B.V.; Dombale, V.D. Histopathological study of salivary gland tumors. *J. Oral. Maxillofac. Pathol.* **2017**, *21*, 46–50. [CrossRef]
2. Rohini, R.K.; Avinash, D.S.; Rajesh, A.K.; Umarji, B.N. Histochemical Study of Mucosubstances of Normal Human Parotid Salivary Gland. *J. Evol. Med. Dent. Sci.* **2014**, *3*, 13079–13085.
3. Naag, S.; Adi, R.P. Histochemical Study of Salivary Mucins in Normal and Neoplastic Salivary Glands. *J. Clin. Diagn. Res.* **2010**, *4*, 3450–3458.
4. Bhatia, R.; Gautam, S.K.; Cannon, A.; Thompson, C.; Hall, B.R.; Aithal, A.; Banerjee, K.; Jain, M.; Solheim, J.C.; Kumar, S.; et al. Cancer-associated Mucins: Role in Immune Modulation and Metastasis. *Cancer Metastasis Rev.* **2019**, *38*, 223–236. [CrossRef]
5. Ashok, K.D.; Xinxin, S.; Herbert, J.Z.; Zong, S.G.; Yong, J.L.; David, L.B.; Haroon, A.C. Mitogen-activated Protein Kinase Inhibition Reduces Mucin 2 Production and Mucinous Tumor Growth. *Transl. Res.* **2015**, *166*, 344–354.
6. Miletich, I. Introduction to Salivary Glands: Structure, Function and Embryonic Development. Salivary Glands. Development, Adaptations and Disease. *Front. Oral. Biol.* **2010**, *14*, 1–20. [PubMed]
7. Rekthman, N.; Bishop, J.A. *Quick Refernce Handbook for Surgical Pathologists*; Springer: Berlin/Heidelberg, Germany; Dordrecht, The Netherlands; London, UK; New York, NY, USA, 2011; pp. 69–75.
8. Lam, K.Y.; Loke, S.L.; Ma, L.T. Histochemistry of Mucin Secreting Components in Mucoepidermoid and Adenosquamous Carcinoma of Oesophagus. *J. Clin. Pathol.* **1993**, *46*, 1011–1015. [CrossRef]
9. Toida, M.; Takeuchi, J.; Tsukidate, K.; Akao, S.; Fukatsu, T.; Nakashima, N. Histochemical Studies on Pseudocyst in Adenoid Cystic Carcinoma of the Human Salivary Gland. *Histochem. J.* **1985**, *17*, 913–924. [CrossRef] [PubMed]
10. Panicker, N.; Jariwala, P.; Buch, A.; Joshi, M. The Utility Periodic Acid Schiff with Diastase and Alcian Blue Stains on Fine Needle Aspirates of Breast and Salivary Gland Neoplasms. *J. Cytol.* **2012**, *29*, 221–225.
11. Mowry, R.W. Alcian Blue Technics for the Histochemical Study of Acid Carbohydrates. *J. Histochem.* **1956**, *4*, 407.
12. Spicer, S.S.; Meyer, D.B. Histochemical Differentiation of Acid Mucopolysaccharides By Means of Combined Aldehyde Fuchsin-Alcian Blue Staining. *Am. J. Clin. Pathol.* **1960**, *33*, 453–460. [CrossRef]
13. Filipe, M.I.; Branfoot, A.C. Abnormal Patterns of Mucus Secretion in Apparently Normal Mucosa of Large Intestine with Carcinoma. *Cancer* **1974**, *34*, 282–290. [CrossRef] [PubMed]
14. Hamada, T.; Matsukita, S.; Goto, M.; Kitajima, S.; Batra, S.K.; Irimura, T.; Sueyoshi, K.; Sugihara, K.; Yonezawa, S. Mucin Expression in Pleomorphic Adenoma of Salivary Gland: A Potential Role for MUC1 as a Marker to Predict Recurrence. *J. Clin. Pathol.* **2004**, *57*, 813–821. [CrossRef] [PubMed]
15. Weed, D.T.; Gomez-Fernandez, C.; Bonfante, E.; Lee, T.D.; Pacheco, J.; Carvajal, M.E.; Carraway, K.L. MUC4 (Sialomucin Complex) Expression in Salivary Gland Tumors and Squamous Cell Carcinoma of the Upper Aerodigestive Tract. *Otolaryngol.—Head. Neck Surg.* **2016**, *124*, 127–141. [CrossRef] [PubMed]
16. Histochemical Study of Salivary Gland Tumors. *J. Pathol. Transl. Med.* **1981**, *15*, 53–61.
17. Peel, R. Diseases of salivary glands. In *Surgical Pathology of the Head and Neck*; Barnes, L., Ed.; Marcel Dekker Inc.: New York, NY, USA, 2001; pp. 634–757.
18. Jain, P.; Mondal, S.K.; Sinha, S.K.; Mukhopadhyay, M.; Chakraborty, I. Diagnostic and Prognostic Significance of Different Mucin Expression, Preoperative CEA, and CA-125 in Colorectal Carcinoma: A Clinicopathological Study. *J. Nat. Sci. Biol. Med.* **2014**, *5*, 404–408. [PubMed]
19. Gad, A. Pathophysiology of GIT mucins. *Adv. Physio Sci.* **1982**, *29*, 161–163.
20. Alos, L.; Lujan, B.; Castillo, M.; Nadal, A.; Carreras, M.; Caballero, M.; Cardesa, A. Expression of Membrane-Bound Mucins (MUC1 and MUC4) and Secreted Mucins (MUC2, MUC5AC, MUC5B, MUC6 and MUC7) in Mucoepidermoid Carcinomas of Salivary Glands. *Am. J. Surg. Pathol.* **2005**, *29*, 806–813. [CrossRef] [PubMed]
21. Agrawal, B.; Krantz, M.J.; Reddish, M.A.; Longenecker, B.M. Cancer-associated MUCl Mucin Inhibits Human T-cell Proliferation, Which is Reversible by IL-2. *Nat. Med.* **1998**, *4*, 43–49. [CrossRef]
22. Satpathy, Y.; Spadigam, A.E.; Dhupar, A.; Syed, S. Epithelial and Stromal Patterns of Pleomorphic Adenoma of Minor Salivary Glands: A Histopathological and Histochemical study. *J. Oral Maxillofac. Pathol. JOMFP* **2014**, *18*, 379–385. [CrossRef]
23. Lombardi, M.; Socciarelli, F.; Fini, G.; Leonardi, A.; Bartolazzi, A. Schwannoma-like Pleomorphic Adenoma: A Case Report with Review of the Literature. *Head Neck Pathol.* **2014**, *8*, 178–181. [CrossRef] [PubMed]
24. Huszno, J.; Mrochen-Domin, I.; Zembala-Nozynska, E.; Tukiendorf, A.; Lange, D.; Nowara, E. Mucin Secretion Activity of Gastric Cancer as a Prognostic Factor: A Clinicopathological Analysis. *Contemp. Oncol.* **2012**, *16*, 159–164. [CrossRef] [PubMed]
25. Badger, C.D.; Benito, D.A.; Joshi, A.S. Incorporating Sialendoscopy into the Otolaryngology Clinic. *Otolaryngol. Clin. N. Am.* **2021**, *54*, 509–520. [CrossRef] [PubMed]
26. Lopez, J.-M. Different Types of Papillae and Their Treatment. In *Sialendoscopy. The Hands-On Book*; Marchal, F., Ed.; Artcast Medical: Annecy, France, 2015; Volume 1, pp. 144–145.

medicina

MDPI

Article

Prelacrimal Recess Approach in Unilateral Maxillary Sinus Lesions: What Is the Impact and Efficacy?

Mohamed Abdulla [1], Osama Refaat [1], Mohamed Alahmer [1], Ayman Yehia [1], Hesham Abdelsalam [1], Khaled Abdelaal [2,*] and Mohamed Shams Eldin [1,*]

1 Department of Otorhinolaryngology, Faculty of Medicine, Al-Azhar University, Cairo 11675, Egypt
2 EPCRS Excellence Center, Plant Pathology and Biotechnology Lab., Faculty of Agriculture, Kafrelsheikh University, Kafr El-Sheikh 33516, Egypt
* Correspondence: khaled.elhaies@gmail.com (K.A.); shamsent@azhar.edu.eg (M.S.E.)

Abstract: *Background and Objectives*: Chronic sinusitis is a commonly encountered diagnosis for otorhinolaryngologists. The profound negative effect of rhinosinusitis on patients' quality of life is frequently overlooked, and surgical lines of treatment are numerous. The aim of the study was to assess the comparative efficacy of endoscopic middle meatal antrostomy with the endoscopic prelacrimal recess approach, combined with middle meatal antrostomy in the treatment of unilateral chronic maxillary sinus lesion. *Materials and Methods*: Thirty patients with unilateral chronic maxillary sinus lesions enrolled in the study at Alahsa hospital. Patients were divided into two groups: 15 treated through a middle meatal antrostomy and 15 treated via a combined middle meatal antrostomy and prelacrimal recess approach. Demographic and clinical information of the patients, including the medical history, CT scan findings, diagnosis, recurrence, and complications, were gathered and analyzed. Pre- and postoperative clinical findings were graded utilizing the Lund–Kennedy Endoscopic Scoring System. *Results*: The enrolled patients varied in age from 18 to 56, with 60% being male and 40% being female. Antrochoanal polyp, maxillary sinus mucocele, and unilateral allergic fungal sinusitis were among the pathological diagnoses. The follow-up period averaged 14.3 months. Following surgery, two patients in Group II encountered nasal discomfort, which included synechia and epiphora. The success rate for preserving a patient's disease-free condition was 86.7%. A statistically significant difference in disease-free incidence was observed among the patients in group II. In group I, recurrence was identified in 26.7% of the patients. The postoperative symptoms diminished considerably, and the VAS score was reduced substantially. In Group II patients, however, there was no significant difference in scarring. Clinically significant differences were observed in the mean total Lund–Kennedy Endoscopic scores when compared to their preoperative values. *Conclusions*: Achieving endoscopic access to the sinus's anterior, lateral, inferior, and inferomedial regions is facilitated by operating via the prelacrimal recess, which is the most advantageous approach. This approach facilitates rapid mucosal healing by maintaining the integrity of the nasolacrimal duct and mucosal covering. The specific pathology, surgical objectives, surgeon expertise, and equipment accessibility influence the choice of endoscopic surgical technique.

Keywords: prelacrimal recess approach; endoscopic sinus surgery; Lund–Kennedy Endoscopic Scoring System

1. Introduction

Due to the placement of the natural ostium and the difficult ascending mucociliary outflow, the maxillary sinus is the sinus most typically impacted by pathology. The function of the maxillary sinus is to significantly warm and humidify the air. Moreover, the maxillary sinus and its floor are utilized in a variety of regenerative procedures that produce a new volume of bone tissue in order to treat bone atrophy [1]. It is also frequently affected by odontogenic infection neoplastic, traumatic, and allergy disorders. Chronic rhinosinusitis

(CRS) represents one of the most prevalent diagnoses seen by an otorhinolaryngologist on a daily basis. Chronic sinusitis refers to repeated episodes of inflammation in the sinus membrane that lines the paranasal canal. This condition lasts for a minimum of 8–12 weeks and is characterized by symptoms such as congested airways, rhinorrhea, facial pain, and a disturbed sense of smell [2]. The significant detrimental impact of rhinosinusitis on patients' quality of life is often underestimated and neglected. Many people were previously informed that they simply had to "live with" their sinus disease [3]. The socioeconomic effect of rhinosinusitis is an increasing subject of study. Conservative estimates US CRS expenses at over USD 30 billion per year, including USD 20 billion in indirect costs. Direct expenditures include medical visits, prescription medications, and surgery, whereas indirect costs entail lost productivity in rhinosinusitis patients [4]. Current recommendations provide precise therapeutic indications for the treatment of CRS. Regarding surgical indication, sinus surgery should be considered for individuals with CRS who are resistant to medicinal therapy. The choice to operate should be considered in patients with symptomatic illness, excluding those with real or imminent complications, according to the recent guidelines [5]. Since the 1980s, functional endoscopic sinus surgery (FESS) has had several designations to describe its surgical spectrum. The minimally invasive sinus technique, first published in 1996, involves simple sinus ventilation and has been shown to alleviate situations even with severe disease [5]. FESS offers the benefit of maintaining sinus ventilation and mucociliary clearance in cases involving inflammation or infection of the sinuses. Resection of the attachment site should be performed in cases of benign sinonasal tumors, such as inverted papillomas or recurrent antrochoanal polyps, in order to prevent earlier recurrence [6]. In basic situations, a routine uncinectomy and middle meatal antrostomy may be enough for disease visualization and clearance. However, we all too often encounter situations in which we can see substantial maxillary sinus pathology that we do not have a way to eradicate. There are few alternative options in such cases when the usual uncinectomy and middle meatal antrostomy are insufficient [7]. Complete removal of the lesion is frequently challenging due to the instrument's restricted reach, despite the improved visibility provided by a 70° or 90° endoscope, particularly in cases involving lesions located in the anterior or inferior wall. [8] The removal in such case may be executed utilizing either the conventional Caldwell–Luc approach (CLA) or a canine fossa puncture. In total, 75% of patients have experienced complications associated with the canine fossa approach, which comprise pain, dental complications, and facial numbness [9]. The Caldwell–Luc approach unfortunately, did not provide adequate access to specific maxillary sinus areas and may have resulted in infraorbital nerve injury [10]. Due to the fact that even with specific curved equipment and angled endoscopes or a wide antrostomy diffuse disease in the maxillary sinus, such as recurring polyposis and pathologies originating from the floor or anterior wall of the maxillary sinus, cannot be eliminated fully endoscopically by middle meatal antrostomy [11], Zhou and colleagues introduced the endoscopic intranasal prelacrimal recess approach (PLRA) to the maxillary sinus in 2007. This approach allows for broad access to the walls and recesses of the maxillary sinus while preserving the inferior turbinate and nasolacrimal duct [12]. It affords an uninterrupted view of almost all interior maxillary linings. This enhanced visibility of the operative field may lessen the inherent limitations of endoscopic techniques. PLRA entails surgically generating a passageway by constructing a gap in the medial wall of the prelacrimal recess, which is often one of the most difficult sites to manipulate during conventional middle meatal antrostomy [13]. The aim of this study was to assess the efficacy of endoscopic middle meatal antrostomy versus endoscopic prelacrimal recess approach and middle meatal antrostomy in the treatment of unilateral chronic maxillary sinusitis.

2. Materials and Methods

The study was conducted in the Department of Otorhinolaryngology, (Alahsa hospital) after obtaining the approval of the local ethics committee, and all patients provided informed consent for permission before enrolment in this study. Between November 2019 and December 2022, all selected patients had unilateral chronic maxillary sinusitis and underwent endoscopic sinus surgery. Patients with bilateral sinonasal pathology, sinusitis with complications, allergic rhinosinusitis with nasal polyposis or malignant sinonasal lesions were excluded from the study. Thirty patients were enrolled in the study. They were classified into two groups. Group I included 15 patients treated endoscopically through only a middle meatal antrostomy (MMA), and Group II included 15 patients who were treated via a combined middle meatal antrostomy and prelacrimal recess approach (PLRA). The postoperative care was implemented over a period of 11–23 months, utilizing a nasal endoscope at regular intervals to remove the crust, blood clot, and dry discharge until adequate healing and epithelization were accomplished. Topical nasal corticosteroid and routine saline irrigation were advised for 4 to 6 months after surgery. The demographic profile of the patients as well as their clinical data were obtained including history taking, a local examination, diagnostic nasal endoscopy findings, CT scan findings (Figures 1–3), pathological diagnosis, recurrence, and complications.

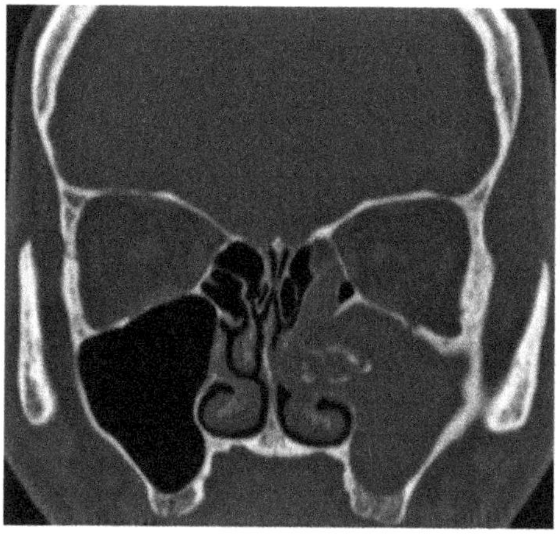

Figure 1. Coronal CT scan of the paranasal sinuses shows the left maxillary and ethmoidal sinuses were completely heterogonous opacified, with linear calcifications and hypertrophy of the maxillary sinus wall; fungal sinusitis.

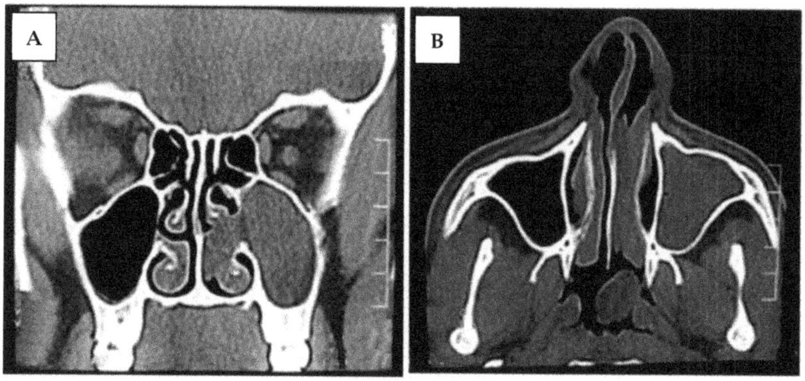

Figure 2. Coronal and axial CT image of an antrochoanal polyp on the left side with extension of the polyp to the nasopharynx (**A**): coronal and (**B**): axial CT image.

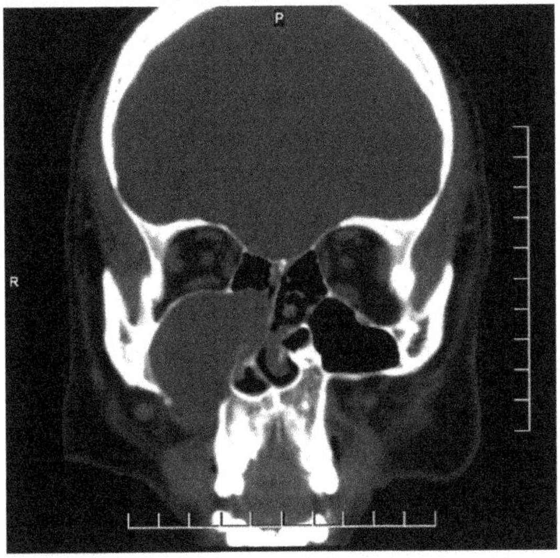

Figure 3. CT scan reveals a right opacified maxillary sinus with medial expansion leading to obstruction of the right nasal cavity and superior bulging causing encroachment on the floor of the orbit.

The 5 main cardinal symptoms were assessed preoperatively, 2 months following the surgery and in the late follow up period ranging from 11 to 23 months including facial pain, headache, nasal obstruction, nasal discharge, and olfactory disturbance. The assessment was conducted using a simple Visual Analogue Scale (VAS), where the patient was asked to give a score of 0 if there were no symptoms and 10 for maximum severity of the symptoms. The score increased from 0 to 10 according to the subjective severity of the symptoms. Preoperative and postoperative findings were also compared in the same sessions regarding scarring degree, crust, mucosal edema, polyps, and nasal discharge depending on the "Lund–Kennedy Endoscopic Scoring System." These findings were scored from 0 to 2, where a score of 0 was given in the case of no presence, 1 in a mild degree, and 2 in a severe degree of the findings. Both groups' data were compared at the end of the follow-up period (ranging from 11 to 23 months), and the results were statistically analyzed.

Surgical Technique

Surgery was conducted under general anesthesia in all instances. Nasal endoscopic surgery started after initial preparation of the nasal cavity by nasal packing with cotton pledges containing Xylometazoline as a topical vasoconstrictor; then, the lateral wall of the nose was infiltrated with 1% lidocaine with 1:100,000 adrenaline solution. It was applied to the lateral nasal wall including the head of the inferior turbinate, inferior meatus, the nasal aperture, the uncinate process, and face of the middle turbinate. A standard uncinectomy with middle meatal antrostomy was performed for patients of both groups with removal of all inflammatory pathological lesions from the maxillary sinus and osteomeatal unit using a 30- and 0-degree endoscope. The prelacrimal recess approach started with a curved mucosal incision (Figure 4A) on the lateral wall of the nasal cavity between the anterior head of the inferior turbinate and the nasal surface of the pyriform aperture and deepened down to the bone, extending from the anterior border of the nasolacrimal dust into the inferior meatus. A mucoperiosteal flap was created and elevated between the inferior meatal wall and lateral nasal wall up to the bony attachment of the inferior turbinate (Figure 4B). At this step, the Hasner's valve could be identified and preserved. A bony cut was made vertically with an osteotomy passing through the lateral nasal wall starting at the bony insertion site of the inferior turbinate (Figure 4C); then, the cut passed posterosuperiorly to the nasolacrimal duct (NLD) with disconnection of the bony attachment of the inferior turbinate. Once the mucoperiosteum was elevated posteriorly, the bony orifice of the NLD could be considered as a landmark from which the medial part of the prelacrimal recess (PLR), which constitutes the anterior part of the medial wall of the maxillary sinus, was chiseled off. After chiseling the bone posteriorly, the performed flap was medialized exposing the maxillary sinus mucosal wall (Figure 4D). At this this step, the (PLR) was entered by removing the anterior or anteromedial maxillary wall (Figure 4E,F), according to the extension of the present pathology that could be dealt with endoscopically with a wide view that ensured complete and successful interaction. The mucosal flap was then repositioned and closed with vicryl 4 /0 with packing of the nasal cavity using Merocel® nasal pack.

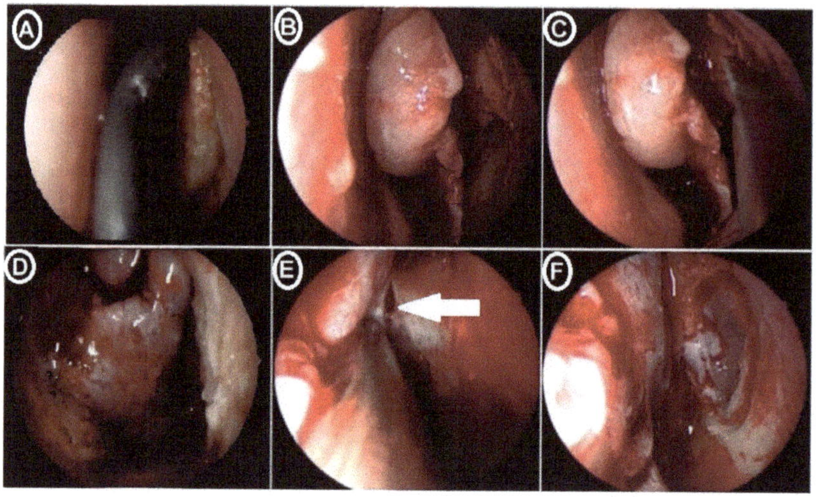

Figure 4. Surgical steps of the prelacrimal recess approach. A c-shaped mucosal incision on the lateral wall of the nasal cavity around the anterior attachment of the inferior turbinate concha (**A**); the mucosa was elevated posteriorly to the insertion site of the inferior turbinate concha (**B**); an osteotomy was performed at the inferior turbinate concha insertion site (**C**); the mucosal flap of the inferior turbinate was sutured to the nasal septum (**D**); the opening of the nasolacrimal duct (labeled with an arrow) was exposed, and the mucosa was left intact (**E**); the maxillary sinus was entered through the antrostomy made at the prelacrimal recess (**F**).

The Statistical Package for the Social Sciences, version 25.0 (IBM SPSS, Armonk, NY, USA: IBM Corp., New York, NY, USA) was used throughout the data analysis process. When it was acceptable to do so, descriptive statistics were given using counts, proportions (percentages), and the mean ± the standard deviation. The chi-square test was used to make a comparison between the middle meatal antrostomy and the middle meatal antrostomy coupled with prelacrimal recess methods among the baseline features of the patients. When calculating statistical significance, a p value cutoff point of 0.05 was utilized at 95% confidence intervals. The tests used were the X mean, SD standard deviation: to measure the central tendency of data and the distribution of data around the mean; Student's t-test: for testing the statistically significant difference between means of two samples; X2 test (chi-square test) to test the statistical relation between different variable or grades (qualitative data). Methods of Statistical Analysis: (i) arithmetic mean: (X) $X = \frac{\Sigma x}{n}$, where Σ = sum, x = value of observation, and n = number of observations; (ii) standard deviation = SD, $SD = \sqrt{\frac{\Sigma(X-X)^2}{n-1}}$, where X = observation, X = mean of the group, and n = number; (iii) Student's "*t*" test: $t = \frac{X_1 - X_2}{\sqrt{SD_1{}^2/n_1 + SD_2{}^2/n_2}}$, where X1 = mean of first group, X2 = mean of the second group, SD1 = standard deviation of the first group, SD2 = standard deviation of the second group, n1= no. of first group, and n2 = no. of second group.

3. Results

We conducted research on thirty individuals who had endoscopic sinus surgery after being diagnosed with unilateral chronic maxillary sinusitis and were impacted by the disease. Patients with unilateral chronic maxillary opacity who underwent endoscopic sinus surgery were classified according to the performed endoscopic procedure into Group I, where 15 patients underwent endoscopic sinus surgery using the middle meatal antrostomy approach, Group II, where 15 patients were managed endoscopically through combined approaches (middle meatal antrostomy combined with prelacrimal recess). Following the splitting of the patients participating in this research into two groups, an analysis of their data was carried out. The ages ranged from 18 to 56 years old, with the mean of 39.5 ± 11.5 years old. The most prevalent range of age for people to have surgery for either of these groups was between the ages of 20 and 35. Males made up 60% of the total population, while females only made up 40%. The pathological diagnosis was distributed as follows: unilateral allergic fungal sinusitis (46.7%), maxillary sinus mucocele (40%), and antrochoanal polyp (13.3%) (Figure 5). The mean duration of follow-up following surgeries was 14.3 months (range 11–23 months). In Group II, the inferior turbinate was unstable in two patients after surgery (13.3%), and these patients had nasal discomfort, which improved in the late follow-up. One patient had chronic epiphora, while one other patient had anterior nasal synechia (6.6%). The operation time expanded by 37 min on average when group II was operated on. The thirty patients' initial demographics and clinical data are presented in (Tables 1 and 2).

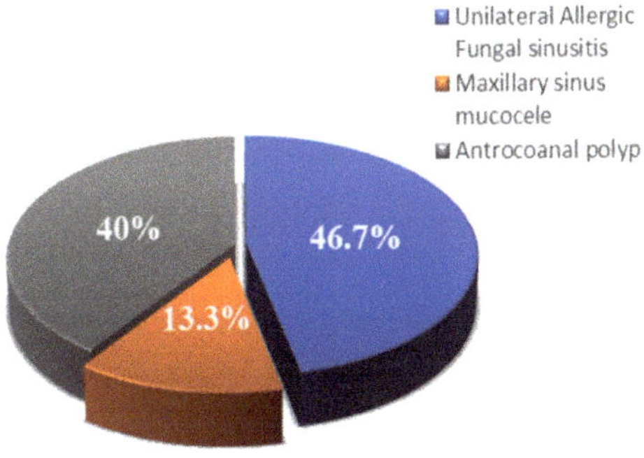

Figure 5. Distribution of the studied cases in relation to their pathological diagnosis.

The postoperative period was uneventful for patients in both groups. Overall, an 86.7% success rate was shown in the studied cases of both groups in terms of maintaining a patient's disease-free status following the procedure. Four patients out of fifteen (26.7%) in group I had recurrence after surgery, but none of the patients in group II showed evidence of recurrence. When compared to Group I, Group II exhibited a statistically significant difference in the incidence of individuals who were disease-free ($p = 0.032$). In group I, the maxillary sinus walls could not be seen to their full extent in eight patients (53.3%), whereas in group II, only two cases (13.3%) presented difficulty with seeing the maxillary sinus in its entirety. In most cases of Group II, the combined prelacrimal and middle meatal antrostomy techniques allowed for complete visualization of the maxillary sinus pathology. Postoperative symptoms were decreased in both approaches, and a significant reduction in the VAS score was obtained in both groups. The improvement in the mean of the symptoms of facial pain, nasal obstruction, nasal discharge, and olfactory disturbance following the combined approach showed a significant statistical difference when compared to that obtained following the endoscopic middle meatal antrostomy approach only. When compared to their preoperative values, the postoperative mean total VAS scores of patients in group I demonstrated a statistically significant and clinically meaningful difference ($p < 0.0001$). According to Table 2, a similar result was seen in patients from group II as well ($p < 0.0001$); however, the postoperative improvement shown in the group II patients was more statistically significant than that seen in the group I patients ($p = 0.0072$), as shown in Tables 3 and 4. These results indicate a considerable increase in the quality of life after endoscopic surgery, with higher outcomes in favor of patients who utilized a combined approach.

Table 1. Clinicopathological features of the study population ($n = 30$).

Study Variables	*N* (%)
Study group	
• Group I	15 (50.0%)
• Group II	15 (50.0%)
Age in years (mean ± SD)	39.5 ± 11.5
Sex	
• Male	18 (60.0%)
• Female	12 (40.0%)
Pathology	
• Unilateral allergic fungal sinusitis	14 (46.7%)
• Antrochoanal polyp	12 (40.0%)
• Maxillary sinus mucocele	04 (13.3%)
Complication	
• Yes	0
• No	30 (100%)
Outcome	
• Disease free	26 (86.7%)
• Recurrence	04 (13.3%)

Table 2. Comparison between Group I and Group II of the baseline characteristics of the patients ($n = 30$).

Factor	Study Group		*p* Value
	Group I *N* (%) ($n = 15$)	**Group II** *N* (%) ($n = 15$)	**0.715**
Age in years			
• <40 years	07 (46.7%)	08 (53.3%)	1.000
• ≥40 years	08 (53.3%)	07 (46.7%)	
Sex			
• Male	09 (60.0%)	09 (60.0%)	1.000
• Female	06 (40.0%)	06 (40.0%)	
Pathology			
• Unilateral allergic fungal sinusitis	07 (46.7%)	07 (46.7%)	
• Maxillary sinus mucocele	02 (13.3%)	02 (13.3%)	0.032 **
• Antrochoanal polyp	06 (40.0%)	06 (40.0%)	
Outcome			0.715
• Disease free	11 (73.3%)	15 (100%)	
• Recurrence	04 (26.7%)	0	

** Significant at the $p < 0.05$ level.

Table 3. Visual analogue score means of the compared groups.

Visual Analogue Score		Facial Pain	Headache	Nasal Obstruction	Nasal Discharge	Olfactory Disturbance	Total VAS
Group (I)	Preoperative	5.1 ± 1.9	4.68 ± 1.51	6.85 ± 1.67	5.61 ± 1.51	3.78 ± 1.33	27.13 ± 5.79
	Postoperative	3.68 ± 1.56	2.09 ± 0.91	2.10 ± 1.29	2.11 ± 1.54	1.8 ± 1.06	12.47 ± 3.68
p Value		0.0348 *	<0.0001 **	<0.0001 **	<0.0001 **	0.0001 **	<0.0001 **
Group (II)	Preoperative	5.46 ± 1.76	5.73 ± 1.27	7.73 ± 1.38	5.73 ± 1.83	5.4 ± 1.88	30.06 ± 3.30
	Postoperative	1.73 ± 1.27	1.26 ± 0.96	1.27 ± 1.03	1.87 ± 1.06	2.13 ± 1.35	8.67 ± 3.5
p Value		<0.000 **	<0.0001 **	<0.0001 **	<0.0001 **	<0.0001 **	<0.0001 **

* Significant difference, ** highly Significant at the $p < 0.05$ level.

Table 4. Comparison between the postoperative VAS means of the studied groups.

	Mean	SD	*t*-Test	*p* Value	SE	95% CI	
						Lower	Upper
GROUP (I)	12.47	±3.68	−2.898	*p* = 0.0072 **	1.311	1.1139	6.4861
GROUP (II)	8.67	±3.5					

** Significant at the $p < 0.05$ level.

The Lund–Kennedy Endoscopic Scoring System was used to grade the endoscopic findings in the postoperative period. Postoperative changes in nasal discharge and nasal polyps were significantly reduced in both techniques, with a highly statistically significant reduction as compared to the preoperative data ($p < 0.0001$).

Crust and mucosal edema were similarly decreased in the surgical follow-up period of the two groups with a significant statistical difference, although the scarring in the lateral nasal wall in Group II patients revealed no significant statistical difference. The postoperative mean total Lund–Kennedy Endoscopic scores of patients in Group I exhibited a highly statistically significant and clinically relevant difference when compared to their preoperative values ($p < 0.0001$), as shown in Table 5. A similar finding was obtained in group II patients; however, the postoperative improvement shown in the group II patients was statistically significantly greater than that seen in the group I patients (Table 6) ($p = 0.0323$).

Table 5. Lund–Kennedy Endoscopic Scoring System of the compared groups.

Lund-Kennedy Endoscopic Scoring System		Scarring	Crust	Mucosal Edema	Polyps	Nasal Discharge	Total Score
Group (I)	Preoperative	0.47 ± 0.64	0.33 ± 0.49	1.53 ± 0.52	1.6 ± 0.83	1.73 ± 0.46	5.66 ± 1.39
	Postoperative	0.93 ± 0.59	0.47 ± 0.52	0.53 ± 0.55	0.4 ± 0.51	0.6 ± 0.51	2.93 ± 0.96
p Value		=0.0502 *	=0.4543 *	<0.0001 **	0.0001 **	<0.0001 **	<0.0001 **
Group (II)	Preoperative	0.33 ± 0.49	0.47 ± 0.52	1.73 ± 0.46	1.8 ± 0.41	1.87 ± 0.35	6.2 ± 0.86
	Postoperative	0.53 ± 0.52	0.93 ± 0.6	1.33 ± 0.49	0.27 ± 0.46	0.8 ± 0.41	3.87 ± 1.3
p Value		0.2876	=0.0329 *	=0.0288 *	<0.0001**	<0.0001 **	<0.0001 **

* Significant difference, ** Significant at the $p < 0.05$ level.

Table 6. Comparison between the postoperative means of the Lund–Kennedy Endoscopic Scoring System in the studied groups.

	Mean	SD	*t*-Test	*p* Value	SE	95% CI	
						Lower	Upper
Group (I)	2.93	±0.96	−2.253	0.0323 *	0.417	0.0853	1.7947
Group (II)	3.87	±1.3					

* Significant difference, at the $p < 0.05$ level.

4. Discussion

Sinonasal disorders could be treated surgically by endoscopic sinus surgery through traditional middle meatal antrostomy as the most basic utilized technique. However, this may not be enough alone, even with an experienced sinus surgeon, as it cannot easily address the entirety of the walls of the maxillary sinus [14]. By combining the prelacrimal approach, which offers enhanced visualization of the maxillary sinus cavity and walls, with middle meatal antrostomy, it is possible to achieve complete eradication of the sinus pathology without any residual pathology. This procedure has the benefit of direct access to the anterior wall of the maxillary sinus without the need to relocate or remove the nasolacrimal duct. Moreover, the inferior turbinate may be restored to its former anatomical position at the completion of the procedure, therefore minimizing the functional complications linked to the excision of the lateral nasal wall. The present research conducted a comparative study of the middle meatal antrostomy and the combination middle meatal antrostomy with prelacrimal recess approach for treating patients with unilateral chronic maxillary sinusitis.

The combination of endoscopic middle meatal antrostomy (EMMA) and prelacrimal recess approach (EMMA-PRA) is more useful than EMMA alone in the treatment of chronic maxillary sinusitis. EMMA had a moderate degree of diagnostic accuracy in patients with acute or chronic sinusitis, according to a study by Kim et al. However, the combined approach of EMMA-PRA produced superior results [15]. It is considered a good option for reaching the infratemporal fossa and lateral part of the pterygopalatine fossa, as well as the anterior maxillary wall and alveolar recess [7]. However, it may not be suitable for direct visualization of the medial part of the pterygopalatine fossa [10]. Following Zhou et al.'s 2007 introduction of PLRA as an innovative technique for managing specific lesions of the maxillary sinus while preserving the NLD and inferior turbinate, the procedure's efficacy and decreased morbidity have been described and discussed in detail [16]. The prelacrimal approach to maxillary sinus lesions is an excellent method, according to the findings of another study, particularly for pathologies that manifest in the inferior and anterior walls of the maxillary sinus [17].

In the examined cases of both groups, the overall success rate in preserving a patient's disease-free status after the procedure was 86.7%. Recurrence was observed in four out of fifteen patients (26.7%) in group I following surgery, whereas in group II, no patients exhibited any indications of recurrence. In contrast to Group I, Group II demonstrated a statistically significant disparity in the prevalence of disease-free individuals. (p = 0.032) Group I comprised eight patients (53.3%) who exhibited incomplete visibility of the maxillary sinus walls. Conversely, group II comprised only two cases (13.3%) whose surgeons encountered challenges in observing the maxillary sinus in its totality. These findings are close to that obtained in another study where the role of the prelacrimal recess approach in the complete removal of anterior maxillary sinus lesions was evaluated. They conclude that, on using a 0° rigid endoscope, it was possible to observe and control every area. Due to the preservation of the lateral nasal wall, nasal physiological functions, including preserving humidity, warmth, and cleanliness is possible. Their preliminary clinical study revealed that in the concealed regions of the maxillary sinus, remnants would be overlooked in 45% of cases in the absence of the PLRA. Consequently, it is an optimal and minimally invasive method for addressing the challenges associated with the maxillary sinus. [11] Consistent with our research, Line et al. [18] compared endoscopic sinus surgery performed through the prelacrimal recess approach in conjunction with middle meatal antrostomy to conventional middle meatal antrostomy. They found that the prelacrimal recess approach to endoscopic sinus operations did not result in any postoperative complications, including but not limited to facial or cheek puffiness or pyriform aperture stenosis. In some instances, granulations formed at the site of the incision at the head of the inferior turbinate; however, these lesions resolved rapidly [18].

In the current study, postoperative symptoms showed a significant reduction in VAS in both groups of the current study. When compared to the endoscopic middle meatal antrostomy technique alone, the improvement in the mean of the symptoms of face discomfort, nasal blockage, nasal discharge, and olfactory pain after the combination treatment revealed a significant statistical difference. The postoperative mean total VAS scores of patients in Group I revealed a statistically significant and clinically relevant difference when compared to their preoperative values. A similar finding was seen in group II patients; however, the postoperative improvement found in group II patients was statistically significantly higher than that seen in group I patients. The findings demonstrate a significant improvement in the quality of life after endoscopic surgery, particularly for individuals who used a combination strategy. Recent research found that both the middle meatal antrostomy and prelacrimal recess approach considerably decreased postoperative symptoms. However, there was no statistically significant difference between the two procedures in terms of symptom reduction. Complete visualization of maxillary sinus pathology was not possible in 14 (46%) patients who underwent middle meatal antrostomy for maxillary sinus lesions. Conversely, this limitation was observed in six (20%) patients who were treated with the endoscopic prelacrimal approach. Most of the time, the prelacrimal approach successfully achieved the comprehensive visualization of the maxillary sinus pathology. Follow-up results revealed epiphora and numbness in three patients (10%) of the prelacrimal approach group. Postoperative facial pain was reported by five patients (16.6%), while facial edema and swelling were observed in three patients (10%) [17].

The complications encountered in the current study during the mean follow-up time of 14.3 months (range 11–23 months) were seen in group II patients, where the inferior turbinate was unstable in two patients after surgery (13.3%), and these patients had nasal discomfort, which improved in the late follow-up. One patient had chronic epiphora, while one other patient had anterior nasal synechia (6.6%). Acute bleeding, local infections, cosmetic alterations to the nasal ala in the event of substantial bone excision, and disruption to the lacrimal drainage routes with epiphora are all possible consequences of PLRA [19]. Pain or paranesthesia in the ipsilateral sinus and upper incisors accounts for the majority of long-term nasal complications associated with PLRA, with reports ranging from 15.7% to 52.4% of instances [20].

One patient in another series had severe intraoperative bleeding from the maxillary artery, necessitating an immediate switch to a conventional medial maxillectomy for management. Also, seven patients (25%) reported numbness, which improved progressively over the course of four months but did not completely resolve. There were no correlations that were deemed statistically significant between the incidence of postoperative neural morbidity and the osteotomy instrument utilized, the type of pathology treated, the site of origin of the lesion, or the incision of the pyriform aperture. The frequency of early postoperative complications during a 15-day period included cheek swelling in 10% of cases, temporary epiphora, orbital cellulitis, and mild epistaxis in 4% of cases each. All these issues were cured within a month. In contrast, a long-term consequence of this condition was the paresthesia ipsilateral anterior superior alveolar process and teeth. This was recorded in 25% of cases. The symptom exhibited a progressive improvement over the course of a few months in all patients, but it did not completely resolve [21]. The prelacrimal recess technique is an effective method for addressing diseases in the anterior or inferior maxillary wall that are difficult to see using just the middle meatal antrostomy approach. Nevertheless, this method is linked to certain postoperative complications such as postoperative hemorrhage, swelling of the cheeks, numbness of the infraorbital nerve, and epiphora [15].

In the current study, the postoperative endoscopic nasal findings graded by the Lund–Kennedy Endoscopic Scoring System present a highly statistically significant reduction in both groups compared to the preoperative data including nasal discharge, nasal polyps, crust, and mucosal edema. However, patients treated with the combined techniques showed no significant statistical difference in relation to the scarring of the lateral nasal wall. A significant and statistically relevant difference was observed in the postoperative mean total Lund–Kennedy Endoscopic scores of patients in Group I, as compared to their preoperative values. A comparable result was observed in patients of group II; nevertheless, the postoperative recovery observed in this group was more statistically significant than that observed in the patients in group I. It is worth mentioning that the published research does not specifically outline the particular application of the Lund–Kennedy Endoscopic Scoring System with the prelacrimal technique. Further studies will be needed to investigate the potential use of that scoring system in the evaluation of the outcome of the prelacrimal approach. A recent study found a statistically significant difference in postoperative crustations between two groups treated with standard endoscopic sinus surgery (ESS) and the prelacrimal approach (PLA) when comparing their 1-, 3-, and 6-month postoperative follow-up periods [22].

The prelacrimal approach to maxillary sinus lesions is an excellent method, according to the findings of another study, particularly for pathologies that manifest in the inferior and anterior walls of the maxillary sinus. The patient's CT findings, particularly the distance between the anterior maxillary wall and the anterior wall of the lacrimal duct, primarily dictate the approach to the sinus [17].

A number of limitations apply to the present study, including the small sample size and a shortage of prior research on the subject. Furthermore, individual variation is a factor in the subjective character of the variable measurements (VAS score) utilized to compare outcomes. This indicates that a substantial prospective multicenter study is required to supplement our findings.

5. Conclusions

The endoscopic prelacrimal recess approach offers notable advantages in comparison to alternative techniques utilized in maxillary sinus surgery. This is primarily due to its ability to facilitate direct endoscopic entry into the maxillary sinus's anterior, lateral, inferior, and inferomedial regions, thereby granting substantial access to claimed areas. This method also maintains the integrity of the nasolacrimal duct and the mucosal covering, resulting in prompt healing of the mucosa. Furthermore, in situations where the extent of the pneumatization of the maxillary sinus is uncertain, thereby affecting the difficulty of accessing the anterior wall of the sinus via alternative methods, the prelacrimal recess approach may be employed. In general, the utilization of the prelacrimal recess approach together with endoscopic MMA enhances both the accessibility and the results of anterior maxillary sinus surgery. The selection of the endoscopic surgical technique for the maxillary sinus is based on variables such as the particular pathology, surgical objectives, the surgeon's proficiency and expertise, and the availability of the appropriate equipment.

Author Contributions: Conceptualization, M.A. (Mohamed Abdalla), M.A. (Mohamed Alahmer), O.R., H.A., A.Y. and M.S.E.; Data curation, M.A. (Mohamed Alahmer) and M.S.E.; Formal analysis, M.A. (Mohamed Abdalla), M.A. (Mohamed Alahmer), H.A. and M.S.E.; Funding acquisition, O.R. and M.S.E.; Investigation, O.R., A.Y. and M.S.E.; Methodology, M.A. (Mohamed Abdalla), M.A. (Mohamed Alahmer), O.R., H.A., A.Y. and M.S.E.; Project administration, M.A. (Mohamed Abdalla). A.Y. and M.S.E.; Software, M.A. (Mohamed Abdalla)., H.A., A.Y. and M.S.E.; Supervision, M.A. (Mohamed Abdalla)., H.A. and O.R.; Visualization, M.A. (Mohamed Alahmer) and M.S.E.; Writing—original draft, M.A. (Mohamed Abdalla) and M.S.E.; Writing—review and editing, M.A. (Mohamed Abdalla), M.A. (Mohamed Alahmer), O.R., H.A., K.A. and M.S.E. All authors have read and agreed to the published version of the manuscript.

Funding: This research received no external funding.

Institutional Review Board Statement: The study was conducted according to the guidelines of the Declaration of Helsinki and approved by the Ethics Committee—Al-Ansari Specialized Hospital, Approval Code:02/19_07_1. Approval Date: 20 September 2019.

Informed Consent Statement: Informed consent was obtained from all subjects involved in the study.

Data Availability Statement: The data presented in this study are available on request from the corresponding author. The data are not publicly available due to terms of privacy.

Acknowledgments: The authors would like to acknowledge the deanship of Faculty of Medicine, Al-Azhar University, Cairo. Also, many thanks to EPCRS Excellence Center, Plant Pathology and Biotechnology Laboratory, Faculty of Agriculture, Kafrelsheikh University, Egypt.

Conflicts of Interest: The authors declare no conflicts of interest.

References

1. Gerardi, D.; Santostasi, N.; Torge, D.; Rinaldi, F.; Bernardi, S.; Bianchi, S.; Varvara, G. Regenerative Potential of Platelet-Rich Fibrin in Maxillary Sinus Floor Lift Techniques: A Systematic Review. *J. Biol. Regul. Homeost. Agents* **2023**, *37*, 2357–2369.
2. Alghofaily, M.; Alsufyani, N.; Althumairy, R.I.; AlSuhaibani, A.; Alfawzan, F.; AlSadhan, L. Odontogenic Factors Associated with Maxillary Sinus Schneiderian Membrane Thickness and their Relationship to Chronic Sinonasal Symptoms: An Ambispective Cohort Study. *Diagnostics* **2023**, *13*, 2710. [CrossRef]
3. Mohan, S.; Thejas, S.; Murali, P.; Prakash, S. Comparison between intranasal antrostomy and middle meatal antrostomy in the management of isolated maxillary sinusitis in the Rural Population: A prospective study. *Rom. J. Rhinology.* **2022**, *12*, 78–84. [CrossRef]
4. Rudmik, L. Economics of Chronic Rhinosinusitis. *Curr. Allergy Asthma Rep.* **2017**, *17*, 20. [CrossRef] [PubMed]
5. Fokkens, W.J.; Lund, V.J.; Hopkins, C.; Hellings, P.W.; Kern, R.; Reitsma, S.; Toppila-Salmi, S.; Bernal-Sprekelsen, M.; Mullol, J.; Alobid, I.; et al. European Position Paper on Rhinosinusitis and Nasal Polyps. *Rhinology* **2020**, *58* (Suppl. S29), 1–464. [CrossRef] [PubMed]
6. Lee, J.J.; Ahmad, Z.A.M.; Kim, D.; Ryu, G.; Kim, H.Y.; Dhong, H.J.; Chung, S.K.; Hong, S.D. Comparison Between Endoscopic Prelacrimal Medial Maxillectomy and Caldwell-Luc Approach for Benign Maxillary Sinus Tumors. *Clin. Exp. Otorhinolaryngol.* **2019**, *12*, 287–293. [CrossRef] [PubMed]
7. Koh, L.T.; Dhepnorrarat, R.C. The modified endoscopic pre-lacrimal approach: How I do it. *Aust. J Otolaryngol.* **2018**, *1*, 30. [CrossRef]
8. Ungari, C.; Riccardi, E.; Reale, G.; Agrillo, A.; Rinna, C.; Mitro, V.; Filiaci, F. Management and treatment of sinonasal inverted papilloma. *Ann. Stomatol.* **2016**, *12*, 87–90. [CrossRef]
9. Robinson, S.R.; Baird, R.; Le, T.; Wormald, P.J. The incidence of complications after canine fossa puncture performed during endoscopic sinus surgery. *Am. J. Rhinol.* **2005**, *19*, 203–206. [CrossRef]
10. Datta, R.K.; Viswanatha, B.; Shree Harsha, M. Caldwell Luc Surgery: Revisited. *Indian J. Otolaryngol. Head Neck Surgery.* **2016**, *68*, 90–93. [CrossRef]
11. Al Ayadi, M.A.; Raafat, S.A.; Ateya, K.A.; Gharib, F.M.; Al Murtada, A.M. The role of intranasal prelacrimal recess approach in complete removal of anterior maxillary sinus lesions. *Egypt J. Otolaryngol.* **2015**, *31*, 213–218. [CrossRef]
12. Zhou, B.; Han, D.M.; Cui, S.J.; Huang, Q.; Wang, C.S. Intranasal endoscopic prelacrimal recess approach to maxillary sinus. *Chin. Med. J.* **2013**, *126*, 1276–1280. [CrossRef] [PubMed]
13. Bertazzoni, G.; Accorona, R.; Schreiber, A.; Pietrobon, G.; Karligkiotis, A.; Fazio, E.; Castelnuovo, P.; Nicolai, P. Postoperative long-term morbidity of extended endoscopic maxillectomy for inverted papilloma. *Rhinology.* **2017**, *55*, 319–325. [CrossRef] [PubMed]
14. Morrissey, D.K.; Wormald, P.J.; Psaltis, A.J. Prelacrimal approach to the maxillary sinus. *Int. Forum Allergy Rhinol.* **2016**, *6*, 214–218. [CrossRef]
15. Zhao, Y.; Jiang, C.; Wu, Q.; Shi, R. Effects of Endoscopic Sinus Surgery Combined with Budesonide Treatment on Nasal Cavity Function and Serum Inflammatory Factors in Patients with Chronic Sinusitis. *J. Health Eng.* **2022**, *2022*, 4140682. [CrossRef] [PubMed]
16. Zhou, B.; Han, D.M.; Cui, S.J.; Huang, Q.; Wei, Y.X.; Liu, H.C.; Liu, M. Endoscopic nasal lateral wall dissection approach to maxillary sinus. *Chin. J. Otorhinolaryngol. Head Neck Surg.* **2007**, *42*, 743–748.
17. Mohankumar, V.; Kannan, D.S.; Narendrakumar, V.; Kuppuswamy, S.; Baby, A.N. A Comparative Study between Endoscopic Prelacrimal Approach and Middle Meatal Antrostomy for Maxillary Sinus Pathologies. Indian journal of otolaryngology and head and neck surgery. *Off. Publ. Assoc. Otolaryngol. India* **2022**, *74*, 90–95. [CrossRef]
18. Lin, Y.T.; Lin, C.F.; Yeh, T.H. Application of the endoscopic prelacrimal recess approach to the maxillary sinus in unilateral maxillary diseases. *Int. Forum Allergy Rhinol.* **2018**, *8*, 530–536. [CrossRef]
19. Chen, Z.; Wang, J.; Wang, Q.; Lu, Q.; Zheng, Z. Assessment of the prelacrimal recess in maxillary sinus in different sex and age groups using cone beam computed tomography (CBCT). *Eur. Arch. Otorhinolaryngol.* **2020**, *277*, 777–783. [CrossRef]
20. Lin, Y.H.; Chen, W.C. Clinical outcome of endonasal endoscopic prelacrimal approach in managing different maxillary pathologies. *Peer J.* **2020**, *8*, e8331. [CrossRef]
21. Arosio, A.D.; Valentini, M.; Canevari, F.R. Endoscopic Endonasal Prelacrimal Approach: Radiological Considerations, Morbidity, and Outcomes. *Laryngoscope* **2021**, *131*, 1715–1721. [CrossRef] [PubMed]
22. Ras, A.; El-Bahy, A.; Abdelsamie, A. Role of Prelacrimal Recess Approach Assisted Middle Meatal Antrostomy in Primary Antrocoanal Polyp. *Benha Med. J.* **2023**, *40*, 336–349.

medicina

MDPI

Article

Esthetic Surgery of the Chin in Cis- and Transgender Patients—Application of T-Genioplasty vs. Single-Piece Segment Lateralization

Rafał Pokrowiecki [1,*], Barbora Šufliarsky [2] and Maciej Jagielak [3]

1 Prive Esthetic and Facial Feminization Surgery Centre, 02-640 Warsaw, Poland
2 Department of Oral and Maxillofacial Surgery, Faculty of Medicine, Comenius University in Bratislava and University Hospital, 81372 Bratislava, Slovakia; barbora.sufliarsky@gmail.com
3 Orthognatic, Private Practice, 05-090 Warsaw, Poland; recepcja@ortognatyka.pl
* Correspondence: dr.pokrowiecki@gmail.com; Tel.: +48-691226414

Abstract: *Background and Objectives:* Correction of lower face asymmetry still remains challenging in maxillofacial surgery. This report describes techniques for the lateral transposition of the symphyseal segment to restore lower face symmetry while maintaining gender-related features in cis- and transgender patients. *Materials and Methods:* A retrospective review of medical records of 31 patients who attended for esthetic corrective surgery after orthodontic camouflage or orthognathic treatment, or during facial feminization of the lower face between June 2021 and June 2023 was performed. *Result:* All patients underwent lateralization genioplasty (with or without advancement or setback), either with or without narrowing T-osteotomy supplemented with necessary procedures in order to obtain proper facial balance and desired esthetical effects, such as bichectomy, liposuction, and face and neck lift. The mean asymmetry of the chin was 5.15 mm and was surgically corrected either by single segment lateralization or T-shape narrowing genioplasty depending on the gender and esthetical requirements. No complications were reported. *Conclusions:* Lateral shift genioplasty serves as a powerful tool in primary and secondary corrective surgery for lower face asymmetry that maintains gender-specific facial features. It may serve either as an additive to orthodontic camouflage or a way to correct previous orthognathic surgery pitfalls. The surgeon performing esthetic genioplasty associated with gender-specific expectations must be trained in facelift and facial liposculpting techniques in order to provide the best results and properly choose the right procedures for the right patients.

Keywords: facial feminization; gender-affirmation surgery; genioplasty; plastic surgery; craniofacial surgery; orthognathic surgery

1. Introduction

Esthetic considerations of the lower third of the face are one of the most commonly encountered problems among cis- and transgender patients. The chin, as a central part of the face, and the nose are responsible for one to be considered symmetrical or not. In esthetical perception, the nose is regarded as a "chief seat" of the face. Nevertheless, chin projection, shape, and interplay with proportions of the whole face play equal roles in facial esthetic surgery.

In clinical reality, there are numerous causes of lower face asymmetry resulting from congenital factors, malocclusion, trauma, incorrect dental treatment, functional factors, or tumors. However, patients being referred for revision surgery or supplemental procedures that focus on the chin symmetrization have usually had either camouflage orthodontics without jaw surgery and/or esthetic dental camouflage or have undergone orthodontic or plastic surgery procedures that failed to fully resolve the initial problem. The second issue associated with lower face esthetics is rooted in gender-related requirements. Cis-

and transgender women usually wish to have a heart-shaped face with a smaller nose and tapered chin [1] Biological and transgender males prefer to have sharp, long, straight noses, as well as prominent jawlines and gonial angles [2]. Consequently, the position and shape of the chin determine the thickness and projection of the overlying soft tissues, which play crucial roles in facial esthetics. The relationship between soft and hard tissues may vary between males and females [3]. It has a significant impact on the individualized treatment plans as desires and expectations may differ between cis- and transgender individuals.

Sliding genioplasty is an established surgical technique for the correction of sagittal dental skeletal malocclusion. However, its application as corrective surgery of lower face asymmetry in complicated cases is rarely reported. This study encompasses the utility of genioplasty techniques in chin symmetrization with regard to gender-identity requirements along with supplemental procedures involving surrounding soft tissues for the best esthetic results.

2. Materials and Methods

A retrospective review of medical records of patients who attended for esthetic corrective surgery of the lower face between June 2021 and June 2023 was conducted. Inclusion criteria were patients who complained of chin asymmetry followed by orthodontic/orthognathic procedures and/or transgender women who attended for feminization surgery of the lower face. Exclusion criteria included incomplete files and adolescents. This study aimed to analyze the previously performed procedures in the lower face performed elsewhere, complications, and reasons for revision surgery. This study was conducted in accordance with the principles of Helsinki. Written informed consent was acquired from the individuals whose pictures are presented within this manuscript.

3. Results

A total of 31 patients were referred for midline chin osteotomy between December 2021 and November 2023. Common complaints reported by patients were chin asymmetry and/or hypoplasia after orthodontic camouflage (n = 20) or orthognathic surgery (n = 6). Eleven patients were referred for facial feminization of the lower third as a part of their male-to-female transition procedures. Nineteen patients presented significant chin deviation which required symmetrization surgery. The average chin asymmetry, concerning the midline, ranged from 3.46 mm to 8.45 mm (average 5.15 mm) (Table 1). Fifteen patients decided on feminizing chin mandibuloplasty (twelve transgender females and three cisgender females). In these patients, variants of T-shape genioplasty were performed (Tables 2 and 3) (Figures 1–4) (Video S1). In cases where the deviation ranged up to 4.5 mm, no lateralization of the segment was required (n = 11) (Figure 3). Additional lateralization of the chin after T-genioplasty was required in cis- and transgender females when the deviation was >4.5 mm (n = 7) (Figure 3).

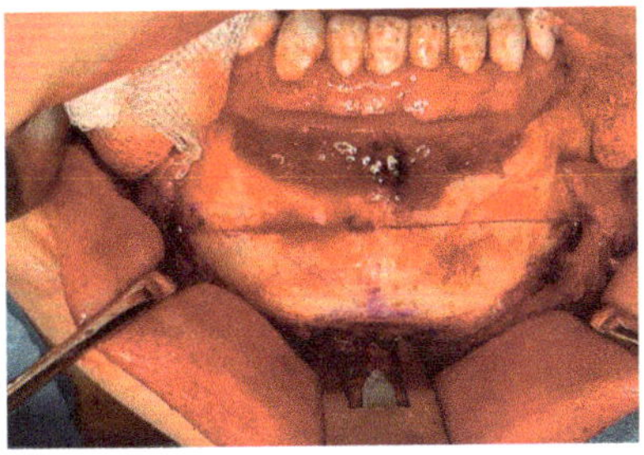

(A)

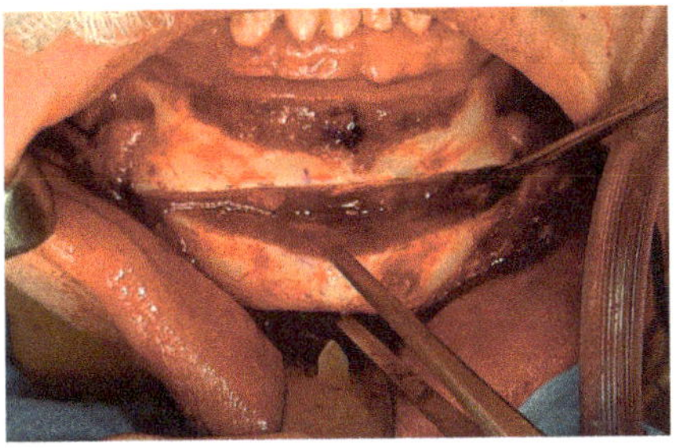

(B)

Figure 1. *Cont.*

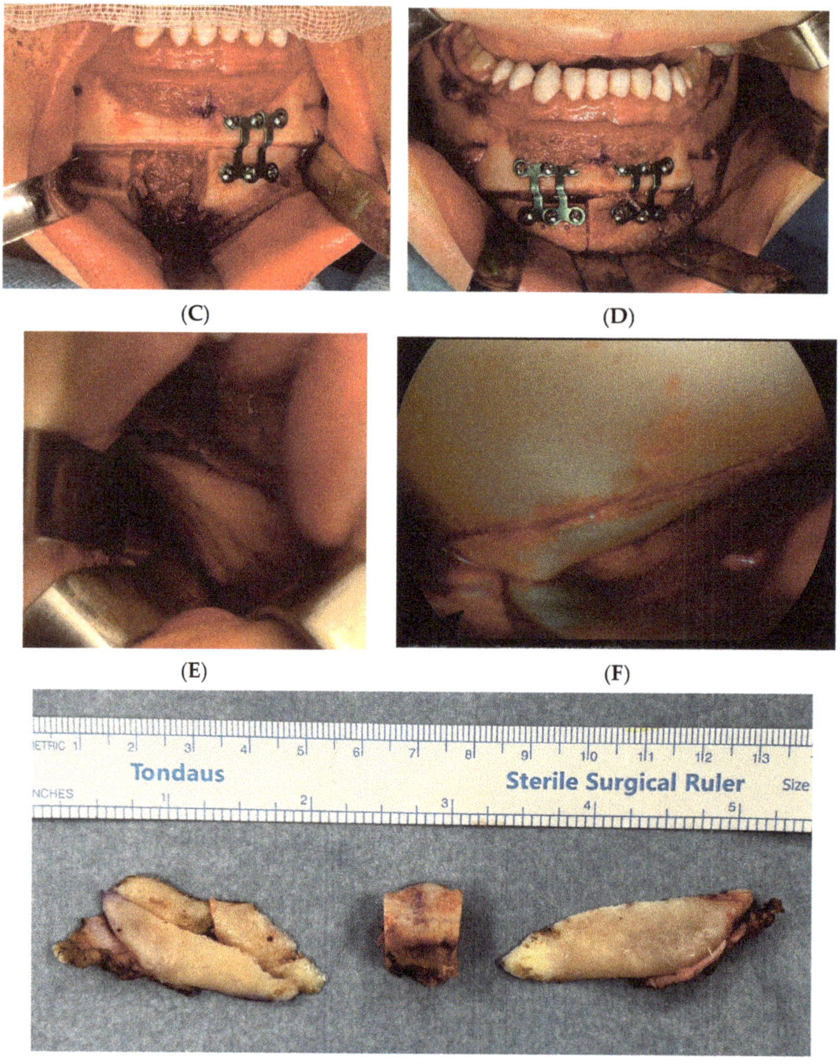

Figure 1. Intraoperative photographs of horizontal T-shape genioplasty, which was most commonly performed in feminization surgery procedures. (**A**,**B**) Horizontal osteotomy and bone segment detachment. In cases with lateralization, bone segment was transpositioned contra-laterally to the deviation, and bone steps and irregularities were burred down with diamond burr. (**C**,**D**) Bone segment sectioned in the midline into two pieces with resection of the central bone block (Video S1). Bone segments were stabilized with 2.0 mm titanium plates (ChM, Poland) (in this particular case, 3 mm setback was necessary to reduce protruding chin but no deviation was diagnosed). (**E**,**F**) V-shape surgery for the purposes of mandible feminization was supplemented with endoscopy-assisted bilateral resection of the mandibular angles, which was performed in a way resembling bilateral sagittal split osteotomy with additional sections and osteoplasty that enabled sufficient narrowing of the mandible. (**G**) Photograph of the resected mandibular angles along with partial resection of the masseter and central genial bone block.

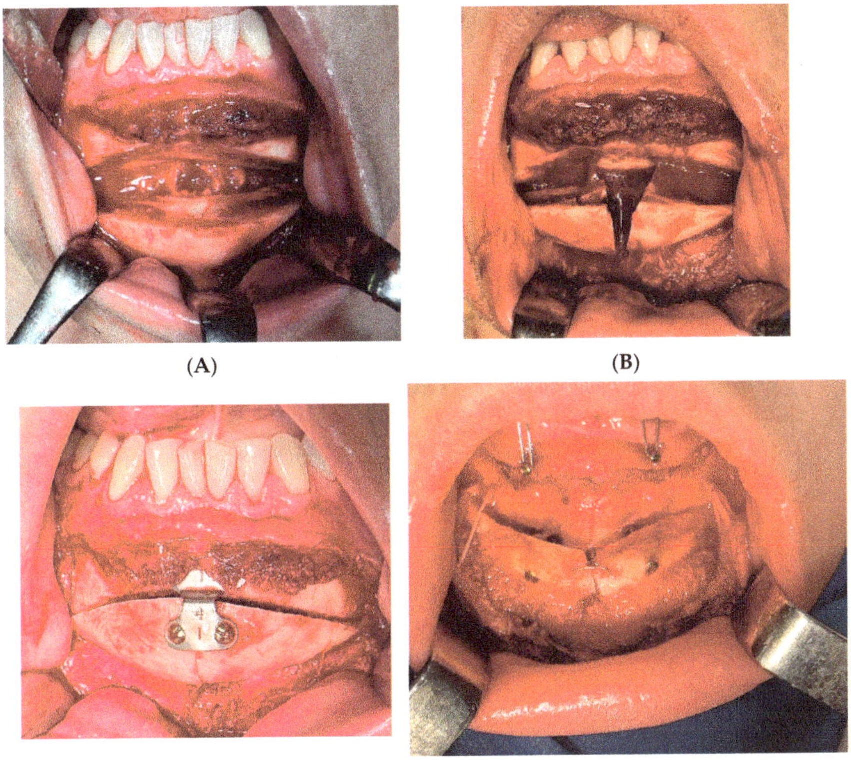

(A) (B) (C) (D)

Figure 2. Examples of T-shape genioplasty variants other than horizontal performed in the presented material. (**A–C**) M-genioplasty. In this case, frontal advancement of 4 mm was necessary and bone segments were stabilized with single 2.0 titanium plate. (**D**) T-shape genioplasty originally described by Greme and Blenkisopp (1990) modified by Jagielak's application of 2 compression screws (2.0 × 20 mm, Medartis, CHF), which allowed for advancements larger than 10 mm with preservation of bone continuity and stable fixation without necessity of mandibular sagittal split osteotomy.

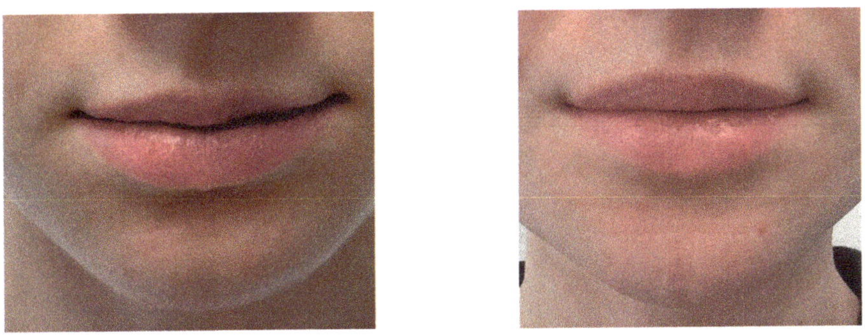

(A) (B)

Figure 3. *Cont.*

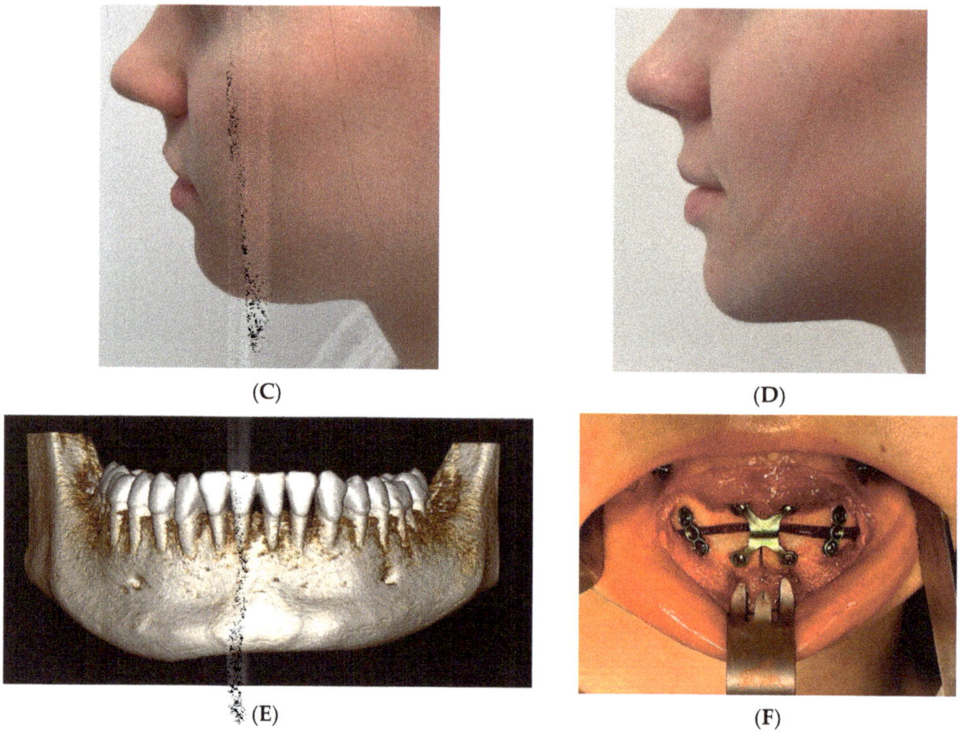

Figure 3. Example of 23-year-old cis-gender female who complained of vertical asymmetry and receded chin. In this case, T-shape genioplasty with advancement supplemented with submental liposuction and non-surgical neck lift (VASER) was performed, which restored symmetry and feminine and youthful look of the lower third. (**A**) Frontal photograph before surgery, (**B**) frontal photograph after the surgery. (**C**) Lateral view before and (**D**) after the surgery. (**E**) Three-dimensional reconstruction showing vertical asymmetry. (**F**) Interoperative view of the reduced, transpositioned, and advanced bone segments (ChM, Lewickie, Poland).

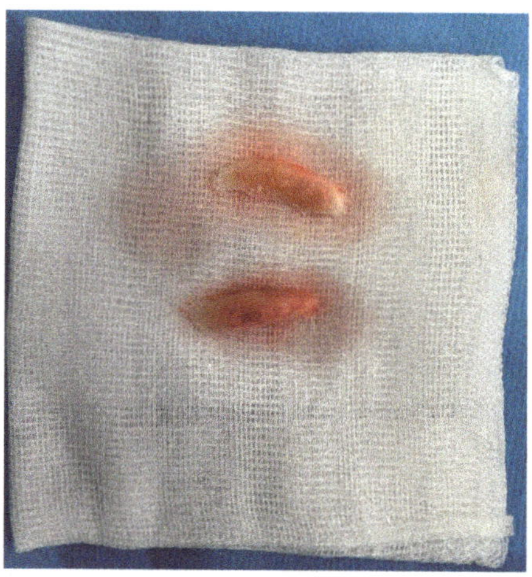

(**A**)

Figure 4. *Cont.*

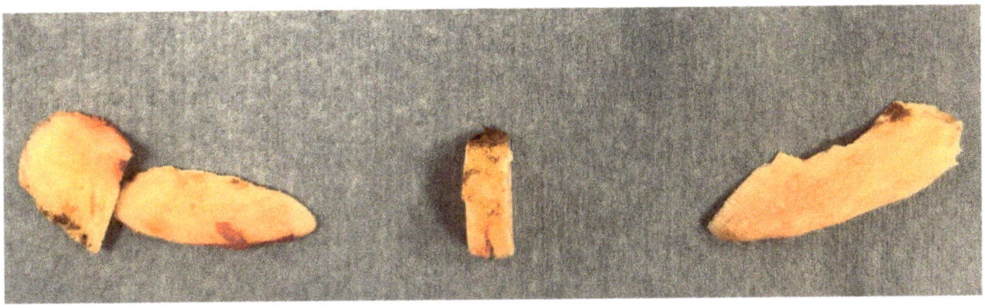

(B)

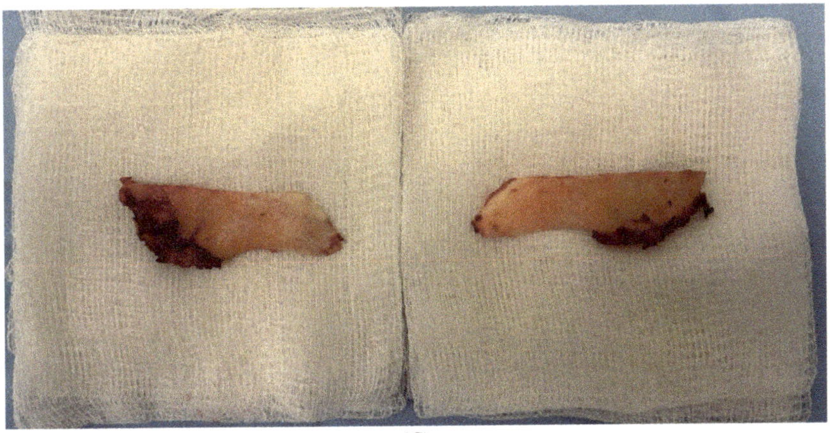

(C)

Figure 4. Intraoperative photographs of the resected mandibular angles in different patients. (**A**) A very conservative resection of the lateral aspects of the gonial angles performed in cisgender woman. (**B**) Intermediate resection involving gonial angles and partial ramus and mandibular body (note 5 mm central block of the bone from the T-genioplasty) (cisgender woman with square lower third), (**C**) extended resection of the angles involving cortical bone of the ramus and body and partial resection of the pterygoid–masseteric sling (transgender woman—facial feminization procedure).

Table 1. Characteristics of the patients referred for the correction of the chin due to symmetry and/or gender-confirming features. F—cis female, F′—trans-female, M—male.

Patient	Gender	Age	Orthodontic	Orthognathic	Cosmetic Dentistry	Chin Deviation (mm)	Site
1	F	24	yes	no	no	5.87	R
2	M	32	yes	yes	no	6.72	R
3	F	39	yes	no	no	8.45	R
4	M	23	yes	yes	no	5.23	L
5	F′	31	yes	no	yes	3.46	R
6	M	32	yes	yes	no	4.67	R
7	M	53	yes	no	yes	7.12	L
8	F	23	yes	no	yes	4.31	L
9	M	53	yes	no	no	5.23	R
10	F	34	yes	no	yes	4.15	L
11	M	23	yes	no	no	4.56	R
12	F′	36	yes	yes	yes	6.64	L

Table 1. *Cont.*

Patient	Gender	Age	Orthodontic	Orthognathic	Cosmetic Dentistry	Chin Deviation (mm)	Site
13	F	21	yes	no	no	7.32	R
14	M	32	yes	no	no	6.57	R
15	F	38	yes	yes	yes	5.21	L
16	M	27	yes	no	no	3.96	R
17	F	22	yes	no	yes	5.12	R
18	M	19	yes	no	no	7.57	L
19	F	34	yes	yes	yes	7.43	R
20	F′	19	no	no	yes	1.1	L
21	F′	21	no	no	yes	0	N/A
22	F′	47	no	no	yes	0	N/A
23	F′	35	no	no	yes	2.1	R
24	F′	28	no	no	yes	0.5	L
25	F′	20	no	no	yes	0	N/A
26	F′	22	no	no	yes	0	N/A
27	F	27	no	no	no	0	N/A
28	F	35	yes	no	no	0	N/A
29	F′	42	no	no	yes	0	N/A
30	F	36	no	no	no	0	N/A
31	F′	37	no	no	no	0	N/A

Table 2. Type of genioplasty and adjuvant procedures performed in order to correct asymmetry and to feminize or masculinize lower third of the face.

Patient	Genioplasty	T-Genioplasty	Feminization	Masculinization	Symmetrization	Angle Resection	Angle Implants
1	no	yes	no	no	yes	no	no
2	yes	no	no	no	yes	no	no
3	no	yes	yes	no	yes	no	no
4	yes	no	no	yes	no	no	yes
5	yes	no	yes	no	yes	no	no
6	yes	no	no	no	yes	no	no
7	yes	no	no	yes	yes	no	yes
8	yes	no	no	no	yes	yes	no
9	yes	no	no	no	yes	no	no
10	yes	no	no	no	yes	no	no
11	yes	no	no	no	yes	no	no
12	no	yes	yes	no	yes	yes	no
13	no	yes	no	no	yes	yes	no
14	yes	no	no	no	yes	no	no
15	no	yes	no	no	yes	no	no
16	yes	no	no	no	yes	no	no
17	no	yes	yes	no	yes	no	no
18	yes	no	no	no	yes	no	no
19	no	yes	no	no	yes	no	no

Table 2. *Cont.*

Patient	Genioplasty	T-Genioplasty	Feminization	Masculinization	Symmetrization	Angle Resection	Angle Implants
20	no	yes	yes	no	no	yes	no
21	no	yes	yes	no	no	yes	no
22	no	yes	yes	no	no	yes	no
23	no	yes	yes	no	no	yes	no
24	no	yes	yes	no	no	yes	no
25	no	yes	yes	no	no	yes	no
26	no	yes	yes	no	no	yes	no
27	yes	no	no	yes	no	no	yes
28	yes	no	yes	no	no	no	no
29	no	yes	yes	no	no	no	no
30	no	yes	yes	no	no	yes	no
31	no	yes	yes	no	no	yes	no

Table 3. Types of osteotomies performed in the patients who underwent T-shape genioplasty.

Patient	T-Genioplasty	Type
1	yes	Horizontal (advancement)
3	yes	M-shape (advancement)
12	yes	Horizontal
13	yes	Horizontal
15	yes	M-shape (advancement)
17	yes	Horizontal (advancement)
19	yes	Horizontal
20	yes	Horizontal
21	yes	M-shape
22	yes	Horizontal
23	yes	Horizontal
24	yes	M-shape
25	yes	Horizontal
26	yes	Horizontal (setback)
29	yes	Horizontal
30	yes	Horizontal (advancement)
31	yes	Horizontal

Also, additional endoscopy-assisted feminization surgery of the mandible (V-shape ostectomy) was performed in 12 cases (three cisgender females, nine transgender females) (Table 2) (Figure 1). In cisgender females, conservative ostectomy was performed, while transgender patients required more aggressive ostectomy with partial resection of the masseter (Figure 4).

Five males desired symmetrization and single-segment lateral shift genioplasty was performed followed by osteoplasty/ostectomy of the residual bone at the lower border of the mandible. In three males, additional masculinization of the mandibular angles with 3D Virtual Surgical Planning and custom implants was performed (Figures 4 and 5).

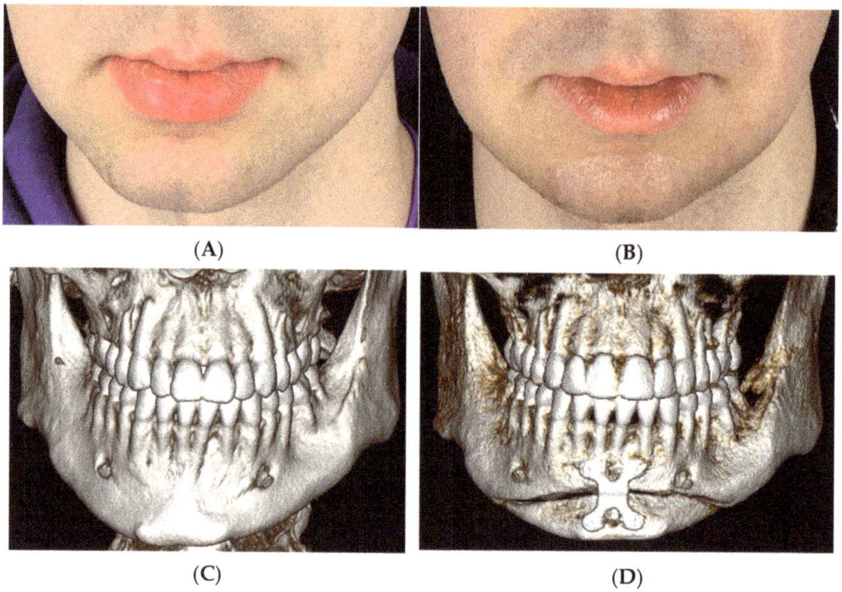

Figure 5. A 27-year-old male who referred for chin symmetrization after orthodontic treatment and bimaxillary surgery performed elsewhere. He did not opt for corrective orthodontic surgery and revision orthognathic surgery. In this case, segmental chin lateralization with 3 mm setback and lower border recontouring were performed.

In order to obtain optimal esthetic results, preserve skin elasticity, and reduce fat tissue from the chin and neck, additional procedures were performed. These included bichectomy (n = 9), liposuction (n = 12), Vibration Amplification of Sound Energy at Resonance liposuction (Vaser, Sound Surgical Technologies, Louisville, CO, USA) (n = 10), central neck lift (n = 5), which were performed simultaneously. Six patients required a supplementary facelift, which was performed simultaneously or 3–6 months after bone recontouring procedures. The techniques used were patient-specific and included Minimal Access Cranial Suspension (MACS) lift (n = 1), deep-plane face and neck lift (n = 4), and endoscopic assisted full facelift (ponytail facelift) (n = 2) (Table 4). No complications after the surgery were reported apart from transient lower lip numbness, which resolved after 3–6 months in all presented cases.

Table 4. Adjuvant procedures performed 3–6 months after bone recontouring. DPF—deep-plane facelift, MACSL—Minimal Access Cranial Suspension Lift, CNL—central neck lift, Endoscopic—full endoscopic ponytail facelift.

Patient	Bichectomy	Liposuction	VASER	Surgical Neck Lift	Face Lift	Type
1	no	no	no	no	no	x
2	no	no	no	no	no	x
3	no	no	no	no	no	x
4	no	no	no	no	no	x
5	no	no	no	no	no	x
6	no	no	no	no	no	x
7	yes	yes	yes	no	no	x

Table 4. *Cont.*

Patient	Bichectomy	Liposuction	VASER	Surgical Neck Lift	Face Lift	Type
8	yes	yes	yes	no	no	x
9	no	no	no	yes	yes	DPFL
10	no	yes	yes	no	no	x
11	no	no	no	no	no	x
12	yes	yes	yes	no	yes	MACSL
13	no	yes	yes	yes	no	CNL
14	no	yes	yes	yes	no	CNL
15	yes	yes	yes	yes	no	CNL
16	no	no	no	no	no	x
17	no	no	no	no	no	x
18	no	no	no	no	no	x
19	yes	no	no	no	no	x
20	yes	yes	yes	no	yes	Endoscopic
21	no	no	no	no	no	x
22	no	no	no	yes	yes	DPFL
23	yes	no	no	yes	yes	DPFL
24	no	no	no	yes	no	CNL
25	yes	yes	no	yes	yes	Endoscopic
26	no	no	no	no	no	x
27	no	no	no	no	no	x
28	no	no	no	no	no	no
29	no	yes	no	yes	no	CNL
30	no	yes	yes	no	no	x
31	yes	yes	yes	no	yes	DPFL

4. Discussion

This study described a simplified midline osteotomy for the correction of facial esthetics in a group of patients complaining about lower third asymmetry following orthodontic compensation. Midline osteotomy techniques of the chin as adjuvant surgery have been reported since 1960. The first osteotomies were based on resection of the midline single bone block and mandible constriction in the treatment of dentofacial deformities. They have been reported to be effective and require significant postoperative downtime. A 10 mm bone segment resection is considered safe for mandibular constriction, without periodontal or temporomandibular joint function contraindications [4,5]. Modified T-shape osteotomy for the correction of asymmetry and advancement was further described by Grime and Bleinkinsopp in 1990 [6]. Midline osteotomy is still considered to be an adjuvant in orthognathic surgery where transverse discrepancy must be corrected [7].

In our opinion, the maximal width of 10 mm of resected chin midline segment is accurate from the point of view of classic orthognathic surgery and not exactly in transgender facial surgery. In our study, resection of the chin segment was followed by its lateral reposition (asymmetries less than 4.5 mm) or followed by T-shape genioplasty based on central bone block resection. The latter was performed in cis- and transgender women and hence, the volume of the bone block corresponded to the deviation extent and feminizing desires of the patients. In our material, blocks wider than 10 mm may be safely resected in feminizing procedures without any harm to periodontal tissues and jawline projection (Figure 1). However, lateral bone fragments should not be totally detached from the surrounding tissues due to the risk of resorption.

There are numerous techniques for chin augmentation osteotomies. In our study, we performed horizontal T-shape osteotomies (n = 13). Two of them were modified T-shape osteotomies with advancement described by Grime and Blenkisopp (1990) [6] stabilized with centrally placed bone wire and two 20 × 2.0 mm compression screws (Jagielak's modification) (Table 3) (Figure 2). This technique allows for the correction of asymmetry and two-stage advancement, which, in some cases, is troublesome to obtain with stock titanium plates. Most of the cases did not require significant advancements and hence, rigid fixation plates and screws were applied after performing chin narrowing and shift correcting the asymmetry. There were two cases where M-osteotomy was performed according to the technique of Lee et al. (2018) where no vertical augmentation was indicated [8]. Another two cases required modified M-osteotomy of the chin with additional advancement according to [9].

In the presented study, cisgender females had usually been previously treated orthodontically followed by cosmetic dentistry procedures such as porcelain veneers or composite work-up (bonding). Among these patients, symmetrization of the chin was a common problem. Patients were not informed by their orthodontist about facial asymmetry and indications for orthognathic surgery in the first place. Patients refused to undergo secondary orthodontic treatment and subsequent orthognathic surgery. Therefore, they were qualified for esthetic corrective treatment either with single-segment lateral shift mandibuloplasty or T-shape genioplasty.

On the contrary, transgender females have usually chosen cosmetic dentistry camouflage instead of orthodontic treatment before scheduling an appointment for corrective surgery. In transgender females, it is commonly seen that they choose the "fast" esthetic effect as transition is a long process and they usually choose shorter ways to enhance feminine features from the "esthetic" point of view but not necessarily in the functional aspect (malocclusion, dentofacial abnormalities requiring orthognathic surgery, etc.). Orthodontic treatment usually lasts 3–4 years and such a period of time is frequently unacceptable for transgender women. Moreover, as facial feminization surgery is not usually covered by national health insurance in many countries, patients seeking gender confirmation procedures try to save as many funds as possible to be able to pursue other FFS procedures. Last but not least, transgender oral healthcare still needs development and adaptation for the special needs of the transgender community. Hormone replacement therapy (HRT) (Estradiol) may affect or even impede orthodontic treatment or dental implant therapy, hence requiring reduction or modification of the hormone dosage. Therefore, patients usually choose a treatment plan that does not require a decrease in HRT [10].

Transgender women usually underwent reduction T-genioplasty and endoscope-assisted mandibular angle reduction. There were two cisgender women who wanted an angle reduction procedure along with chin correction. In these cases, more conservative resection was performed when compared to transgender patients so as not to over-resect the angles (Figure 4A).

Cisgender males were referred for simple correction of asymmetry and/or advancement after orthodontic treatment. They did not perform additional cosmetic dentistry such as veneers or bonding. Three patients wished to masculinize their faces by mandible augmentation with individual 3D custom implants (Figure 6). A total of six patients decided on symmetrization of the residual chin asymmetry that persisted after orthognathic surgery performed elsewhere. Chin symmetrization in cisgender males with or without masculinization (angle implants) was based on one-piece segment lateralization. It is advised not to perform T-genioplasty among cisgender males due to the feminization effect of such a procedure. Another interesting technique described by Raffaini and Sesenna in 1995 was based on the hemi-genioplasty technique for the correction of chin asymmetry [11]. However, as this technique is based on chin sagittal split osteotomy and lateralization on only the mobilized half of the chin, such a technique, in our opinion, is beneficial for cis-

and transgender males as by that movement, the chin may be significantly wider. Moreover, such osteotomy does not provide possibilities for eventual advancement or setback, making this technique straightforward and simple, yet restricted to very specific indications [11]. In our study, we opted for full chin osteotomy and repositioning as it provided better control, soft tissue management, and advancement/setback when necessary.

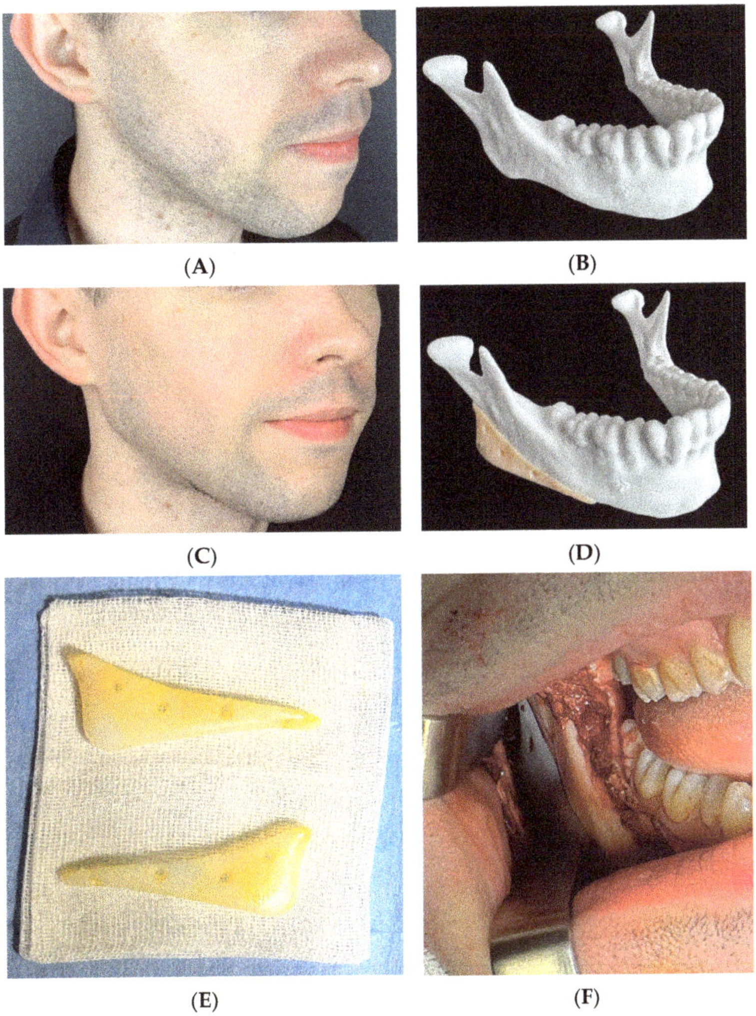

Figure 6. A 26-year-old male after orthodontic camouflage. He did not opt for corrective orthodontic surgery and revision orthognathic surgery. Patient wanted to correct receded chin and to masculinize hypoplastic mandibular angles which were caused by gonial deficiency resulting from class II malocclusion. Advancement genioplasty (5 mm forward, no asymmetry correction needed) and 3DVSP individual mandibular implants were performed. (**A**) Photograph before surgery, (**B**) 3D printed model of the mandible before surgery, (**C**) photograph after surgery, (**D**) mandible model with planned templates. (**E**) Implants (PTFE) before implantation, (**F**) intraoperative view of the right angle implant placed on the gonial angle and then stabilized with 5 × 2.0 mm titanium screws in order to provide stable fixation, preventing movement and hence encapsulation or infections.

This study also showed that asymmetries of the chin where the deviation is less than 4.5 mm may be corrected by single-segment chin lateralization and conservative mandibular shaving. Asymmetries more than 4.5 mm in cis- or transgender women may be sufficiently corrected with T-genioplasty. Resection of the central segment enables for a smooth shift of the chin and by narrowing, it offers a feminizing effect in both of these genders. It also reduces the risk of irregularities at the lower border of the mandibular body and provides a smooth transition between the shifted chin and the mandibular body.

Mandibular angle reduction was initially introduced into Korean facial surgery where patients desired less prominent mandibular angles. This surgery may be performed either as a Korean plastic surgery procedure alone or in combination with orthognathic surgery [12–14].

With time, this procedure was adapted for patients seeking feminization procedures, usually during the male-to-female transition [15–17]. In the study by Lee et al. (2023), a retroauricular approach for mandibular angle reduction was described [18]. In our opinion, this approach may be beneficial in cases where a simultaneous facelift is planned and two procedures may be performed through one access. However, in cases where genioplasty is planned and no facelift is performed, the classic intraoral approach through the oral vestibulum is still the safest; there is no risk of injury to the facial nerves and it leaves no scar on the skin.

In our study, angle resection was performed simultaneously with T-shape genioplasty with endoscopic-assisted angle reduction as it provides direct vision and resection control. Endoscopic-assisted mandible osteoplasty for esthetic purposes was also described in the study by [19].

Similarly to Lee and Singh (2022), we observed the best feminizing effect after complex V-shape surgery consisting of angle reduction and chin feminization [16]. In cases requiring more aggressive resections, we also advocate for extended sagittal split ostectomy of the cortical bone of the ramus, angle, and mandibular body with partial excision of the masseter (Figure 4C) [15,20]. The distal border of the resection is preferably placed below the mental foramen with a smooth transition into the osteotomy of the chin. This reduces the risk of unwanted irregularities and enables conservative osteoplasty of the lower border and muscle attachment preservation. We did not perform total inferior border ostectomy as was described in the study by [21], where this technique was presented as superior to T-genioplasty [21]. The authors described total U-shape ostectomy of the whole mandibular complex en block in wider, more asymmetrical chins. None of our patients required this approach. Despite being useful, in certain cases, such a modification required the complete dissection of the muscle attachments from the inferior border. Detachment of the muscles generates a risk of postoperative chin ptosis, and hence we do not find justification for total muscle resections in esthetic surgery [22].

Facial masculinization surgery procedures are frequently performed in cis- and transgender males. Patients in transition from female to male constitute less than 10% of the transgender individuals. Both cis- and transgender males are groups of patients who usually desire to enhance their masculine features through chin and mandibular angle augmentation. In transgender males, masculinization of the lower third is the most commonly performed procedure and, along with recently described rib-graft Adam's apple augmentation and testosterone HRT, is sufficient in reshaping the face [20,23].

While the chin may be masculinized either by advancement genioplasty or chin implants, mandibular angles require a different approach. As no osteotomy provides vertical augmentation in that particular anatomical area, the placement of stock or custom-made implants is a straightforward, safe, and effective procedure [24–26]. In our study, there were no transgender males; however, two cisgender males opted for masculinization, which shows the increasing interest of biological males in esthetic facial surgery procedures.

Soft tissue projection is crucial for the ultimate esthetic outcome. Surgical correction of the lower third requires addressing potential problems that may mask the osteoplastic procedures. These include buccal fat pad hypertrophy, appearing as visible bulging in the cheek area lateral to the nasolabial grooves, jowling, which may increase after angle resection and lower border marginectomy in certain cases, loose skin of the neck, platysma dehiscence, or contrarily, double chin and deep fat accumulation. Therefore, these conditions must be addressed before any bone recontouring, osteoplasty, or mandibular angle resection [16,27].

In younger individuals, facial liposculpting based on bichectomy and power-assisted liposuction may greatly enhance the V-shape goal of feminizing surgery. When no significant laxity of the skin is present, no additional procedures are indicated. In cases with minimal jowling, a MACS lift (MACSL) may be sufficient as it does not interfere in the area of the skin and is of great value in younger patients who do not want more aggressive facelift procedures at that age [28]. Full endoscopic facelift, currently known as "ponytail face lift", is also of great utility. It is usually indicated in younger individuals without significant loose skin and greatly enhances feminizing procedures. Extended versions of the ponytail facelift may also be used in older patients [29]. However, significant jowling and excess skin present before reduction surgeries such as mandible angle resection or lower border ostectomy may require the traditional lower face and neck lift approach. A preferable technique is a deep-plane facelift as it focuses on re-draping the deeper layers of the face (SMAS and muscles) and not only re-draping and cutting off extra skin. Central neck lift, although a powerful tool in cases with platysma dehiscence and banding, causes accumulation of fat tissue. Power-assisted liposuction with central neck lift along with advancement genioplasty may dramatically re-drape, smoothen, and rejuvenate the neck area without a facelift approach. This approach is advocated in younger patients without significant jowls and skin laxity. These are better addressed by a classic deep-plane facelift or ponytail facelift where platysma tightening is performed at its distal aspect either by plication or transaction and platysma hammock techniques [29,30].

5. Conclusions

The presented study focused on the application of different variants of genioplasty for esthetic purposes in complicated orthodontic/orthognathic patients as well as transgender individuals. It described indications for lateralization of the chin in one segment or application of T-genioplasty variants in both correction of asymmetry and gender-confirmation facial surgery without revision orthodontic treatment nor orthognathic surgery based on bimaxillary surgery. For males, one-piece lateral shift genioplasty is advised. Residual bone at the lower mandible may be smoothened using a bone burr, preserving the male shape of the chin. For females with an asymmetry of <4.5 mm, a similar approach is advised, whereas asymmetries >4.5 mm require T-genioplasty to restore the feminine, triangular shape of the chin.

This is the first study describing procedures such as bichectomy, facial liposculpting, and face-lifting techniques as additive procedures necessary for a satisfying outcome. Endoscopic-assisted minimally invasive bone recontouring surgery procedures supplemented with 3D Virtual Surgical Planning and custom-made implants as well as properly addressing the surrounding soft tissues is undoubtedly the future of modern cosmetic surgery in both cis- and transgender patients.

Supplementary Materials: The following supporting information can be downloaded at: https://www.mdpi.com/article/10.3390/medicina60010139/s1, Video S1.

Author Contributions: Conceptualization, R.P. and M.J.; methodology, R.P., B.Š. and M.J.; software, R.P. and B.Š.; validation, R.P. and B.Š.; formal analysis, M.J.; investigation, R.P.; resources, R.P., B.Š. and M.J.; data curation, R.P., B.Š. and M.J.; writing—original draft preparation, R.P., B.Š. and M.J.; writing—review and editing, R.P., B.Š., M.J., R.P., B.Š. and M.J.; supervision, M.J.; project administration, R.P.; funding acquisition, R.P., B.Š. and M.J. All authors have read and agreed to the published version of the manuscript.

Funding: This study was funded by the Gender Affirmation Surgery (GAS) Foundation, Warsaw, Poland (no. Publication—2023).

Institutional Review Board Statement: This study was conducted in accordance with the Declaration of Helsinki. Ethical review and approval were waived for this study due to the retrospective nature of the research.

Informed Consent Statement: Informed consent was obtained from all subjects involved in the study. Written informed consent has been obtained from the patient(s) to publish this paper.

Data Availability Statement: Data are contained within the article.

Conflicts of Interest: The authors declare no conflicts of interest.

References

1. Somenek, M.; Romero, N.J. Facial Analysis for Gender Affirmation/Gender-Related Facial Analysis. *Facial Plast. Surg. Clin. N. Am.* **2023**, *31*, 341–348. [CrossRef]
2. Balaji, S.; Balaji, P. Psychological Desire of Facial Esthetics in Males. *Ann. Maxillofac. Surg.* **2019**, *9*, 326. [CrossRef] [PubMed]
3. Alhumadi, A.; Al-Khafaji, T.J.; Alyassiri, A.M.H.; Alhamadi, W.W. Gender differences in lower facial soft tissue thickness among different skeletal patterns, based on soft tissue cephalometric analysis. *J. Orthod. Sci.* **2022**, *11*, 54. [CrossRef]
4. Anghinoni, M.L.; Magri, A.S.; Blasio, D.; Tomad, L.; Sesenna, E. Midline mandibular osteotomy in an asymmetric patient. *Angle Orthod.* **2009**, *79*, 1008–1014. [CrossRef] [PubMed]
5. Joondeph, D.R.; Bloomquist, D. Mandibular midline osteotomy for constriction. *Am. J. Orthod. Dentofac. Orthop.* **2004**, *126*, 268–270. [CrossRef] [PubMed]
6. Grime, P.D.; Blenkinsopp, P.T. Horizontal-T genioplasty—(A modified technique for the broad or asymmetrical chin). *Br. J. Oral Maxillofac. Surg.* **1990**, *28*, 215–221. [CrossRef]
7. Ramanathan, M.; Sonoyama-Osako, R.; Shimamura, Y.; Okui, T.; Kanno, T. Mandibular midline osteotomy for correction of bimaxillary transverse discrepancy: A technical note. *J. Korean Assoc. Oral Maxillofac. Surg.* **2023**, *49*, 107–113. [CrossRef]
8. Lee, J.B.; Han, J.W.; Park, J.H.; Min, K.H. Lower facial contouring surgery using a novel method: M-genioplasty. *Arch. Plast. Surg.* **2018**, *45*, 572. [CrossRef]
9. Fariña, R.D.; Valladares-Pérez, S.D.; Navarro-Cuellar, C.D.; Torrealba, R.D.; Fariña-Silva, A.; Fariña-Silva, G. M-shaped Genioplasty: New Findings after 10 Years of Experience. *Plast. Reconstr. Surg.—Glob. Open* **2023**, *11*, e4778. [CrossRef] [PubMed]
10. Delgado-Ruiz, R.; Swanson, P.; Romanos, G. Systematic review of the long-term effects of transgender hormone therapy on bone markers and bone mineral density and their potential effects in implant therapy. *J. Clin. Med.* **2019**, *8*, 784. [CrossRef]
11. Raffaini, M.; Sesenna, E. Hemi-genioplasty: A technique to correct chin asymmetry. *J. Oral Maxillofac. Surg.* **1995**, *53*, 1362–1364. [CrossRef] [PubMed]
12. Han, K.; Kim, J. Reduction mandibuloplasty: Ostectomy of the lateral cortex around the mandibular angle. *J. Craniofacial Surg.* **2001**, *12*, 314–325. [CrossRef] [PubMed]
13. Hwang, K.; Lee, D.K.; Lee, W.J.; Chung, I.H.; Lee, S.I. A split ostectomy of mandibular body and angle reduction. *J. Craniofacial Surg.* **2004**, *15*, 341–346. [CrossRef] [PubMed]
14. Kim, J.-H.; Han, S.-J.; Kim, M.-Y. New method for an evaluation of the esthetical improvements resulting from a mandibular angle reduction. *J. Korean Assoc. Oral Maxillofac. Surg.* **2017**, *43*, 239–246. [CrossRef] [PubMed]
15. Deschamps-Braly, J. Feminization of the Chin: Genioplasty Using Osteotomies. *Facial Plast. Surg. Clin. N. Am.* **2019**, *27*, 243–250. [CrossRef] [PubMed]
16. Lee, H.H.; Singh, M. Jaw Reduction Surgery. *Otolaryngol. Clin. N. Am.* **2022**, *55*, 859–870. [CrossRef] [PubMed]
17. Taskov, C. 3D Sliding Genioplasty and Its Role in Facial Feminization Surgery. *Otolaryngol. Clin. N. Am.* **2022**, *55*, 849–858. [CrossRef]
18. Lee, Y.J.; Park, Y.; Ha, Y.; Kim, S. Mandible Angle Resection with the Retroauricular Approach. *J. Clin. Med.* **2023**, *12*, 2641. [CrossRef]
19. Wu, G.; Zhou, B.; Chen, X.; He, X.; Bi, J. Endoscopic-Assisted Intraoral Three-Dimensional Reduction Mandibuloplasty. *Ann. Plast. Surg.* **2015**, *75*, 10–18. [CrossRef]
20. Deschamps-Braly, J.C. Approach to Feminization Surgery and Facial Masculinization Surgery: Aesthetic Goals and Principles of Management. *J. Craniofacial Surg.* **2019**, *30*, 1352–1358. [CrossRef]
21. Wang, Y.; He, Y.; Al-Watary, M.; Bi, D.; Song, L.; Li, J. Total inferior border ostectomy versus T-shape genioplasty for chin narrowing combined with mandibular contouring. *Int. J. Oral Maxillofac. Surg.* **2022**, *51*, 1549–1555. [CrossRef] [PubMed]
22. Garfein, E.S.; Zide, B.M. Chin Ptosis: Classification, Anatomy, and Correction. *Craniomaxillofacial Trauma Reconstr.* **2008**, *1*, 1. [CrossRef] [PubMed]
23. Deschamps-Braly, J.C.; Sacher, C.L.; Fick, J.; Ousterhout, D.K. First Female-to-Male Facial Confirmation Surgery with Description of a New Procedure for Masculinization of the Thyroid Cartilage (Adam's Apple). *Plast. Reconstr. Surg.* **2017**, *139*, 883e–887e. [CrossRef]
24. Al-Jandan, B.; Marei, H.F. Mandibular angle augmentation using solid silicone implants. *Dent. Med. Probl.* **2018**, *55*, 367–370. [CrossRef]

25. Eppley, B.L. Chin Reshaping in Profileplasty: Augmentative and Reductive Strategies. *Facial Plast. Surg.* **2019**, *35*, 499–515. [CrossRef]
26. Eppley, B.L. Mandibular Angle Implants. *Facial Plast. Surg.* **2019**, *35*, 158–163. [CrossRef] [PubMed]
27. Rochlin, D.H.; Morrison, S.D.M.; Harirah, M.B.; Rohrich, R.J.; Satterwhite, T. Face Lift after Facial Feminization Surgery: Indications and Special Considerations. *Plast. Reconstr. Surg.* **2022**, *149*, 107–115. [CrossRef]
28. Tonnard, P.; Verpaele, A. The MACS-lift short scar rhytidectomy. *Aesthetic Surg. J.* **2007**, *27*, 188–198. [CrossRef]
29. Kao, C.C.; Duscher, D. Advanced Endoscopic Techniques in Asian Facial Rejuvenation. *Clin. Plast. Surg.* **2023**, *50*, 51–60. [CrossRef]
30. Jacono, A.A.; Alemi, A.S.; Harmon, J.J.; Ahmedli, N. The Effect of a Novel Platysma Hammock Flap During Extended Deep Plane Facelift on the Signs of Aging in the Neck. *Aesthetic Surg. J.* **2022**, *42*, 845–857. [CrossRef]

medicina

MDPI

Article

Feminization Surgery of the Upper Face as the Crucial Factor in Gender Confirmation—Pearls and Pitfalls

Rafał Pokrowiecki [1,*], Barbora Šufliarsky [2,*] and Maciej Jagielak [3]

1 Prive Esthetic and Facial Feminization Surgery Centre, 02-640 Warsaw, Poland
2 Department of Oral and Maxillofacial Surgery, Faculty of Medicine, Comenius University in Bratislava and University Hospital, 81372 Bratislava, Slovakia
3 Orthognathic, Private Practice, 05-090 Warsaw, Poland; recepcja@ortognatyka.pl
* Correspondence: dr.pokrowiecki@gmail.com (R.P.); barbora.sufliarsky@gmail.com (B.Š.); Tel.: +48-691226414 (R.P.)

Abstract: *Background*: Upper-face feminization is a frequently executed procedure in sexual reassignment surgery, owing to its ability to influence gender identity through adjustments to the hairline, forehead, and peri-orbital area. The procedure includes reducing the hairline, lifting the brows, shaving the orbital region, and applying specific techniques to reduce the frontal bone. This research aims to assess the outcomes, results, and potential complications associated with this surgery among transgender patients. *Material and Method*: Retrospective review of medical records of 20 patients who attended for facial feminization surgery of the upper face between June 2022 and June 2023, analyzing the previously performed procedures, complications and revision surgery outcomes, and first-time procedures. A literature review was performed for similar studies. *Results*: 20 patients were included in the study. Among the cohort treated elsewhere (n = 11), the primary complaint was insufficient browbone reduction and anterior frontal sinus table setback. They underwent poorly performed Type 1 reduction when full forehead reconstruction (Type 3/4) was indicated (n = 3), or no reduction was performed during hairline advancement (n = 4). Type 3 forehead reduction with orbital shaving and hairline advancement with simultaneous temporal browlift was most commonly performed in both revision and first-time surgical upper face feminization (n = 15) (75%). Type 1 osteoplasty was performed in four patients (10%), one Type 3 revision surgery was performed after insufficient Type 3 reduction, and one case of shock-induced alopecia was reported, treated with PRP/peptides and a FUE hair graft. *Conclusions*: The author's preferred technique, 'whole-in-one' upper face feminization by modified bi-coronal incision with frontal trichophytic hyper-beveled incision, provides sufficient insight into the frontal bone and orbital region, the desired forehead osteoplasty and the most efficient insight into the temporal area, enabling safe dissection between fasciae, ligamentous adhesion removal, and periosteal attachment, providing full soft and hard tissue feminization. Nevertheless, feminization procedures should be meticulously planned, and all concerning issues should be addressed during the first surgery in order to prevent revisions, complications, and patient dissatisfaction.

Keywords: facial feminization; gender affirmation surgery; frontal sinus setback; plastic surgery; craniofacial surgery

1. Introduction

Gender dysphoria is defined as a state where gender identity is incongruent with the sex assigned at the patient's birth. As facial characteristics are very important in gender recognition, feminization surgery is a complex and sequential set of procedures that enable to re-shape the facial features into something more feminine at both the bone- and soft tissue level [1,2]. As such, they are targeted at the distinctive anatomical differences seen between the anthropomorphic male and female skulls. Over 90% of trans-gender patients are in male-to-female transition (MTF). Among other surgeries that are necessary for gender confirmation surgery (e.g., breast augmentation, vaginoplasty, and waist-narrowing surgery), facial feminization surgery (FFS) is one of the most important phases throughout this process, as it is the face that defines the gender in the first place. Acquiring desired features matching the gender improves the self-esteem and social life of these patients, but it also decreases suicidal ideation, psychological distress, alcohol abuse, and smoking. Forehead and brow position are two of the most important factors in gender confirmation surgery, as the upper face represents 35–40% of the face [3,4]. Therefore, forehead feminization, along with rhinoplasty and jawline reshaping, is most commonly chosen by individuals undergoing gender affirmation surgery. Routinely, upper third feminization procedures involve hairline lowering and reshaping, different variants of browlift, reduction of the frontal bossing, and orbital aperture widening [5–7]. Protocols and surgery approaches may differ between the surgery centers providing gender-affirmation procedures. The fronto-glabellar region is the most challenging aspect of facial feminization in the upper third of the face. Douglas Ousterhout was the first to describe a detailed protocol for reshaping the forehead, taking into consideration the frontal bone and sinus anatomy. Type 1 forehead feminization involves the reduction of the frontal cortical bone. This procedure is suitable when the frontal sinus is underdeveloped and the cortical bone is thick enough to achieve both aesthetic goals and bone wall integrity. It typically allows for up to a 10 mm reduction in bone. Type 2 is performed when no setback is needed, but augmentation of the forehead crease is required to create a more feminine slope. Type 3 involves the reconstruction of the forehead with bone setback and stabilization using wires (following Ousterhout's original recommendations) or titanium plates (as in current approaches). Type 4 forehead reconstruction is relatively rarely necessary and involves complete forehead augmentation. This is done when the frontal area is too narrow or the other three types are insufficient to achieve the desired aesthetic [1,3].

The aim of this study was to analyze treatment needs and surgery outcomes in a cohort of transgender patients who recently underwent upper-face feminization procedures. This is also the first multidisciplinary Central-East Europe FFS Team annual report on transfeminine facial surgery.

2. Materials and Methods

A retrospective review of the medical records of patients who attended for facial feminization surgery between June 2022 and June 2023. Inclusion criteria included patients undergoing facial gender-affirming surgery, including the fronto-orbital region, at least 6 months of actual hormone replacement therapy, and patients under the continuous care of a psychologist and sexologist. Exclusion criteria included incomplete files, patients undergoing facial surgeries not including the upper face, and adolescents. The study aimed at analyzing the previously performed procedures in the upper face performed elsewhere, complications, and reasons for revision surgery. This study was conducted in accordance with the principles of Helsinki. Written informed consent was obtained from the individuals whose pictures are presented within the manuscript depicted in this article.

3. Results

Among the 35 transfeminine patients who attended for facial feminization surgery between June 2022 and June 2023 20 were included in the study (Table 1). 11 individuals opted for revision surgery of the fronto-orbital region due to a lack of satisfaction after previous procedures. 15 patients were not included in this study as the FFS procedures planned did not involve the upper face. Common complaints reported by patients were: insufficient reduction/setback of the anterior table of the frontal sinus (n = 7), inadequate or lack of orbital rim widening (n = 8), inadequate or not modified/lowered hairline (n = 7) (Table 1).

Table 1. Patients included into the study and procedures performed before elsewhere and reasons for eventual secondary surgery.

Patient	Age	Type 2	Type 2	Type 3	Type 4	Orbital Shaving	Hairline Advancementt	Browlift	Complaint	Commentary
1	42	yes	no	no	no	no	no	no	yes	insufficient forehead and orbital reduction, hairline
2	23	no	no	no	no	no	no	no	no	no
3	19	no	no	no	no	no	no	no	no	no
4	17	no	no	no	no	no	no	no	no	no
5	20	no	no	no	no	no	no	no	no	no
6	18	no	no	no	no	no	no	no	no	no
7	24	no	no	no	no	no	no	no	no	no
8	31	yes	no	no	no	no	no	no	yes	insufficient forehead and orbital reduction, hairline
9	45	no	no	no	no	no	yes	yes	yes	lack of bone reduction at all
10	23	no	no	no	no	no	no	no	no	no
11	23	no	no	no	no	no	no	no	no	no
12	45	yes	no	no	no	yes	no	no	yes	insufficient forehead and orbital reduction, hairline
13	51	yes	no	no	no	no	no	no	no	hairline
14	34	no	no	no	no	no	no	yes	yes	insufficient forehead and orbital reduction, hairline
15	32	no	no	no	no	no	yes	no	yes	insufficient forehead and orbital reduction, hairline
16	45	no	no	no	no	no	yes	yes	yes	insufficient forehead and orbital reduction, hairline
17	21	no	no	no	no	no	no	no	no	no
18	19	no	no	no	no	no	no	no	no	no
19	35	no	no	no	no	no	no	no	no	no
20	19	no	no	yes	no	no	no	yes	yes	insufficient forehead and orbital reduction, hairline, browlift

A total of 9 patients attended our FFS Team for the first time for consultation, according to the detailed protocol and decision tree (Tables 1–3). A classical coronal pretrichial incision was performed in all the patients that required revision surgery. In 3 cases, a limited pretrichial incision was performed, as no intervention in the temporal area was desired/needed (Figure 1). We did not perform a classic coronal incision in any of the presented cases. This was due to the limited application of such an approach in FFS. It is performed only in cases where bone remodeling is required without any intervention in the hairline. Common surgeries performed in revision cases and primary cases were: hairline advancement, orbital shaving, browlift, and frontal bossing reduction. We performed endoscopic-assisted Type 3 surgery (reconstruction) with orbital shaving in seven patients (Figures 2 and 3) and simple Type 1 osteoplasty (shaving) in three patients (Figure 4). One patient required revision surgery after Type 3 reduction.

Table 2. Patients included into the study and procedures performed at our clinic.

Patient	Type 1	Type 2	Type 3	Type 4	Orbital Shaving	Hairline Advancement	Browlift	Complaint	Complication	Type of Complication
1	no	no	no	no	no	no	no	no	yes	Screw infection
2	yes	no	no	no	yes	yes	yes	no	no	x
3	no	no	yes	no	yes	yes	yes	no	no	x
4	no	no	no	no	yes	yes	yes	no	no	x
5	no	no	yes	no	yes	yes	yes	no	yes	Shock hair loss
6	no	no	yes	no	yes	yes	yes	no	no	x
7	no	no	yes	no	yes	yes	yes	no	no	x
8	no	no	yes	no	yes	yes	yes	no	no	x
9	no	no	yes	no	yes	yes	yes	no	no	x
10	no	no	yes	no	yes	yes	yes	no	no	x
11	yes	no	no	no	yes	yes	yes	no	no	x
12	no	no	yes	no	yes	yes	yes	no	yes	Temporal hematoma
13	no	no	no	no	yes	yes	no	no	no	x
14	no	no	yes	no	yes	yes	yes	no	no	x
15	no	no	yes	no	yes	yes	yes	no	no	x
16	no	no	yes	yes	yes	yes	yes	no	no	x
17	no	no	yes	no	yes	yes	yes	no	no	x
18	no	no	yes	no	yes	yes	yes	no	no	x
19	yes	no	no	no	yes	no	yes	no	no	x
20	no	no	yes	no	yes	yes	yes	no	no	x

Table 3. Detailed upper third FFS procedures decision tree.

Hairline	High	Scalp advancement surgery
	Low	Consider coronal/temporal browlift only
Receding hairline	Yes	Correction during scalp advancement
	No	In case of scalp advancement consider less invasive incision
Widow's peak	Present	Remove for better scar camouflage
	Not Present	x
Medial brow ptosis	Yes	Addressed during scalp advancement and/or coronal browlift
	No	x
Lateral brow ptosis	Yes	Temporal lift during scalp advancement or other closed techniques
	No	x
Negative vector of the eye	Yes	Addressed during temporal lift. Consider canthopexy/canthoplasty along with midface lift and feminizing upper/lower blepharoplasty
	No	Simple upper/lower blepharoplasty if needed
Orbital shaving required	Yes	Osteoplasty with piezosurgery/pineapple bone bur
	No	x
Frontal bossing	Present	Ousterhout Type 1, 2, 3 or 4 forehead procedure
	Not present	x

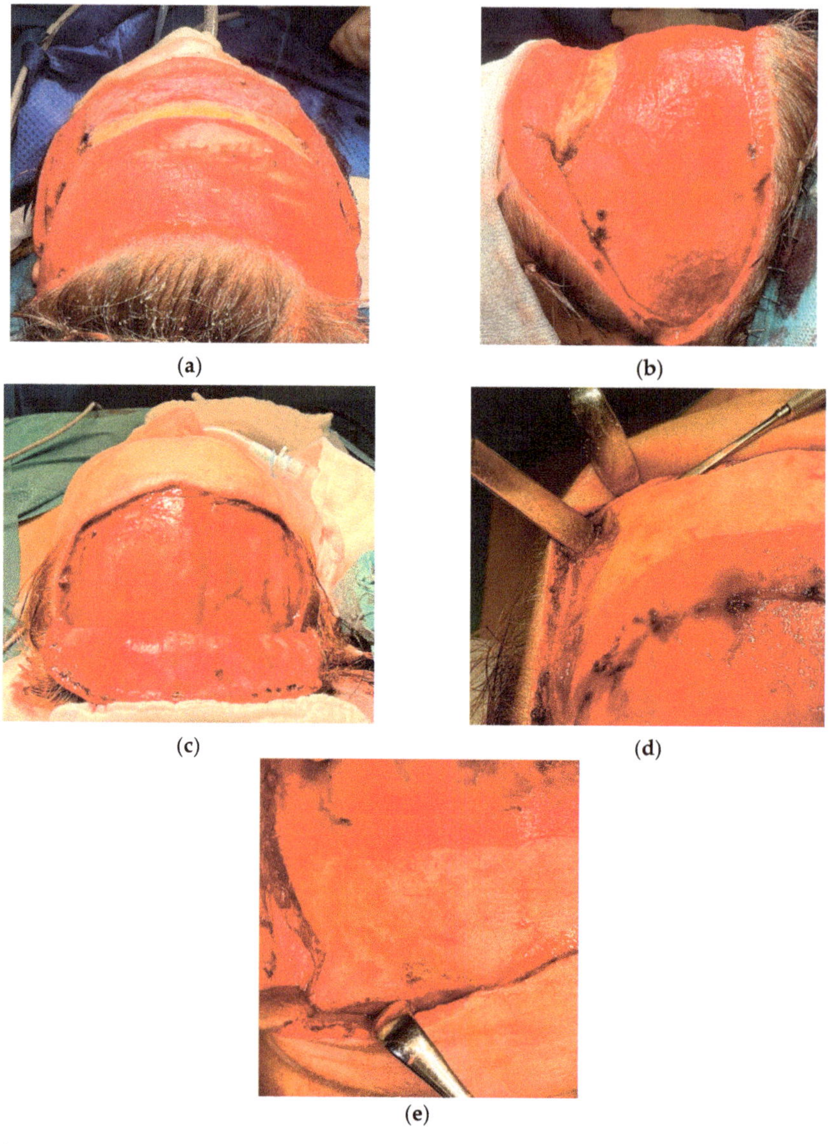

Figure 1. Examples of incision designs and flaps preparation commonly used in our protocol. (**a**,**b**) coronal pretrichial incision recommended in hairline lowering surgery and receding hairline reduction, as well as temporal browlift. This approach was performed in vast majority of the cases. (**c**–**e**) limited pretrichial when hairline lowering is advised but no intervention in temporal area is required. This approach provides comparable possibilities for insight into the peri-orbial area. Both approaches enable midface lift along with canth oplasty and cat eye surgery if desired. We usually do not use classic coronal incision (not shown here) as it does not provide sufficient feminization effects. We use this approach in cases with bone recontouring only and/or in cases without a need to address the hairline. However, coronal approach may also provide temporal and midface lifts if desired.

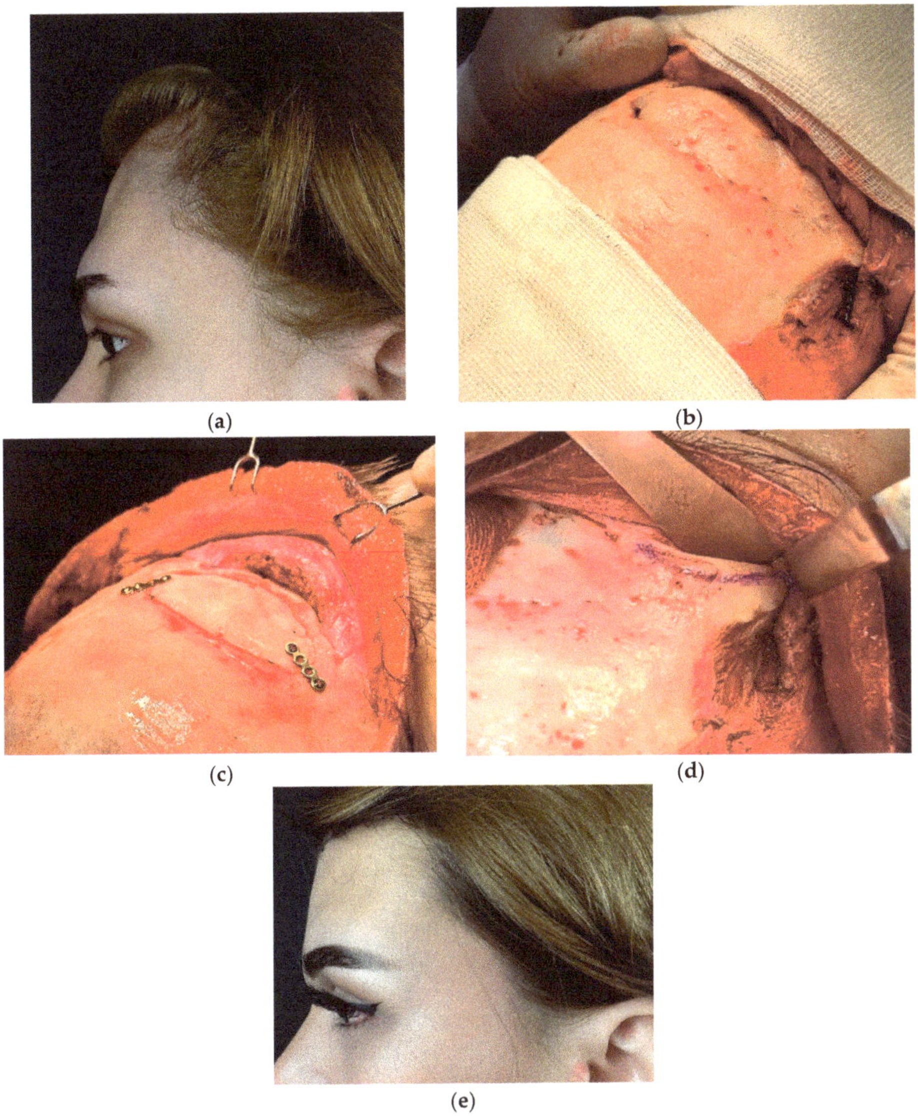

Figure 2. Photographs of the 19-year-old transgender female who attended revision surgery on the upper third. She complained of residual deformity, high hairline, and inadequate browlift. (**a**) lateral view of the forehead. (**b**) intraoperative view of the deformity and bone segment stabilized with Prolene 3.0 suture. (**c**) anterior wall repositioned and stabilized with 1.5 mm titanium plates (ChM, Lewickie, Poland). (**d**) Additional widening orbital rim ostectomy was performed. (**e**) lateral view 10 days post-op.

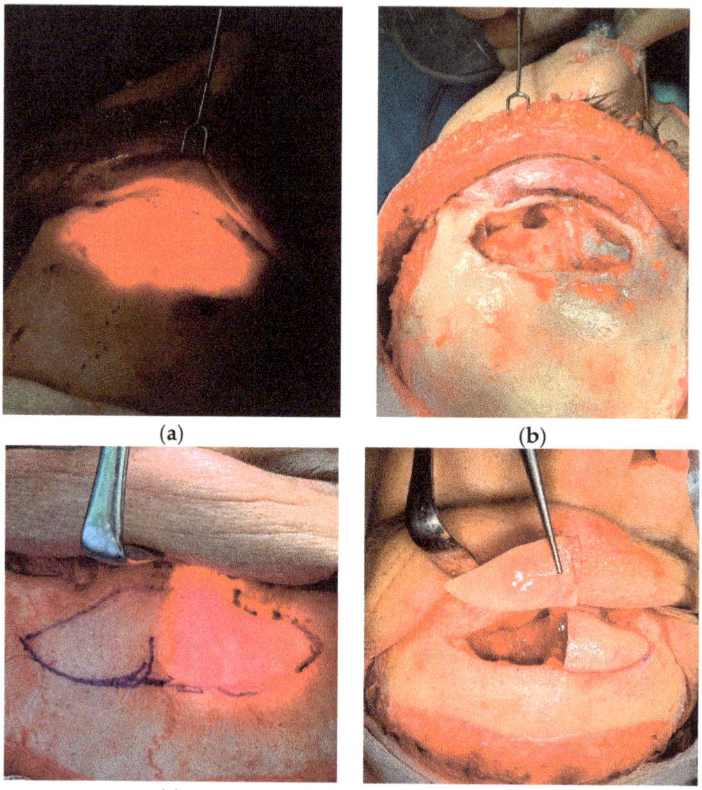

(a) (b) (c) (d)

Figure 3. Intraoperative photograph of endoscopic-assisted transillumination technique of the frontal sinus that enables safe marking of the sinus border before resection and reposition. (**a**) large sinus without septum, where one block resection of the anterior wall was performed. (**b**) view of the frontal sinus after removal of the anterior table. (**c**) Transillumination of the bifid frontal sinus septum. (**d**) two-piece resection of the anterior wall was performed due to thick septum and risk of fracture.

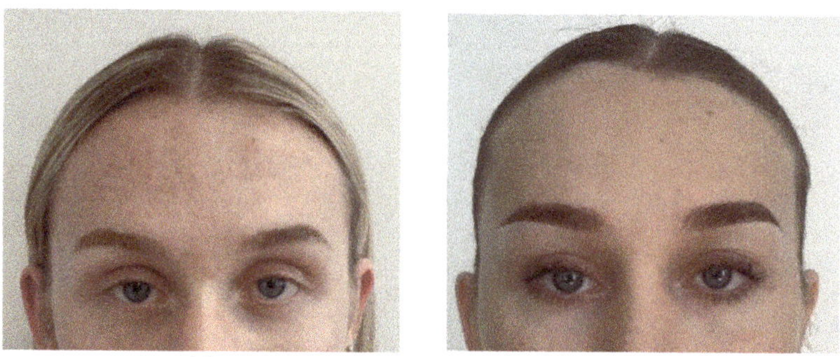

(a) (b)

Figure 4. *Cont.*

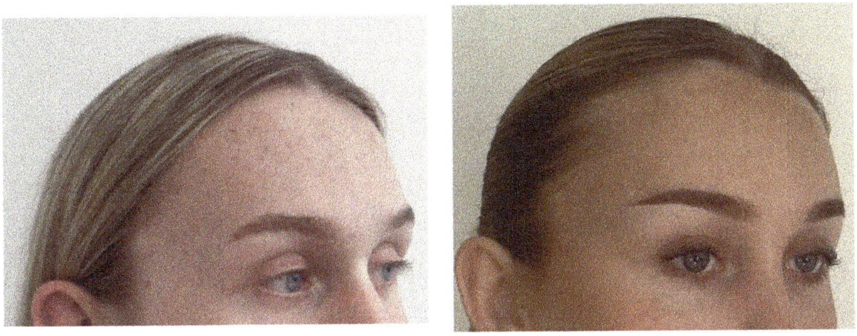

(c) (d)

Figure 4. Photographs of 21-year-old transgender females after primary complex feminization of the upper third: Type 1 frontal bone reduction, extended orbital aperture widening, hairline lowering, temporal browlift. (**a**) before and (**b**) 6 months after the surgery. (**c**) before the surgery, and (**d**) 6 months pot-op.

The complication rate was low and temporary. One patient developed a biomaterial-associated infection of the scalp stabilization screw, which was removed on the 10th day after the surgery. Other patients developed unilateral temporal hematoma, which was drained on the 2nd day post-op (revision case). Shock-induced alopecia was diagnosed in another revision case, which was fully treated within 3 months after 6 rounds of PRF/Peptides injections. Full regrowth of the hair was observed at the time of the follow-up. No incidents of nerve paresthesia, injury to the frontal branch of the facial nerve, mucocele, facial paresis, cerebrospinal fluid leak, palpable contour deformities, or nonunion were reported.

4. Discussion

Facial feminization surgery is a distinctive part of surgical practice as it combines multidisciplinary knowledge and backgrounds rooted in cranio-maxillo-facial, plastic, and reconstructive surgery. Its evolution and form known today were a natural process since Paul Tessier set his miles stones in craniofacial surgery. Ousterchout's research about male/female skull anthropometric differences performed in the 1980s was the first to target the transgender community directly, giving them hope for reaching their identity. Along with the technological development and incorporation of 3D virtual surgical planning procedures, they can be performed in a safer, time-consuming, and elegant manner [8,9] Patients usually do not need a hospital stay longer than 1–2 days. However, not every part of FFS may be calculated and automated. Indeed, reshaping of the skull features requires excellent training in cranio-maxillo-facial surgery. As a safe approach, the use of intraoral and subperiosteal dissections provides safe and reliable osteoplasty of every part of this complex region. "The projection of the soft tissues, understanding the subtle differences between cis-male and cis-female features, position of the brows, shape of the eyelid, canthal position, hairline design, and subdermal fat distribution are equally relevant in the final post-operational results. Therefore, it must be clearly stated that FFS surgery requires an in-depth understanding of clinical anatomy, anthropometry, skills in bone and plastic surgery, as well as artistic and esthetic touch. Transgender patients should be operated on at FFS-targeted centers that provide comprehensive care and a holistic approach [3,4] (Deschamps-Braly, 2019b; Ousterhout & Deschamps-Braly, 2019).

The group of patients presented here confirmed observations made in other research regarding feminization procedures of the upper third of the face. In the retrospective study performed by Rochlin et al. (2022) 25.5% of the cases were revision surgeries consisting of additional procedures due to previous under-correction [10]. In the analyzed material presented, 55% of the cases were revisions requiring additional procedures. However, our analysis was only restricted to the upper third.

When discussing bone remodeling of the upper face, one must take into consideration the proper approach to the skeleton, considering the hairline. In general, there are few approaches used in FFS of the upper third: standard bi-coronal, limited coronal incisions, coronal-pretrichial, and inverted-U trichial incisions [11]. When bone remodeling does not require hairline lowering or brow lifting, the classic coronal approach or limited coronal approach are then performed. This, however, is uncommon, as the vast majority of surgeries performed in FFS require re-shaping of the hairline and lowering and addressing the brows position in order to expose the widened orbits. Thus, the most common approach is pretrichal hyperbeveled coronal incision, and such was usually done in our patients. Pansritum described an inverted U-trichial incision for simple supraorbital ridge shaving with or without augmentation [11]. This is a shortened version of the classical coronal approach and permits simple orbital ridge shaving without reconstruction. As most commonly performed forehead feminization surgeries require reconstruction, in minimal-access cases, we prefer our version of "short" incision, which is also U-shaped but not inverted. This approach provides much better access to the fronto-orbital region, enables reconstruction and not only simple shaving, and provides hairline lowering and/or trichophytic browlift (Figure 1c).

Regardless of the scalp incision design, one must keep in mind to avoid incisions in non-hair-bearing areas of the temples, as it is impossible to camouflage thereafter [10].

Endoscopic-assisted Type 3 forehead reduction with orbital shaving and hairline advancement in different extents with simultaneous temporal browlift with or without deep-plane midface lift was the most commonly performed surgery in our patients. This approach was the method of choice in most first-and-revision cases, as it provided feminization and rejuvenation. The use of trans nasal endoscopic light in order to set the borders of an anterior wall osteotomy minimizes the risk of injury to the dura and post-operational CFS leak reported in different studies (Figure 2) [12].

Scalp advancement requires sequentially performed galeotomies in order to mobilize and push the scalp forward. The general rule of galea scoring involves subgaleal-periosteal dissection up to the nuchal ridge, taking care to avoid injury to the occipital arteries. Galeal scoring is performed in a horizontal manner, and each galeotomy gives 1–2 mm of mobilization of the scalp [13]. The number of galeal scores depends on the extent of the lowering necessary; however, they should be planned judiciously without causing any harm to hair follicles. Usually, galeotomies are performed from the back of the scalp to the front (Video S1).

Video S1. Intraoperative view of the galeotomies. Distance between each should be 1–1.5 cm. Incisions should be made in a horizontal manner with care not to violate the skin and hair follicles. Each galeotomy provides 1–2 mm of scalp advancement.

Forehead reduction in transgender facial surgery is commonly discussed in various publications. We do, however, prefer the classic approach described by Ousterhout. Type 3 surgery (reconstruction) was necessary in 75% of the cases. Surprisingly, revision cases were previously wrongly qualified patients for Type 1 reduction (bone burr). This was probably due to common undercorrection of the forehead, where Type 3 was really needed, but an unexperienced surgeon chose to burr down the cortical bone in a way not to open the sinus, leaving a thin wall. This was a frequently reported mistake, as Type 1 is only justified by an underdeveloped or lack of frontal sinus (Figure 4) [1]. In our cohort, only 10% of cases were Type 1 reduction, which generally agrees with the statistics published in other studies (Figure 5) [1,7,14,15].

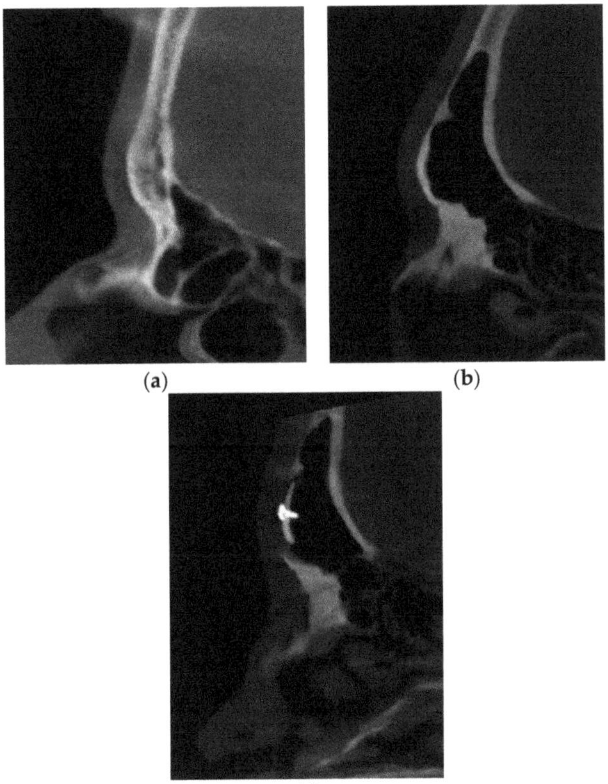

(a) (b) (c)

Figure 5. Sagittal sections of the frontal sinuses of two different patients who attended for the feminization of the upper third (not revision cases). (**a**) agenesis of the frontal sinus, which allowed for Type 1 forehead reduction. (**b**) large pneumatic frontal sinus, which required resection, remodeling, 5 mm setback, and osteosynthesis stabilization (Type 3). (**c**) the same sinus after feminization.

We prefer conservative fixation of the anterior table with miniplates and miniscrews (typically micro-systems 1.2–1.5 mm for upper third reconstruction) as it provides sufficient stabilization and reduces the risk of nonunion. We do not use wires to stabilize the bone fragments, as was originally advised by Ousterhout, due to the undisputable superiority of stable osteosynthesis with regard to bone fragment stabilization. Similar observations were presented in the work of Lee et al. (2022). However, we opt for minimal use of biomaterials needed for stable fixation in order not to increase the risk of biomaterial-associated infections (preferably 2 miniplastes). We also do not find using titanium meshes in Type 3 surgery justified in other cases, which are more complicated, which is in contrast to the approach proposed by Bonapace–Potvin et al. (2022) [16]. In the work of Telang (2020), meshes were described as a substitute material for the reconstruction of the hypertrophic sinuses, where the anterior was resected and the defect closed with mesh only [15]. We do not support this technique, as leaving the sinus open without any bony anterior wall is completely unjustified, especially in aesthetic-reconstructive surgery. Meshes are also avoided in the protocol described by Maggio (2019) [14]. The author, however, prefers using wire fixation, as was originally postulated by Ousterhout. Maggio (2019) uses miniplates only when stabilization is not achieved by wires, showing that the topic of bone fragment stabilization in the non-mobile forehead is rather based on each author's preferences and experience. If patients wish not to use titanium biomaterials, resorbable osteosynthesis is an option In selected cases.

We aim to preserve the frontal sinus mucosa by leaving the open nasofrontal duct. We ablate the sinus only in cases with a small sinus and an increased risk of mucocele and infections. In the presented report, no complications regarding the frontal sinus were reported.

Orbital shaving is as important as frontal bone setback. Male orbital volume is generally larger; however, women have a larger orbital opening compared to the rest of the face [17]. Undercorrection has been reported in the cohort of revision cases presented here and must have been addressed in secondary surgeries. Thus, much attention should be paid to the periorbital area when forehead osteoplasty procedures are planned. We aim at resecting the upper and upper-lateral orbital rim apertures. Similar to Maggio (2019), we are strongly convinced that burring down the upper aspect of the orbital rim may not provide sufficient feminization [14]. Especially as a properly dissected fronto-temporal area provides safe access to the upper and lateral aspects of the orbital aperture, wider resection is possible, which gives more feminine and balanced orbital widening than resection of the upper part only. More aggressive shaving of the upper-lateral part of the orbital aperture greatly enhances the effect of the temporal browlift during FFS. In our cohort, 7 patients who attended revision surgery complained about under resection of the orbital aperture, which was successfully corrected during revisions.

We advocate using suction drains. Some authors also do not use them, which, in our opinion, should be discussed [16]. We put at least 2 transverse suction drains: one under the frontal flap (in front of the incision) and a second caudally to the incision for 24–48 h. This prevents subgaleal hematoma and thus significantly reduces the incidence of traumatic alopecia and scalp necrosis [18].

Scalp stabilization after its reposition usually requires some tension, and screw-based stabilization is always required. Closure should be firm; however, tension should be restricted to galea. The skin should be tensionless, while the galea should be stabilized in the calvarium. Otherwise, wound rupture, scarring, and hair loss may occur [13]. Generally, there are two commonly used techniques of scalp stabilization. The first is performed with the use of cranially fixated titanium screws piercing the skin-galeal flap 1.5–2 cm caudally to the incision line. These screws are kept for a period of 2–3 weeks, and then, after the scalp settlement, the screws are removed by a screwdriver (Figure 6). The second technique uses miniscrews placed on the calvarium. Sutures are placed subcutaneously, and tension is placed only on the galea. The first technique may be used in advancements with low to moderate tension, as stabilization and screw removal are straightforward. However, if scalp advancement is significant and increased tension is to be expected, calvarium-based miniscrews are advised (Figure 5). This reduces the risk of necrosis, alopecia, infection, and bad scars. Alternative fixations are endotines or cortical tunnels [17].

Another observation made in this analysis was that browlift procedures were not specifically addressed in the cohort who attended revision surgery. It was surprising, as browlifting is an inherent part of facial feminization. The position of the brows and their lateral tails is one of the most important factors distinguishing the male and female peri-orbital areas, even without bone reduction surgery. Osteoplasty of the upper and upper-lateral orbital rim is performed in order to widen the orbital aperture and expose the eyeballs, but without any form of browlift, this effect cannot be achieved as soft tissues will remain in their place or will even droop due to bone deficiency after reduction. Surprisingly, 9 out of 11 revision cases required a browlift during their second surgery. We usually perform temporal browlifts during scalp transection and hairline advancement with deep-plane cheek lifts, canthoplasty, and eyelid surgery. We performed both hard and soft tissue feminization during one-stage surgery, similarly to the protocol described by Maggio (2019) [14]. However, we do not advise a hair transplant at the time of the main surgery, as injury to the scalp and frontal flap may affect graft healing and stability. This is in contrast to the study published by Capitain et al. (2017), as they encourage performing

FUE grafting at the time of the facial surgery [6]. The authors justify this technique by introducing the posterior-coronal flap, which in theory provides hairline lowering and the simultaneous use of strip hair follicles. This seems illogical, as resection of the skin behind the hairline can produce nothing but forehead lengthening, which is then masked by grafts. Careful planning of the hairline incision with regards to the full-feminization plan is crucial. It is completely unjustified to perform a coronal incision placed behind a hairline if the patient requires hairline-lowering surgery. Especially in revision cases, the risk of alopecia between two incisions is increased. Such observations were described in the report of Dechamps–Braly (2019) [10] (2 cases), and so they were diagnosed in one of our patients, where revision of the Type 3 surgery was necessary due to insufficient setback, deformity, and a lack of addressing the hairline during the first surgery. Shock hair loss may develop in 10% of scalp advancement cases, but it increases significantly in secondary procedures. Especially when a second, different incision design is necessary for hairline lowering, which results in the formation of two scars that impede blood supply to the hair follicles. Therefore, it is an absolute must to address all the issues judicially during the first surgery and not increase the risk of unwanted complications. Shock hair loss is usually temporary, and hair regrowth is expected after a few weeks or months. Platelet-rich fibrin (PRF) and hair-stimulating peptide injections every two weeks provide sufficient boosters for regrowth, as was fortunately observed in our patient.

We do advise hair transplants 6–12 months after scalp advancement for a more predictable outcome and better addressing the temple hollowing and potential scar, similarly to the protocols described by Dechamps–Braly (2019) [3,4]. Last but not least, the gold standard of hair grafting is the follicular unit extraction (FUE) technique. As such, it requires the patient's prone position for follicular harvesting from the occipital area. Not only would it require changing the patient's position during feminization surgery (supine position), but it would also result in the unjustified elongation of general anesthesia. Taking into account all the aforementioned arguments, delayed hair transplant as an adjunctive treatment that can be comfortably performed under local anesthesia is the most advantageous, effective, and safest.

Soft and hard tissue relationships are of great importance in any facial surgery. However, in FFS, one must aim at the feminine aspect by reducing osteoplasties and, hence, considering the physiology and anatomy of the aging face. Issues related to anti-aging procedures go beyond the scope of this manuscript. What is more, upper-third feminization surgery is usually also a solution for aging processes in the upper face through browlifts. Nevertheless, a few remarks should be made regarding lifting procedures as such. Contrary to the protocols described by Maggio, we advise addressing the mid- and lower face and neck soft tissues 6–12 months after bone remodeling and not simultaneously [14]. Especially in the aging face. In our experience, face and neck lifts, liposculpting, and other surgeries are far more powerful after the final settlement of these tissues on the remodeled bone framework, and by that, the risk of under correction (typically in facelifts) is far less plausible. When considering facial feminization surgery, upper-third feminization may greatly deal with aging in this area during one-stage surgery. However, in the case of the lower third, we strongly recommend a 2-stage approach for better re-draping of the soft tissues after bone reduction procedures.

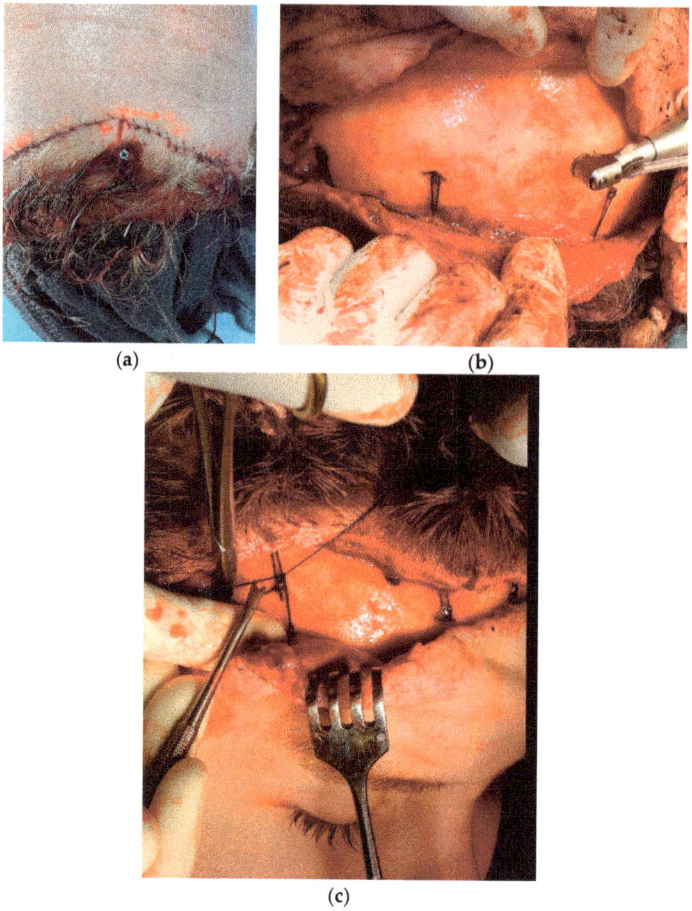

Figure 6. Intraoperative view of the two different techniques for scalp stabilization. (**a**) transcutaneous titanium screws placed temporarily directly on calvarial bone, 1.5–2 cm caudally to the incision line. Usually 4–5 screws of 2.0 × 15 mm are used. These can be easily identified and then removed 10–14 days later under local anesthesia. (**b**) permanent miniscrews placed monocortically under the skin-galea flap. Such screws may be used as both anchor points for scalp fixation sutures and browlift suspension sutures (**c**).

5. Conclusions

The authors' preferred technique, 'whole-in-one' upper face feminization by modified bi-coronal incision with frontal trichophytic hyper-beveled incision, provides sufficient insight into the frontal bone and orbital region, the desired forehead osteoplasty, and the most efficient insight into the temporal area, enabling safe dissection between fasciae, ligamentous adhesion removal, and periosteal attachment, providing full soft and hard tissue feminization during one surgery. The approach is suitable for revision surgery as it is for the first-time upper-face full feminization. The study's findings highlight the importance of additional training in facial surgery for transgender patients in order to offer them comprehensive care within a single surgical facility. This will have a significant impact on patient safety, aesthetic outcomes, and overall satisfaction.

Supplementary Materials: The following supporting information can be downloaded at: https://www.mdpi.com/article/10.3390/medicina60010120/s1, Video S1.

Author Contributions: Conceptualization, R.P. and M.J.; methodology, R.P., B.Š. and M.J.; software, R.P., B.Š. and M.J.; validation, R.P. and M.J.; formal analysis, R.P.; investigation, R.P.; resources R.P., B.Š. and M.J.; data curation, R.P., B.Š. and M.J.; writing, R.P., B.Š. and M.J.; supervision, M.J.; project administration, R.P.; funding acquisition, R.P., B.Š. and M.J. All authors have read and agreed to the published version of the manuscript.

Funding: The study was funded by the Gender Affirmation Surgery (GAS) Foundation, Warsaw, Poland (Publication-2023).

Institutional Review Board Statement: The study was conducted in accordance with the Declaration of Helsinki. Ethical review and approval were waived for this study due to the retrospective nature of the manuscript.

Informed Consent Statement: Informed consent was obtained from all subjects involved in the study. Written informed consent has been obtained from the patient(s) to publish this paper.

Data Availability Statement: Data are contained within the article.

Conflicts of Interest: The authors declare no conflicts of interest.

References

1. Altman, K. Facial Feminization Surgery: The Forehead. Surgical Techniques and Analysis of Results. *Plast. Reconstr. Surg.* **2015**, *136*, 301–318. [CrossRef]
2. Glorion, A.; Perrillat, A.; Foletti, J.M.; Cristofari, S. Surgical techniques used in chin feminization: Literature review and knowledge update. *J. Stomatol. Oral Maxillofac. Surg.* **2022**, *123*, 883–887. [CrossRef] [PubMed]
3. Ousterhout, D.K.; Deschamps-Braly, J.C. Special Edition on Transgender Facial Surgery. *J. Craniofacial Surg.* **2019**, *30*, 1326–1327. [CrossRef] [PubMed]
4. Deschamps-Braly, J.C. Approach to Feminization Surgery and Facial Masculinization Surgery: Aesthetic Goals and Principles of Management. *J. Craniofacial Surg.* **2019**, *30*, 1352–1358. [CrossRef] [PubMed]
5. Altman, K. Facial feminization surgery. In *The Transgender Handbook: A Guide for Transgender People, Their Families and Professionals*; Nova Science Publishers, Inc.: Hauppauge, NY, USA, 2017; pp. 301–318. [CrossRef]
6. Capitán, L.; Simon, D.; Meyer, T.; Alcaide, A.; Wells, A.; Bailón, C.; Bellinga, R.J.; Tenório, T.; Capitán-Cañadas, F. Facial Feminization Surgery: Simultaneous Hair Transplant during Forehead Reconstruction. *Plast. Reconstr. Surg.* **2017**, *139*, 573–584. [CrossRef] [PubMed]
7. Dang, B.N.; Hu, A.C.; Bertrand, A.A.; Chan, C.H.; Jain, N.S.; Pfaff, M.J.; Lee, J.C.; Lee, J.C. Evaluation and treatment of facial feminization surgery: Part i. forehead, orbits, eyebrows, eyes, and nose. *Arch. Plast. Surg.* **2021**, *48*, 503–510. [CrossRef] [PubMed]
8. Efanov, J.I.; Roy, A.A.; Huang, K.N.; Borsuk, D.E. Virtual surgical planning: The Pearls and pitfalls. *Plast. Reconstr. Surg. Glob. Open* **2018**, *6*, e1143. [CrossRef] [PubMed]
9. Ganry, L.; Comert, M. Low-cost and simple frontal sinus surgical cutting guide modeling for anterior cranioplasty in facial feminization surgery: How to do it. *J. Craniofacial Surg.* **2022**, *33*, E84–E87. [CrossRef]
10. Rochlin, D.H.; Chaya, B.F.; Rodriguez Colon, R.; Onuh, O.; Rojas, A.; Rodriguez, E.D. Secondary Surgery in Facial Feminization: Reasons and Recommendations. *Ann. Plast. Surg.* **2022**, *89*, 652–655. [CrossRef] [PubMed]
11. Pansritum, K. Forehead and Hairline Surgery for Gender Affirmation. *Plast. Reconstr. Surg. Glob. Open* **2021**, *9*, E3486. [CrossRef] [PubMed]
12. Capitán, L.; Simon, D.; Kaye, K.; Tenorio, T. Facial feminization surgery: The forehead. Surgical techniques and analysis of results. *Plast. Reconstr. Surg.* **2014**, *134*, 609–619. [CrossRef] [PubMed]
13. Öreroglu, A.R. Forehead Reduction and Hairline Lowering Surgery Aesthetic Implications. *Turk. J. Plast. Surg.* **2022**, *30*, 108–114. [CrossRef]
14. Di Maggio, M. Forehead and Orbital Rim Remodeling. In *Facial Plastic Surgery Clinics of North America*; W.B. Saunders: Philadelphia, PA, USA, 2019; Volume 27, pp. 207–220. [CrossRef]
15. Telang, P.S. Review of Facial Feminization Surgery Telang Facial Feminization Surgery: A Review of 220 Consecutive Patients. *Indian J. Plast. Surg.* **2020**, *53*, 244–253. [CrossRef] [PubMed]
16. Bonapace-Potvin, M.; Pepin, M.; Navals, P.; Medor, M.C.; Lorange, E.; Bensimon, É. Facial Gender-Affirming Surgery: Frontal Bossing Surgical Techniques, Outcomes and Safety. *Aesthetic Plast. Surg.* **2023**, *47*, 1353–1361. [CrossRef] [PubMed]
17. Louis, M.; Travieso, R.; Oles, N.; Coon, D. Narrative review of facial gender surgery: Approaches and techniques for the frontal sinus and upper third of the face. *Ann. Transl. Med.* **2021**, *9*, 606. [CrossRef] [PubMed]
18. Rachidi, S.; Bender, A.M.; Cohen, B.A. Disorders of the hair and nails. *Pediatr. Dermatol.* **2022**, *2022*, 227–259. [CrossRef]

medicina

MDPI

Article

Physical Conditions Prevailing in the Nasal and Maxillary Sinus Cavities Based on Numerical Simulation

Monika Morawska-Kochman [1], Ziemowit Miłosz Malecha [2,*], Krzysztof Zub [1,*], Jakub Kielar [2], Krzysztof Dudek [3], Kamil Nelke [4,5] and Tomasz Zatonski [1]

1 Department of Otolaryngology, Head and Neck Surgery, Medical University, Borowska 213, 50-556 Wroclaw, Poland; monika.morawka-kochman@umw.edu.pl (M.M.-K.); tomasz.zatonski@umw.edu.pl (T.Z.)
2 Department of Cryogenics and Aerospace Engineering, Wroclaw University of Science and Technology, Wybrzeze Wyspianskiego 27, 50-370 Wroclaw, Poland; jakub.kielar@pwr.edu.pl
3 Statistical Analysis Centre, Wroclaw Medical University, 50-368 Wroclaw, Poland; krzysztof.dudek@pwr.edu.pl
4 Maxillofacial Surgery Ward, EMC Hospital, Pilczycka 144, 54-144 Wroclaw, Poland
5 Health Department, Academy of Applied Sciences, Academy of Silesius, Zamkowa 4, 58-300 Walbrzych, Poland
* Correspondence: ziemowit.malecha@pwr.edu.pl (Z.M.M.); krzysztof.zub@umw.edu.pl (K.Z.)

Abstract: *Background and Objectives*: This paper presents a unique study that links the physical conditions in the nasal passage with conditions that favour the development of bacterial strains and the colonization of the mucous membranes of the nose and paranasal sinuses. The physical parameters considered were air flow, pressure, humidity, and temperature. *Materials and Methods*: Numerical models of the human nose and maxillary sinus were retrospectively reconstructed from CT images of generally healthy young subjects. The state-of-the-art numerical methods and tools were then used to determine the temperature, humidity, airflow velocity, and pressure at specific anatomical locations. *Results*: The results were compared with optimal conditions for bacterial growth in the nose and sinuses. *Conclusions*: Temperature, humidity, air velocity, and pressure were shown to play critical roles in the selection and distribution of microorganisms. Furthermore, certain combinations of physical parameters can favour mucosal colonisation by various strains of bacteria.

Keywords: airflow; nasal cavity; sinus cavity; computational fluid dynamics; temperature; humidity; microorganisms

1. Introduction

The question of the development and role of paranasal sinuses in humans remains open. The most popular theories come from three hypotheses: structural, evolutionary, and functional. The structural hypothesis assumes that sinus cavities reduce the weight of the face and relieve the muscles of the head and neck, optimizing balance. Evolutionary theory claims that its development resulted from adapting to maintaining airways outside the aquatic environment. Finally, the functional hypothesis assumes that paranasal sinuses are a voice resonator, thermal insulator, and protector against brain injury and increase the surface area of the mucous membrane that humidifies inhaled air [1–4].

The anatomical variability of the shape and volume of the nasal cavity and sinuses affects the prevailing physical conditions. Factors such as temperature, humidity, airflow, and air pressure can simultaneously play a significant role in their proper functioning [5]. They can also indirectly shape the selection and distribution of microorganisms on the mucous membrane [6]. The available literature lacks research results describing the relationships between physical conditions and environmental requirements of bacteria colonizing the nasal cavity and sinuses. The use of computer modelling techniques have proved to be helpful. Three-dimensional geometric modelling has opened up new possibilities for physical and digital airflow simulations in the nasal cavity based on anatomically precise computer models [7]. Measurements based on computational fluid dynamics (CFD) have been the subject of studies demonstrating the method's effectiveness [8–11]. Numerical analysis has been used in various studies such as airflow diagnostics in patients with sleep apnoea, deposition fraction, and drug delivery efficiency [12,13]. Recent research has confirmed that the use of numerical modelling to analyse airflow through the nasal cavity (virtual rhinomanometry) can be considered a reliable method [14]. Many studies have shown that simulations and numerical modelling, particularly numerical fluid dynamics (CFD), are mature and reliable enough to be treated as part of personalized medicine. Computational fluid dynamics (CFD) has been a valuable diagnostic tool used in numerical simulations and to analyse data related to the interactions of liquid and gas particles whose movements are also limited by solid surfaces, to evaluate heat and moisture exchange [15,16]. Several studies have investigated the use of CFD in paranasal sinus modelling, e.g., to investigate the effect of nasal anatomical deformations on airflow [17] or to simulate the distribution of inhaled particles within the sinuses [18]. The CFD method has also been used to study air flow, and heat and moisture exchange in healthy and diseased noses and sinuses after surgical procedures or to investigate intranasal medicine deposition [16,19–23]. In addition, as stated in the work [24], numerical simulations may become part of personalized medicine, especially when appropriate software is developed to shorten the tedious calculations.

Evolution has led to complex relationships between microorganisms that form ecosystems and their specific host organism [25]. Due to the different environmental requirements, their distribution varies between regions of the human body. For example, the upper respiratory tract provides suitable conditions for the colonisation of bacteria, which also depend on various external factors (such as temperature and humidity) and internal factors (such as diseases or immune responses) [26].

Summarizing the above review of the literature, it can be stated that numerical calculations can be a reliable and detailed source of information on the physical conditions prevailing in the nasal passage. It allows researchers to analyse a wide spectrum of data from anywhere in the nasal cavity and paranasal sinuses without performing invasive and uncomfortable in vivo procedures. On the other hand, a thorough knowledge of these conditions can help to better understand the formation of conditions favourable for the development of bacterial colonies and infections.

The aim of this study was to determine and compare, using state-of-the-art CFD calculation methods, the values of temperature, humidity, airflow velocity, and air pressure in healthy individuals in three clinically significant locations: the inferior nasal meatus, the area near the opening of the ostiomeatal complex, and the maxillary sinus cavity. To our knowledge, no study published so far has simultaneously considered all clinically significant characteristics of nasal airflow, such as pressure, humidity, velocity and temperature, at the locations investigated in the present study. Moreover, no study to date has attempted to link these flow characteristics, obtained on the basis of calculations, with the requirements of bacterial strains colonizing the mucous membranes of the nose and paranasal sinuses.

2. Material and Methods

The presented study utilized Computer Tomography (CT) images to reconstruct realistic human nose and maxillary sinus models. The CT images comprised 100 cross-sections, each with a 512 × 512 pixels resolution in DICOM format. Ten young and generally healthy subjects (four women and six men) were retrospectively analysed (mean age = 27 years; SD = 3.46; min. = 23; max. = 34). All individuals included in the analysis never reported nasal or sinus complaints and showed no imaging evidence of sinusitis. The CT examinations were performed previously as part of the preparation for orthognathic surgery. Therefore, the inclusion criteria were patients without symptoms and signs of sinonasal mucosal inflammation selected for orthognathic surgery treatment. Exclusion criteria consisted of patients under 18 years of age and older than 35 years of age, with acute or chronic rhinosinusitis, with previous nose/sinus surgery, with allergic rhinitis or smokers. The patients should not be on medication for one month before the CT scan. The study was approved by the Bioethics Committee at the local Medical University and conducted according to the principles of the Declaration of Helsinki (KB-545/2015).

After the reconstruction of the ethmoid labyrinth, the sphenoid and frontal sinuses were bilaterally excluded from the computation, and calculations were performed for the two most extensive maxillary sinuses. Based on anatomical and clinical considerations, three locations were selected for analysis: the inferior nasal duct, the area around the issue of the ostiomeatal complex, and the maxillary sinus floor. These sites were chosen due to the routine collection of swab cultures for microbiological testing [27–29].

3. Numerical Simulation Methods

To maintain natural airflow entering the nasal cavity and ensure the numerical stability of the model, an additional computational area was created that was connected to the nasal openings. This area was shaped like a 60 mm × 60 mm × 65 mm cuboid and simulated the external environment, as shown in Figure 1. This approach has also been used in other papers [30]. In addition, an additional 50 mm extension piece was attached to the end of each model's nasopharyngeal section to ensure numerical stability and prevent flow reversal at the nasopharyngeal outlet.

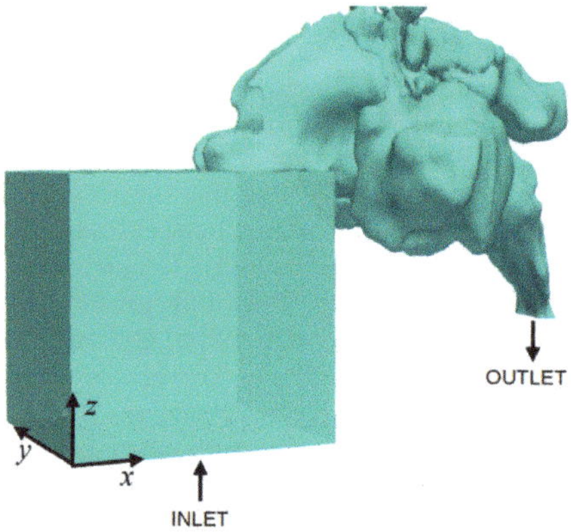

Figure 1. The computational domain of one of the cases consists of the nasal cavity reconstructed from CT images and a box simulating the outside environment.

Following the reasoning presented in a series of papers regarding the modelling of airflow in the nasal cavity [30–33], it was assumed that the flow was incompressible, laminar, and steady:

$$\nabla \cdot u = 0 \tag{1}$$

$$\nabla \cdot (\rho u u) = -\nabla p + \nabla \cdot \mu \nabla u \tag{2}$$

$$\rho C_p (u \cdot \nabla T) = k \nabla^2 T \tag{3}$$

$$u \cdot \nabla C = D \nabla^2 C \tag{4}$$

The velocity vector is represented by $u = (u_x, u_y, u_z)$, while p represents the pressure in Pa, T represents temperature, C represents the concentration of water vapour, ρ represents the density, μ represents the dynamic viscosity, C_p represents the specific heat, and k represents the thermal conductivity of air. Finally, D represents the mass diffusion coefficient of the water vapour into the air.

Equation (1) is the principle of mass conservation; Equation (2) is the Navier–Stokes equation for incompressible fluids and describes the principle of conservation of momentum; Equation (3) is the principle of conservation of energy in the flow; and Equation (4) describes the process of diffusion and transportation of moisture in the flow.

Similarly, as in [9,30], a two-film theory was adopted to determine the mass fraction of water in the nasal cavity. Therefore, the transport of vapour from the walls of the nasal cavity to the interior was simulated using the following boundary condition.

$$-D\frac{\partial C}{\partial n} = \frac{C_a - C_b}{R} \tag{5}$$

In Equation (5), C_a = 0.032 represents the mass fraction of the vapour at the interface between the organ and mucous (ambient mass fraction of the vapour), and n indicates a normal direction towards the nearest wall. The value of C_a is constant because the mucous is constantly supplied with water by the capillary layer, C_b is the mass fraction of vapour on the surface of the nasal cavity wall, and R is the cumulative mass diffusion resistance:

$$R = \frac{D_{bl}}{\delta_{bl}} + \frac{D_{memb}}{\delta_{memb}} \tag{6}$$

$D_{bl} = 3 \cdot 10^{-5}\ \mathrm{m^2/s}$ and $D_{memb} = 2.6 \cdot 10^{-5}\ \mathrm{m^2/s}$ are the mass diffusion coefficient of the boundary layer and mucous membrane [14]. The thickness of the boundary layer and the mucous membrane layer thickness is $\delta_{bl} = 0.3$ mm and $\delta_{memb} = 0.5$ mm, respectively [34].

Equations (1) through (4) were discretised using the finite volume method (FVM) and solved numerically using the OpenFOAM (Open Source Field Operation and Manipulation) software [35] along with the SIMPLE (Semi-Implicit Method for Pressure-Linked Equations) algorithm [36,37]. Table 1 shows the boundary conditions used in the created numerical model illustrated in Figure 1. All boundaries of the box simulating the external environment, except for the inlet, are called "box walls", and the outer boundaries of the nasal cavity are called "nasal walls".

Table 1. Boundary conditions used in the numerical calculations of the model illustrated in Figure 1. "Nasal wall" corresponds to all the walls of the nasal cavity, "Box walls" correspond to the boundaries of the external environment (apart from the "Inlet" boundary).

Physical Conditions	Inlet	Outlet	Nasal Wall	Box Walls
Velocity, l/min	15	15	No-slip	slip
Temperature, °C	25	36.6	34	25
Vapour, %	0.007	$\frac{\partial C}{\partial n} = 0$	Equation (5)	0.007
Pressure, Pa	100,000	$\frac{\partial p}{\partial n} = 0$	$\frac{\partial p}{\partial n} = 0$	$\frac{\partial p}{\partial n} = 0$

Table 2 displays the information regarding the numerical grid used in the simulations. The grid was composed primarily of hexagonal and polyhedral cells, with a total of approximately 6 million grid cells, consistent with the quantity utilized in previous numerical grid studies [30]. In addition, the mesh cells were progressively reduced in size near the walls to ensure an accurate representation of the intricate shape of the nasal cavity wall.

Table 2. Resolution and shape details of the computational mesh used in the study.

Number of Mesh Cells and Their Shape			Min Volume of Cell	Max Volume of Cell
hexahedra	polyhedra	total number	m^3	m^3
~4 million	~2 million	~6 million	$\sim 10^{-13}$	$\sim 10^{-8}$

Figure 2 presents a cross-section through the calculation domain from Figure 1 and shows the structure of the numerical grid. It can be seen that the mesh very closely reproduces the actual shape of the nasal cavity, and the mesh cells became smaller as they neared the wall. In addition, the narrow channels contained a sufficiently large number of grid cells to represent the flow profile. These features ensure the physical behaviour of the flow and heat and mass transfer at the walls and reliable calculation results.

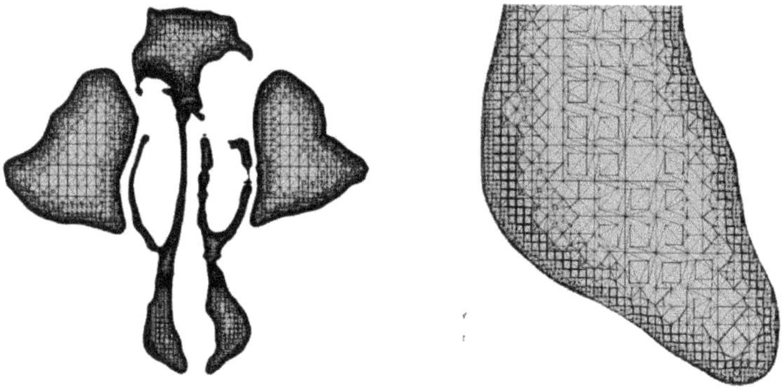

Figure 2. An example of the numerical mesh structure. (**Left**) Cross-section in the y-z plane just above the nostrils; (**Right**) enlarged section of inlet into the right nostril.

4. Results

Figure 3 shows example computational results of the humidity in the nasal cavity (of one of the considered geometries reproduced from the CT images), along with the selected measurement locations for further analysis: the area around the ostiomeatal complex (A1, A2), the inferior nasal duct (B1, B2), and the maxillary sinus floor (C1, C2). It was ensured that the measurement locations on the left and right sides of the nasal cavity were as anatomically similar as possible. It can be seen that the mass fraction of the vapour in the area representing the external environment was 0.007%. After air flows into the nasal passage, its humidity increased and in places where the flow is very low or close to zero (maxillary sinuses), the mass fraction of the vapour in the air increased to 0.032%, which corresponds to the vapour content in the mucous membranes.

Table 3 presents the temperature and humidity, and Table 4 presents the mean velocity and pressure magnitude, in the selected locations. It can be observed that the remaining differences between the nose's right and left sides were insignificant. A comparison of individual parameters in different areas showed that the p-value was greater than 0.05. Consequently, the averaged values were used in further analyses and discussions.

Table 3. Humidity and temperature of the air flowing through three selected anatomical locations.

Location	Side	Temperature (°C)	Humidity (%)
Inferior nasal meatus	Right	33.15 (32.35 ÷ 33.95)	0.022 (0.018 ÷ 0.031)
	Left	32.05 (31.05 ÷ 33.75)	0.019 (0.015 ÷ 0.024)
	R vs. L	p-value = 0.126	p-value = 0.094
Ostiomeatal complex	Right	33.85 (33.55 ÷ 33.95)	0.027 (0.026 ÷ 0.031)
	Left	33.65 (33.65 ÷ 33.95)	0.026 (0.022 ÷ 0.028)
	R vs. L	p-value = 0.827	p-value = 0.275
Maxillary sinus floor	Right	34.05 (34.05 ÷ 34.05)	0.032 (0.032 ÷ 0.032)
	Left	34.05 (34.05 ÷ 34.05)	0.032 (0.032 ÷ 0.032)
	R vs. L	p-value = 0.827	p-value = 0.716

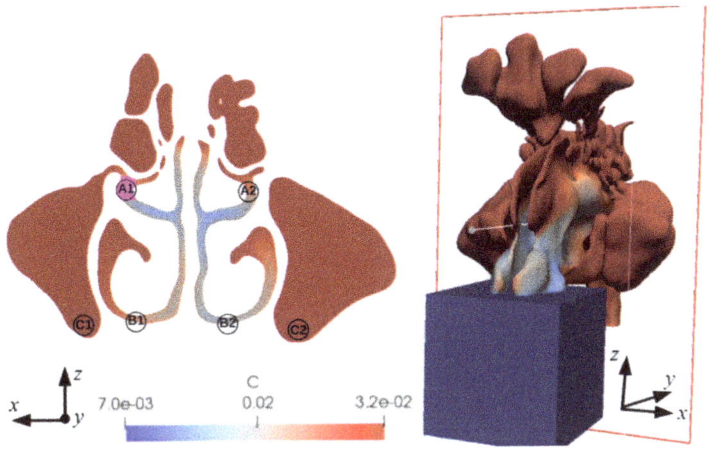

Figure 3. (**Left**) Cross-section through the nostrils indicating the measurement locations: A1, A2—the area around the ostiomeatal complex, B1, B2—the inferior nasal duct, C1, C2—maxillary sinus floor. (**Right**) General view of the 3D geometry of the nostrils with a sectional plane. The colour map indicates the humidity (C) in the nostrils.

Table 4. The magnitude of velocity and the pressure of air in three selected anatomical locations.

Location	Side	$\mathbf{\vert V_{avg} \vert}$ (m/s)	Pressure (Pa)
Inferior nasal meatus	Right	0.512 (0.127 ÷ 1.140)	99,978 (99,946 ÷ 99,990)
	Left	1.258 (1.056 ÷ 2.165)	99,975 (99,973 ÷ 99,990)
	R vs. L	p-value = 0.062	p-value = 0.846
Ostiomeatal complex	Right	0.491 (0.031 ÷ 0.646)	99,981 (99,962 ÷ 99,989)
	Left	0.542 (0.092 ÷ 0.857)	99,982 (99,966 ÷ 99,989)
	R vs. L	p-value = 0.320	p-value = 0.903
Maxillary sinus floor	Right	0.000 (0.000 ÷ 0.002)	99,980 (99,961 ÷ 99,989)
	Left	0.000 (0.000 ÷ 0.000)	99,974 (99,963 ÷ 99,988)
	R vs. L	p-value = 0.942	p-value = 0.961

Figure 4 presents the comparison of temperature, humidity, flow velocity, and pressure values at the selected locations in the nose and sinuses. It should be noted that the obtained empirical distributions of the variables significantly deviated from the theoretical normal distribution (verified using the Shapiro–Wilk test). Therefore, the results shown in Figure 4 are presented as the median (Me) and the interquartile range IQR (Q1 and Q3). Nonparametric tests (Wilcoxon, Kruskal–Wallis, and Friedman) were used to compare the average values between the groups.

Analysing the results from Figure 4, it can be seen that statistically significant differences were observed in the three examined locations for all evaluated parameters except for pressure, which had similar values at every location. The highest air temperature and humidity were recorded in the maxillary sinus lumen and the lowest in the inferior nasal meatus. The air flow had almost zero velocity at the bottom of the maxillary sinus.

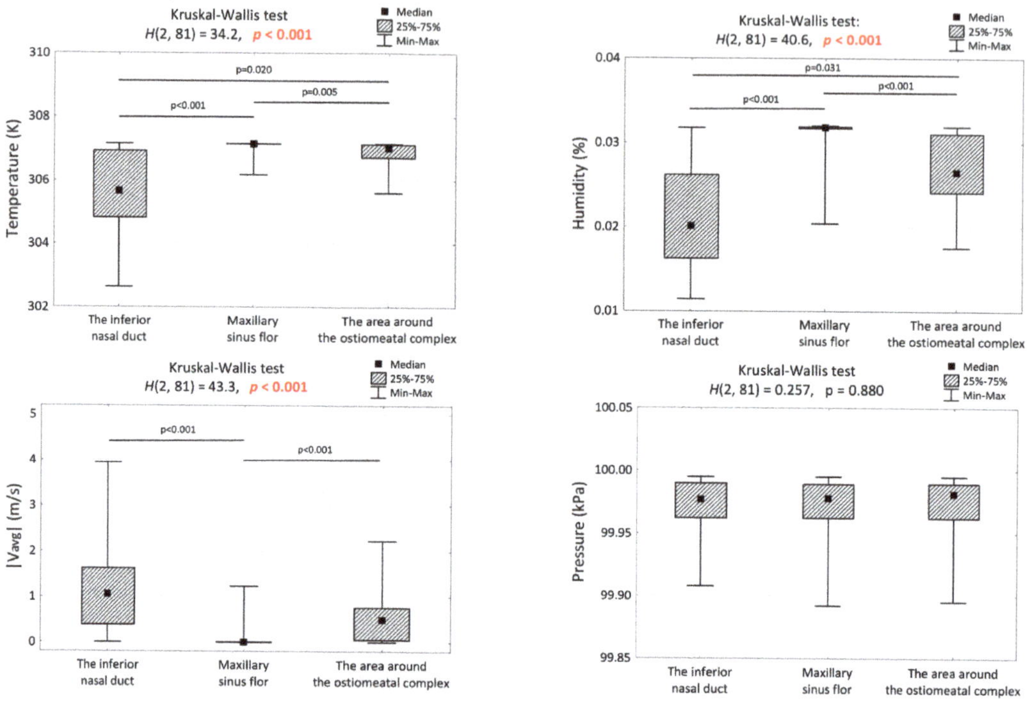

Figure 4. Comparison of temperature, humidity, flow velocity, and pressure values at selected locations for the nose and sinuses.

5. Discussion

The nasal cavity connects the external environment, full of various pollutants and of variable physical parameters, with the upper and lower respiratory tract's protected and regulated internal environment. The primary functions of the nasal cavity are to transport, clean, heat, and humidify inhaled air. Disorders of airflow through the nose caused by anatomical anomalies can alter the regulation of heat and moisture, which is believed to harm the physiology of the respiratory tract, predisposing to, among others, sinus inflammatory conditions [3]. The question arises as to whether modified physical conditions at different locations will favour the colonisation of pathogenic bacteria with requirements that differ from those of physiological flora.

The most clinically significant locations should be selected to determine the conditions conducive to bacterial colonization in the nose and sinuses. The preferred sampling sites include the anterior nares, middle meatus, nasopharynx, and occasionally the sinuses themselves [38–40]. The middle meatus is the most commonly chosen site. With the introduction of FESS, swabs have replaced sinus puncture aspirates as the standard sampling technique [41]. However, for the sinus microflora, a mid-meatus swab may not be as representative as is currently believed [42]. The results of this research do not accurately reflect the local sinus microbiome, and the data from the literature do not provide a uniform opinion about the microbiota. According to Yan et al., there are microenvironment-dependent interactions between *Corynebacterium accolens*, *C. pseudodiphtheriticum*, and *S. aureus*. They suggest that humidity is a favourable factor for the *Corynebacterium* and *Staphylococcus* species and may explain their abundant presence in the nasal mucosa [43].

Comparing swabs from the inferior and middle nasal meatuses in the same patient showed significant individual variability in the microbiota and similar intrapersonal profiles. Furthermore, the middle nasal meatus had a lower microbiological diversity in the same patient than the inferior nasal meatus [38]. Recently, a so-called "core microbiome" has been identified for the mucous membrane of the maxillary sinuses. Although the individual microbiome is variable, it usually consists of species such as *Corynebacterium*, *Staphylococcus*, *Streptococcus*, *Haemophilus*, and *Moraxella*. Comparing the results of microbiological studies from the nasal mucosa and the interior of the maxillary sinuses, a statistically significant correlation was found between the type and location of eight microorganisms, especially *Propionibacterium acnes*, which was identified only in the sinus cavities [42,44].

We measured the temperature, humidity, air velocity, and air pressure in three locations in reference to our earlier studies [45]. The average air temperature between 32 and 34 °C did not differ statistically between the right and left sides. The lowest temperature was found on the floor of the nasal cavity, while the highest was in the lumen of the sinus. However, it was similar to that of the ostiomeatal complex region. Although the differences were statistically significant, the temperature never exceeded 34.05 °C.

Similarly, Zang et al.'s calculations indicate higher maxillary sinus temperatures values than those of the middle nasal meatus. This phenomenon is explained by the low airflow velocity through the sinus, which prolongs its contact time with the mucosa [46]. The calculation results are consistent with the in vivo measurements conducted by Lindeman et al. In the inferior meatus, at the anterior edge of the inferior turbinate, they obtained values ranging from 30.2 to 32.2 °C [47]. Similar results were presented by Keck et al. for healthy individuals. The temperature was measured with a miniaturised thermocouple in the nasal vestibule, at the nasal valve, in the anterior part of the middle turbinate, and in the nasopharynx. A logarithmic increase in air temperature was observed from the anterior nostril to the nasopharynx, where it reached about 34 °C [48]. Therefore, our numerical calculations based on CT scans correspond to the values obtained from in vivo studies.

The temperature values impact the bacterial flora on the mucous membrane, as shown in Table 5. A good example is bacteria of the *Streptococcus* genus, which colonize the respiratory tract and are subject to the effects of varying temperature, oxygen, and pressure levels depending on their location. At an average temperature of around 33 °C in the nasopharynx, they remain part of the physiological flora. During viral infections and when the tissue barrier is breached, the temperature to which they are exposed increases to 37 °C or greater [49]. In the work of Tóthpál et al., the effect of temperature and oxygen level changes on the growth of different strains and serotypes of *Streptococcus pneumoniae* was studied. They grew at the highest density and had the shortest lag phase under conditions similar to the nasopharynx temperature, that is, around 30 °C, rather than under laboratory conditions of around 37 °C.

Table 5. Optimal temperature values for the growth of selected bacterial strains identified on the mucous membrane of the nose and sinuses, based on the published literature.

Bacterial Strain	Oxygen Requirements	Optimal Growth Temperature Ranges	Reference(s)
Streptococcus spp.	aerobic	35–37 °C, maximal grow at low temperatures (~33 °C)	[45,50]
Corynebacterium spp.	anaerobic, aerobic, and microaerophilic	31–37 °C	[46]
Propionibacterium spp.	anaerobic to aerotolerant	25–35 °C thermotolerant	[47]
Staphylococcus spp.	aerobic or facultatively anaerobic	30° to 37 °C	[48]
Haemophilus spp.	aerobic or facultatively anaerobic	35–37 °C	[49]
Moraxella spp.	aerobic	33–35 °C	[51]

In our calculations, the temperature for all three locations did not exceed 34 °C, which was therefore optimal for most bacteria colonising the nasal mucous membrane and paranasal sinuses. Of course, in addition to an increase in temperature during an infection, many other factors, such as different oxygen levels or increased mucus production, also play an important role. Following endoscopic procedures, *Staphylococcus aureus* is the most commonly identified bacterium [50], whose optimal growth temperature ranges between 30 and 37 °C. Therefore, the question arises as to whether a moderate decrease in temperature, due to the broader opening of the sinuses, would enhance the colonization of this bacterium on the mucous membrane.

Another physical factor that we investigated was air humidity. It was the lowest in the inferior nasal meatus and the highest in the maxillary sinus floor, probably due to almost zero airflow through its lumen. However, the differences were not statistically significant. In the results presented by Keck et al., the measured humidity and error ranges were plotted. Both in vivo and simulated values showed the same trend: the relative humidity increased rapidly by 2.5 cm from the anterior nostrils. Then, it rose slowly, but the inhaled air was humidified to nearly 100% [48].

The airflow velocity in the maxillary sinuses is significantly lower than in the nasal meatuses [46,51]. Our research confirmed this finding, although the differences were not statistically significant. Developmental anomalies, such as a deviated nasal septum, can change the airflow pattern, but it has not been proven that this can affect, for example, heating [52].

In our study, based on examination results from healthy people, the pressure differences between the interior of the sinus, the inferior nasal meatus, and the ostiomeatal complex were not statistically significant. According to Xiong et al. [51], the air pressure is simultaneously high in the anterior part of the inferior and middle nasal meatuses and the uncinate process (ostiomeatal complex). As in our study, a slight pressure difference was observed between the interior of the maxillary sinus and the nasal meatuses, allowing for perceptible air exchange [51]. At the same time, it should be emphasized that various biological factors always come into play, including symbiosis or inter-species competition [53,54].

The limitation of our work was the small group of healthy subjects who were referred for CT scans. All patients were qualified only for cosmetic orthognathic surgery. In addition, the calculations performed for one person were quite time consuming and it would be necessary to prepare calculation applications to facilitate the work.

In summary, CFD modelling methods can provide reliable information about the anatomical structure and physical conditions in the nose and paranasal sinuses. However, it can also be the basis for studying their relationships and the bacterial flora inhabiting this section of the respiratory tract. The study confirmed that different conditions prevail in the nasal and sinus cavities (in other locations). It can be assumed that a chronic inflammatory process that causes oedema and hypertrophy of the mucous membrane will change the parameters of airflow. This will also affect the humidity and temperature, which may be favourable or unfavourable for the growth of certain bacteria. In fact, this cannot be the only significant factor in the complex chronic inflammatory process of the sinonasal mucous membrane. However, this method may contribute to the precise treatment planning for chronic rhinosinusitis.

6. Conclusions

The main findings of the presented study can be summarized as follows:

- Physical conditions may promote the colonisation of the mucous membrane by various bacterial strains.
- The CFD method enables the determination of airflow, heat exchange, and humidity values in the nose and sinuses, and the results are consistent with other in vivo studies.
- These findings highlight the variations in air temperature, humidity, and airflow patterns within the nasal cavity, specifically emphasizing the distinct characteristics of the maxillary sinus and the inferior nasal meatus.
- Our study may initiate further exploration of the relationship between nasal and sinus conditions and the requirements of colonising bacteria.

Author Contributions: Conceptualization, M.M.-K.; methodology, M.M.-K., Z.M.M., K.Z. and J.K.; software, Z.M.M., K.Z., J.K. and K.D.; validation, M.M.-K., Z.M.M. and K.Z.; formal analysis, K.D.; investigation, M.M.-K., Z.M.M. and K.Z.; resources, M.M.-K., Z.M.M. and K.Z.; data curation, M.M.-K., Z.M.M. and K.Z.; writing—original draft preparation, M.M.-K. and Z.M.M.; writing—review and editing, M.M.-K., Z.M.M. and K.Z.; visualization, M.M.-K. and Z.M.M.; supervision, M.M.-K., Z.M.M., K.N. and T.Z.; project administration, K.N.; funding acquisition, no funding. All authors have read and agreed to the published version of the manuscript.

Funding: This research received no external funding.

Institutional Review Board Statement: The study was approved by the Bioethics Committee at the local Medical University and conducted according to the principles of the Declaration of Helsinki (KB-545/2015).

Informed Consent Statement: Informed consent was obtained from all subjects involved in the study.

Data Availability Statement: Data sharing is not applicable to this article.

Conflicts of Interest: The authors declare no conflict of interest.

References

1. Amorosa, L.; Latini, G. Maxillary Sinus: The Role of the Otolaryngologist. In *Computer-Guided Applications for Dental Implants, Bone Grafting, and Reconstructive Surgery*; Elsevier: Amsterdam, The Netherlands, 2016; pp. 124–134.
2. Havel, M.; Kornes, T.; Weitzberg, E.; Lundberg, J.O.; Sundberg, J. Eliminating Paranasal Sinus Resonance and Its Effects on Acoustic Properties of the Nasal Tract. *Logop. Phoniatr. Vocol.* **2016**, *41*, 33–40. [CrossRef] [PubMed]
3. Koo, S.K.; Kwon, S.B.; Chon, K.M.; Kim, Y.J.; Kim, Y.J. The Role of the Maxillary Sinus on the Voice. *Eur. Arch. Oto-Rhino-Laryngol.* **2014**, *272*, 2347–2350. [CrossRef] [PubMed]
4. Ahmed, S.; Naik, P. Physiology of the Nose and Paranasal Sinuses. In *Scott-Brown's Essential Otorhinolaryngology*; Taylor & Francis: Abingdon, UK, 2022; pp. 145–147.
5. Noback, M.L.; Harvati, K.; Spoor, F. Climate-Related Variation of the Human Nasal Cavity. *Am. J. Phys. Anthropol.* **2011**, *145*, 599–614. [CrossRef] [PubMed]
6. Qiu, Y.; Zhou, Y.; Chang, Y.; Liang, X.; Zhang, H.; Lin, X.; Qing, K.; Zhou, X.; Luo, Z. The Effects of Ventilation, Humidity, and Temperature on Bacterial Growth and Bacterial Genera Distribution. *Int. J. Environ. Res. Public Health* **2022**, *19*, 15345. [CrossRef] [PubMed]
7. Burgos, M.A.; Sanmiguel-Rojas, E.; Martín-Alcántara, A.; Hidalgo-Martínez, M. Effects of the Ambient Temperature on the Airflow across a Caucasian Nasal Cavity. *Int. J. Numer. Method Biomed. Eng.* **2014**, *30*, 430–445. [CrossRef] [PubMed]
8. Guo, Y.; Yu, S.; Wang, J.; Jin, W.; Yang, Y.I. A Numerical Model of the Inuence of Maxillary Sinus Ostium Size on the Distribution of Nitric Oxide Concentration in the Nasal Cavity and Sinuses. *Res. Sq.* **2021**. [CrossRef]
9. Kumahata, K.; Mori, F.; Ishikawa, S.; Matsuzawa, T. Nasal Flow Simulation Using Heat and Humidity Models. *J. Biomech. Sci. Eng.* **2010**, *5*, 565–577. [CrossRef]
10. Finck, M.; Hänel, D.; Wlokas, I. Simulation of Nasal Flow by Lattice Boltzmann Methods. *Comput. Biol. Med.* **2007**, *37*, 739–749. [CrossRef]
11. Lee, J.H.; Na, Y.; Kim, S.K.; Chung, S.K. Unsteady Flow Characteristics through a Human Nasal Airway. *Respir. Physiol. Neurobiol.* **2010**, *172*, 136–146. [CrossRef]
12. Larimi, M.M.; Babamiri, A.; Biglarian, M.; Ramiar, A.; Tabe, R.; Inthavong, K.; Farnoud, A. Numerical and Experimental Analysis of Drug Inhalation in Realistic Human Upper Airway Model. *Pharmaceuticals* **2023**, *16*, 406. [CrossRef]
13. Hisagai, S.; Li, K.K.; Iwasaki, T.; Tsujii, T.; Sakoda-Iwata, R.; Oku, Y.; Ban, Y.; Sato, H.; Yamasaki, Y. Exploring the Widespread Effectiveness of Maxillomandibular Advancement. *J. Oral Health Biosci.* **2023**, *35*, 71–79.
14. Karbowski, K.; Kopiczak, B.; Chrzan, R.; Gawlik, J.; Szaleniec, J. Accuracy of Virtual Rhinomanometry. *Pol. J. Med. Phys. Eng.* **2023**, *29*, 59–72. [CrossRef]
15. Bailie, N.; Hanna, B.; Watterson, J.; Gallagher, G. An Overview of Numerical Modelling of Nasal Airflow. *Rhinology* **2006**, *44*, 53–57.
16. Leite, S.H.P.; Jain, R.; Douglas, R.G. The Clinical Implications of Computerised Fluid Dynamic Modelling in Rhinology. *Rhinology* **2019**, *57*, 2–9. [CrossRef]
17. Kepler, G.M.; Richardson, R.B.; Morgan, K.T.; Kimbell, J.S. Computer Simulation of Inspiratory Nasal Airflow and Inhaled Gas Uptake in a Rhesus Monkey. *Toxicol. Appl. Pharmacol.* **1998**, *150*, 1–11. [CrossRef]
18. Xi, J.; Kim, J.; Si, X.A. Computational Fluid Dynamics Modelling of Nasal Cavity Heat and Moisture Exchange: Toward Treatment Planning for Sinonasal Diseases. *Ann. Biomed. Eng.* **2010**, *38*, 3804–3820.
19. Chen, X.B.; Lee, H.P.; Chong, V.F.H.; Wang, D.Y. Drug Delivery in the Nasal Cavity after Functional Endoscopic Sinus Surgery: A Computational Fluid Dynamics Study. *J. Laryngol. Otol.* **2012**, *126*, 487–494. [CrossRef]
20. Xiong, G.X.; Li, J.F.; Jiang, G.L.; Zhan, J.M.; Rong, L.W.; Xu, G. Effect of Endoscopic Sinus Surgery on Airflow of the Nasal Cavity and Paranasal Sinuses: A Computational Fluid Dynamics Study. *Chin. J. Otorhinolaryngol. Head Neck Surg.* **2009**, *44*, 911–917.

21. Saibene, A.M.; Felisati, G.; Pipolo, C.; Bulfamante, A.M.; Quadrio, M.; Covello, V. Partial Preservation of the Inferior Turbinate in Endoscopic Medial Maxillectomy: A Computational Fluid Dynamics Study. *Am. J. Rhinol. Allergy* **2020**, *34*, 409–416. [CrossRef]
22. Khatri, H.; Salati, H.; Wong, E.; Bradshaw, K.; Inthavong, K.; Sacks, R.; Singh, N. Modelling the Effects of Post-FESS Middle Turbinate Synechiae on Sinonasal Physiology: A Computational Fluid Dynamics Study. *Auris Nasus Larynx* 2023, *in press*. [CrossRef]
23. Kleven, M.; Singh, N.P.; Messina, J.C.; Djupesland, P.G.; Inthavong, K. Development of Computational Fluid Dynamics Methodology for Characterization of Exhalation Delivery System Performance in a Nasal Airway with Draf-III Surgery. *J. Aerosol Sci.* **2023**, *169*, 106121. [CrossRef]
24. Xavier, R.; Menger, D.J.; De Carvalho, H.C.; Spratley, J. An Overview of Computational Fluid Dynamics Preoperative Analysis of the Nasal Airway. *Facial Plast. Surg.* **2021**, *37*, 306–316. [CrossRef] [PubMed]
25. Lloyd-Price, J.; Abu-Ali, G.; Huttenhower, C. The Healthy Human Microbiome. *Genome Med.* **2016**, *8*, 51. [CrossRef] [PubMed]
26. Kumpitsch, C.; Koskinen, K.; Schöpf, V.; Moissl-Eichinger, C. The Microbiome of the Upper Respiratory Tract in Health and Disease. *BMC Biol.* **2019**, *17*, 87. [CrossRef] [PubMed]
27. Araujo, E.; Palombini, B.C.; Cantarelli, V.; Pereira, A.; Mariante, A. Microbiology of Middle Meatus in Chronic Rhinosinusitis. *Am. J. Rhinol.* **2018**, *17*, 9–15. [CrossRef]
28. Vogan, J.C.; Bolger, W.E.; Keyes, A.S. Endoscopically Guided Sinonasal Cultures: A Direct Comparison with Maxillary Sinus Aspirate Cultures. *Otolaryngol.-Head Neck Surg.* **2000**, *122*, 370–373. [CrossRef]
29. Szaleniec, J.; Gibała, A.; Hartwich, P.; Hydzik-Sobocińska, K.; Konior, M.; Gosiewski, T.; Szaleniec, M. Challenging the Gold Standard: Methods of Sampling for Microbial Culture in Patients with Chronic Rhinosinusitis. *Eur. Arch. Oto-Rhino-Laryngol.* **2021**, *278*, 4795–4803. [CrossRef]
30. Ma, J.; Dong, J.; Shang, Y.; Inthavong, K.; Tu, J.; Frank-Ito, D.O. Air Conditioning Analysis among Human Nasal Passages with Anterior Anatomical Variations. *Med. Eng. Phys.* **2018**, *57*, 19–28. [CrossRef]
31. Zhao, K.; Scherer, P.W.; Hajiloo, S.A.; Dalton, P. Effect of Anatomy on Human Nasal Air Flow and Odorant Transport Patterns: Implications for Olfaction. *Chem. Senses* **2004**, *29*, 365–379. [CrossRef]
32. Weinhold, I.; Mlynski, G. Numerical Simulation of Airflow in the Human Nose. *Eur. Arch. Oto-Rhino-Laryngol. Head Neck* **2004**, *261*, 452–455. [CrossRef]
33. Croce, C.; Fodil, R.; Durand, M.; Sbirlea-Apiou, G.; Caillibotte, G.; Papon, J.F.; Blondeau, J.R.; Coste, A.; Isabey, D.; Louis, B. In Vitro Experiments and Numerical Simulations of Airflow in Realistic Nasal Airway Geometry. *Ann. Biomed. Eng.* **2006**, *34*, 997–1007. [CrossRef]
34. Lee, C.Y.; Wilke, C.R. Measurements of Vapor Diffusion Coefficient. *Ind. Eng. Chem.* **2002**, *46*, 2381–2387. [CrossRef]
35. User Guide n.d. Available online: https://www.openfoam.com/documentation/user-guide (accessed on 12 February 2023).
36. Issa, R.I.; Gosman, A.D.; Watkins, A.P. The Computation of Compressible and Incompressible Recirculating Flows by a Non-Iterative Implicit Scheme. *J. Comput. Phys.* **1986**, *62*, 66–82. [CrossRef]
37. Ferziger, J.H.; Perić, M.; Street, R.L. *Computational Methods for Fluid Dynamics*, 4th ed.; Springer: Berlin/Heidelberg, Germany, 2019; pp. 1–596.
38. Lal, D.; Keim, P.; Delisle, J.; Barker, B.; Rank, M.A.; Chia, N.; Schupp, J.M.; Gillece, J.D.; Cope, E.K. Mapping and Comparing Bacterial Microbiota in the Sinonasal Cavity of Healthy, Allergic Rhinitis, and Chronic Rhinosinusitis Subjects. *Int. Forum Allergy Rhinol.* **2017**, *7*, 561–569. [CrossRef]
39. Biswas, K.; Hoggard, M.; Jain, R.; Taylor, M.W.; Douglas, R.G. The Nasal Microbiota in Health and Disease: Variation within and between Subjects. *Front. Microbiol.* **2015**, *6*, 134. [CrossRef]
40. Copeland, E.; Leonard, K.; Carney, R.; Kong, J.; Forer, M.; Naidoo, Y.; Oliver, B.G.G.; Seymour, J.R.; Woodcock, S.; Burke, C.M.; et al. Chronic Rhinosinusitis: Potential Role of Microbial Dysbiosis and Recommendations for Sampling Sites. *Front. Cell. Infect. Microbiol.* **2018**, *8*, 57. [CrossRef]
41. Brook, I. Microbiology of Acute Sinusitis of Odontogenic Origin Presenting with Periorbital Cellulitis in Children. *Ann. Otol. Rhinol. Laryngol.* **2007**, *116*, 386–388. [CrossRef]
42. Morawska-Kochman, M.; Jermakow, K.; Nelke, K.; Zub, K.; Pawlak, W.; Dudek, K.; Bochnia, M. The PH Value as a Factor Modifying Bacterial Colonization of Sinonasal Mucosa in Healthy Persons. *Ann. Otol. Rhinol. Laryngol.* **2019**, *128*, 819–828. [CrossRef]
43. Yan, M.; Pamp, S.J.; Fukuyama, J.; Hwang, P.H.; Cho, D.Y.; Holmes, S.; Relman, D.A. Nasal Microenvironments and Interspecific Interactions Influence Nasal Microbiota Complexity and *S. aureus* Carriage. *Cell Host Microbe* **2013**, *14*, 631–640. [CrossRef]
44. Paramasivan, S.; Bassiouni, A.; Shiffer, A.; Dillon, M.R.; Cope, E.K.; Cooksley, C.; Ramezanpour, M.; Moraitis, S.; Ali, M.J.; Bleier, B.; et al. The International Sinonasal Microbiome Study: A Multicentre, Multinational Characterization of Sinonasal Bacterial Ecology. *Allergy* **2020**, *75*, 2037–2049. [CrossRef]
45. Morawska-Kochman, M.; Marycz, K.; Jermakow, K.; Nelke, K.; Pawlak, W.; Bochnia, M. The Presence of Bacterial Microcolonies on the Maxillary Sinus Ciliary Epithelium in Healthy Young Individuals. *PLoS ONE* **2017**, *12*, e0176776. [CrossRef] [PubMed]
46. Zang, H.; Liu, Y.; Han, D.; Zhang, L.; Wang, T.; Sun, X.; Li, L. Airflow and Temperature Distribution inside the Maxillary Sinus: A Computational Fluid Dynamics Simulation. *Acta Oto-Laryngol.* **2012**, *132*, 637–644. [CrossRef] [PubMed]
47. Lindemann, J.; Keck, T.; Scheithauer, M.O.; Leiacker, R.; Wiesmiller, K. Nasal Mucosal Temperature in Relation to Nasal Airflow as Measured by Rhinomanometry. *Am. J. Rhinol.* **2007**, *21*, 46–49. [CrossRef] [PubMed]

48. Keck, T.; Leiacker, R.; Riechelmann, H.; Rettinger, G. Temperature Profile in the Nasal Cavity. *Laryngoscope* **2000**, *110*, 651–654. [CrossRef]
49. Tóthpál, A.; Desobry, K.; Joshi, S.S.; Wyllie, A.L.; Weinberger, D.M. Variation of Growth Characteristics of Pneumococcus with Environmental Conditions. *BMC Microbiol.* **2019**, *19*, 304. [CrossRef]
50. Shah, S.J.; Hawn, V.S.; Zhu, N.; Fang, C.H.; Gao, Q.; Akbar, N.A.; Abuzeid, W.M. Postoperative Infection Rate and Associated Factors Following Endoscopic Sinus Surgery. *Ann. Otol. Rhinol. Laryngol.* **2022**, *131*, 5–11. [CrossRef]
51. Xiong, G.X.; Zhan, J.M.; Jiang, H.Y.; Li, J.F.; Rong, L.W.; Xu, G. Computational Fluid Dynamics Simulation of Airflow in the Normal Nasal Cavity and Paranasal Sinuses. *Am. J. Rhinol.* **2008**, *22*, 477–482. [CrossRef]
52. Li, L.; Zang, H.; Han, D.; London, N.R. Impact of Varying Types of Nasal Septal Deviation on Nasal Airflow Pattern and Warming Function: A Computational Fluid Dynamics Analysis. *Ear Nose Throat J.* **2021**, *100*, NP283–NP289. [CrossRef]
53. Bomar, L.; Brugger, S.D.; Yost, B.H.; Davies, S.S.; Lemon, K.P. Corynebacterium Accolens Releases Antipneumococcal Free Fatty Acids from Human Nostril and Skin Surface Triacylglycerols. *mBio* **2016**, *7*, e01725-15. [CrossRef]
54. Yang, R.; Dong, C.; Chen, Y.; Liu, H.; Zhang, C.; Lai, Y.; Zha, D.; Han, Y. Analysis of the Clinical Features and Surgical Outcomes of First Branchial Cleft Anomalies. *Laryngoscope* **2022**, *132*, 1008–1014. [CrossRef]

medicina

MDPI

Review

Long-Standing Temporomandibular Joint Dislocation: A Comprehensive Review and Proposal of a Treatment Algorithm

Kazuya Yoshida

Department of Oral and Maxillofacial Surgery, National Hospital Organization, Kyoto Medical Center, 1-1 Mukaihata-cho, Fukakusa, Fushimi-ku, Kyoto 612-8555, Japan; yoshida.kazuya.ut@mail.hosp.go.jp; Tel.: +81-75-641-9161

Abstract: *Background and Objectives*: Long-standing or protracted temporomandibular joint dislocation refers to a condition that persists for more than 1 month without reduction. To elucidate the clinical characteristics and treatment results of this condition, this comprehensive review analyzed the available data. *Materials and Methods*: Studies were assessed using electronic medical databases and manual searches from their inception to 31 December 2024. *Results*: Overall, 229 cases (139 women and 81 men; mean age, 52.3 years) from 113 reports were assessed. The proportion of patients with bilateral and unilateral dislocations was 74.7% and 8.7%, respectively. The mean duration since dislocation was 11.9 months. Closed and open reductions were possible in 49 (21.4%) and 175 patients (76.4%), respectively. The mean dislocation duration was significantly ($p = 0.001$) shorter in patients who underwent closed reduction (4.9 months) than in those who underwent open reduction (14.8 months). *Conclusions*: Clinically, it is crucial to diagnose and treat this condition early to prevent it from becoming chronic. However, for cases of long-standing dislocations due to other more serious diseases, conservative treatments such as manual reduction and continuous elastic traction should be attempted first. If reduction fails, surgical treatment should be performed as an alternative.

Keywords: temporomandibular joint dislocation; long-standing; protracted; chronic; reduction; treatment; surgery; algorithm

1. Introduction

Dislocation of the temporomandibular joint (TMJ) refers to displacement of the mandibular condylar head from its normal position in the glenoid fossa. Dislocation of the TMJ is common, with an estimated annual incidence ranging from 2.5 to 25 cases per 100,000 individuals annually [1,2]. TMJ dislocations can be categorized as anterior, posterior, medial, lateral, or superior [3]. Anterior dislocations are the most frequently encountered, whereas posterior, medial, and lateral dislocations are comparatively rare. A systematic review reported 79 acute, 35 chronic, and 311 recurrent cases of TMJ dislocation [3].

The first recorded manual reduction of TMJ dislocations was described in the Edwin Smith papyrus, dating back to the 17th century BC [4]. The Edwin Smith papyrus is a record of a surgical procedure translated into English in 1930 [4]. This reduction method is not significantly different from the current method. Hippocrates also reported the method for anterior dislocations in the *Hippocrates Corpus* in the 5th century BC, which remains widely used today as the Hippocratic method. The Hippocratic method is the most widely recognized technique for manually reducing anterior TMJ dislocations. In this approach, the physician positions the thumbs laterally adjacent to the molars and places the remaining fingers under the mandible, applying downward pressure, followed by backward pressure to reposition the joint [1].

The European Society of Temporomandibular Joint Surgeons recently published consensus- and evidence-based guidelines for managing anterior condylar dislocations [2]. These guidelines recommend that the initial treatment should involve manual reduction using the Hippocratic method. If this approach fails, subsequent attempts may be made with the aid of medications, such as muscle relaxants and/or analgesics, and if required, under sedation or general anesthesia [2]. Securing methods should be considered for patients with recurrent, long-standing, and/or habitual dislocations. Non-surgical methods should be exhausted before attempting minimally invasive or open surgical interventions [2]. Botulinum toxin has been proposed as a potential therapeutic option for managing recurrent TMJ dislocations [5,6]. Indications for open surgical treatment [7–9] should be established only after the failure of conservative treatment and/or minimally invasive therapy for anterior TMJ dislocation [2].

Terms such as chronic, protracted, long-standing, prolonged, and permanent have been used to describe long-term, untreated TMJ dislocations. In this review, the author employs the term "long-standing". No consensus exists regarding the duration after which an untreated dislocation should be considered long-standing. However, as most reports specify 1 or more months, this review adopts this definition.

Although a consensus has been reached regarding the treatment of anterior TMJ dislocation, the incidence of long-standing dislocation is significantly lower than that of acute dislocation, and no consistent treatment method has been established. Therefore, this review comprehensively analyzes all available reports of long-standing TMJ dislocation regarding its causes, symptoms, treatment, and clinical course and proposes a treatment algorithm for long-standing TMJ dislocation.

2. Materials and Methods

2.1. Literature Review

A comprehensive literature search was performed using major electronic medical databases and specific keywords relevant to the topic (["long-standing" OR "chronic" OR "protracted" OR "prolonged" OR "permanent" OR "irreducible" OR "unreduced" OR "persistent"] AND ["temporomandibular joint" OR "mandible" OR "condyle" OR "mandibular condyle"] AND ["dislocation" OR "luxation"] AND ["reduction" OR "treatment" OR "management" OR "approach"]). Additionally, a manual search was conducted to identify articles cited from related sources. All reports identified through electronic databases or manual searches without language restrictions and published up to 31 December 2024 were screened as previously described [10,11]. The inclusion criteria were reports of cases in which TMJ dislocations were not reduced for more than 1 month and that described key patient information including sex, age, etiology, clinical presentation, and treatment. Before 1900, radiography was rarely used to diagnose TMJ dislocations. Therefore, reports published before 1900 were excluded from this review. Duplicate reports of the same case, studies lacking essential diagnostic imaging findings, records with incomplete data, and studies that were irrelevant to the objectives of the study were excluded. All eligible reports were independently assessed and reviewed by the author.

2.2. Analysis

Fundamental clinical data were extracted and evaluated from the selected studies. These included age, sex, affected side, etiology, chief complaint, diagnostic imaging findings, duration of dislocation, maximal mouth opening, presence of an open bite, treatment methods, complications, follow-up periods, and sequelae.

2.3. Statistics

Binomial logistic regression analysis was performed to evaluate whether age, sex, and dislocation duration could serve as potential predictors for selecting the appropriate treatment approach (closed versus open reduction). Two-tailed unpaired *t*-tests and Mann–Whitney U tests were used to evaluate the differences between groups. The ratio of closed and open reduction was analyzed in six groups: 1 month or more but less than 2 months after dislocation, 2 months or more but less than 3 months, 3 months or more but less than 4 months, 4 months or more but less than 5 months, 5 months or more but less than 6 months, and 6 months or more after dislocation. The difference in the duration after dislocation between cases with closed reduction and those with open reduction was analyzed using the Mann–Whitney U test. The etiology was classified as traumatic (e.g., trauma, fall, or motor vehicle accident) or atraumatic (e.g., yawning or dental treatment), and differences were analyzed using an unpaired *t*-test. All statistical analyses were performed using SPSS for Windows (version 24.0; SPSS Japan, Inc., Tokyo, Japan). Statistical significance was set at $p < 0.05$.

3. Results

The number of studies retrieved from electronic databases and registers, assessed for eligibility and included in the comprehensive review, is presented in a flow diagram (Figure 1). Overall, 19,604 articles were retrieved from the following databases: PubMed (313), Google Scholar (19,100), Japan Medical Abstracts Society (41), and J-Stage (150). Forty-two additional records were retrieved through manual searches of relevant papers and books. The search yielded 113 reports [12–124]. Table S1 shows the demographic data of all the patients. The number of evaluated reports categorized by the original language was as follows: English, 74; Japanese, 34; German, 4; and French, 1. The number of reports according to the number of cases was as follows: 1 case, 83; 2 cases, 13; 3 cases, 7; 4 cases, 2; 5 cases, 1; 6 cases, 1; 8 cases, 2; 10 cases, 1; 15 cases, 1; 19 cases, 1; and 20 cases, 1. All studies were case reports or case series.

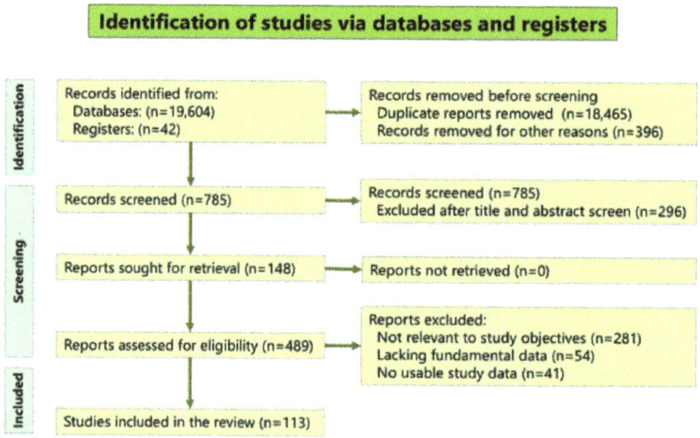

Figure 1. Diagram of the literature search and screening strategy.

3.1. Demographic Data and Diagnoses

A total of 113 articles comprising 229 patients were included in the analysis (mean age ± standard deviation: 52.3 ± 19.5 years; age range: 5–89 years) (Table S1). The demographic characteristics and diagnostic findings are summarized in Table 1. This study included 139 women (60.7%) and 81 men (35.4%). Among them, 171 (74.7%), 11 (4.8%), and 9 (3.9%) were bilateral, left-sided, and right-sided, respectively (Table 1). The mean duration of dislocation was 11.9 months (Table 1).

Table 1. Summary of the demographic data and diagnosis.

Sex, (n [%)]	Women, n = 139 (60.7%); men, n = 81 (35.4%); NR, n = 9 (3.9%)
Age (years), [mean ± SD, range]	52.3 ± 19.5, 5–89
Affected side, (n [%)]	Bilateral, n = 171 (74.7%); left, n = 11 (4.8%); right, n = 9 (3.9%); NR, n = 31 (13.5%)
Duration (months), (mean ± SD, n [%], range)	11.9 ± 34.4, n = 174 (76%), range 1–300
First clinical diagnosis, (n [%])	TMJ dislocation, n = 100 (43.7%); undiagnosed, n = 39 (17%); palsy, n = 4 (1.7%); inflammation, n = 4 (1.7%); neurological diseases, n = 3 (1.3%); normal, n = 3 (1.3%); other, n = 5 (2.2%); NR, n = 71 (31%)
Previous dislocation, (n [%])	Once, n = 14 (6.1%); frequently, n = 6 (2.6%); sometimes, n = 3 (1.3%); N, n = 37 (16.2%); NR, n = 169 (73.8%)
Anamnesis, (n [%])	Psychiatric diseases, n = 19 (8.3%); dementia or mental retardation, n = 15 (6.6%); neurological diseases, n = 10 (4.4%); cerebral infarction, n = 10 (4.4%); cerebral hemorrhage, n = 9 (3.9%); brain injury, n = 4 (1.7%); NR, n = 121 (52.8%)
Diagnostic image, (n [%])	Radiography; n = 165 (72.1%); CT, n = 57 (24.9%); MRI, n = 4 (1.7%); NR, n = 45 (19.7%)

SD, standard deviation; N, no; NR, not reported; CT, computed tomography; TMJ, temporomandibular joint; MRI, magnetic resonance imaging.

The initial clinical diagnosis was TMJ dislocation in 100 patients (43.7%). Additionally, four (1.7%), four (1.7%), and three (1.3%) patients were presented with palsy, inflammation, and neurological disease, respectively (Table 1, Figure 2).

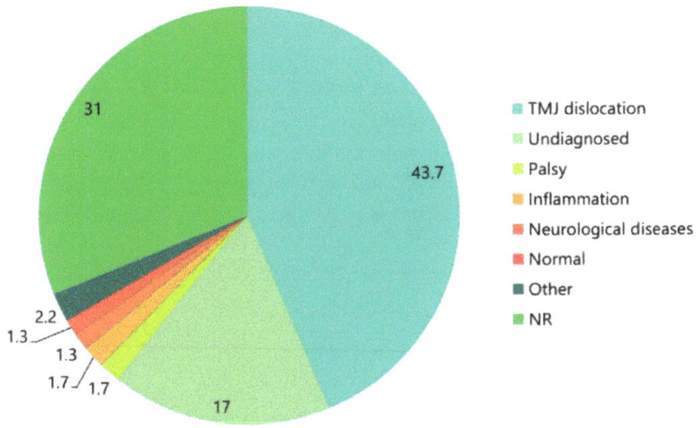

Figure 2. First clinical diagnosis of patients with long-standing TMJ dislocation. The numbers in the pie chart represent percentages. TMJ, temporomandibular joint; NR, not reported.

Previous dislocations were reported once, frequently, and sometimes in 14 (6.1%), 6 (2.6%), and 3 (1.3%) patients, respectively (Table 1). Moreover, 37 patients (16.2%) reported no history of dislocation. In addition, the history of the dislocation itself was not recorded in 169 patients (73.8%).

The psychiatric diseases identified based on anamnesis included dementia or mental retardation, neurological diseases, cerebral infarction, cerebral hemorrhage, and brain injury in 15 (6.6%), 10 (4.4%), 10 (4.4%), 9 (3.9%), and 4 (1.7%) patients, respectively. No relevant neurological or psychiatric history was identified in 121 (52.8%) patients (Table 1).

Radiography was the primary diagnostic imaging modality (72.1%) (Table 1). Computed tomography (CT) and magnetic resonance imaging (MRI) were also performed (Table 1).

3.2. Symptoms and Etiology

The patients' symptoms are summarized in Table 2. The most frequent chief complaints were preauricular pain (26.6%), inability to close the mouth (19.2%), masticatory disturbances (14%), and difficulty in speaking (10.5%) (Table 2).

Table 2. Summary of patient symptoms and etiology.

Chief complaint, (*n* [%])	Preauricular pain, *n* = 61 (26.6%); inability to close mouth, *n* = 44 (19.2%); masticatory disturbance, *n* = 32 (14%); difficulty in speaking, *n* = 24 (10.5%); malocclusion, *n* = 15 (6.6%); facial deformity, *n* = 12 (5.2%); difficulty in swallowing, *n* = 12 (5.2%); other, *n* = 5 (2.2%); NR, *n* = 87 (38%)
Maximal mouth opening (mm), (mean ± SD, *n* [%])	24.6 ± 69.9, *n* = 62 (27.1%); NR, *n* = 167 (72.9%)
Open bite (mm), (mean ± SD, *n* [%])	14.4 ± 6.6, *n* = 26 (11.4%); NR, *n* = 203 (88.6%)
Edentulousness, (*n* [%])	Total edentulous, *n* = 48 (21%); upper or lower, *n* = 8 (3%); N, *n* = 95 (41.5%); NR, *n* = 62 (27.1%)
Etiology, [*n* (%)]	Yawning, *n* = 33 (14.4%); unknown, *n* = 23 (10%); surgical procedures, *n* = 19 (8.3%); neurological diseases, *n* = 15 (6.6%); trauma, *n* = 14 (6.1%); fall, *n* = 13 (5.7%); tooth extraction, *n* = 13 (5.7%); motor vehicle accident, *n* = 12 (5.2%); sleep, *n* = 8 (3.5%); assault; *n* = 4 (1.7%); others, *n* = 4 (1.7%); NR, *n* = 69 (30.1%)

SD, standard deviation; N, no; NR, not reported.

The mean maximum mouth opening at the initial visit was restricted to 24.6 mm. The open bite (a gap between the anterior incisors when biting down) was 14.4 mm; however, it was reported in only 11.4% of the patients (Table 2).

The distribution of etiologies among all patients is shown in Figure 3. The most prevalent etiologies were yawning (14.4%, *n* = 33), surgical procedures (8.3%, *n* = 19), and neurological disorders (6.6%, *n* = 15). In 23 patients (10%), the etiologies were unknown, and 69 cases (30.1%) were not recorded (Table 2, Figure 3).

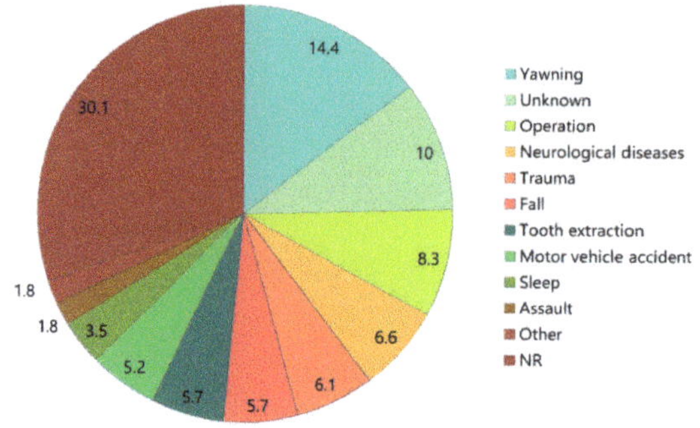

Figure 3. Etiologies of long-standing temporomandibular joint dislocation. NR, not reported.

Patients with traumatic etiology (*n* = 41) were significantly ($p = 0.001$) younger than those with atraumatic etiology (*n* = 72) (39.2 ± 17 years vs. 51.3 ± 39.2 years) (Figure 4).

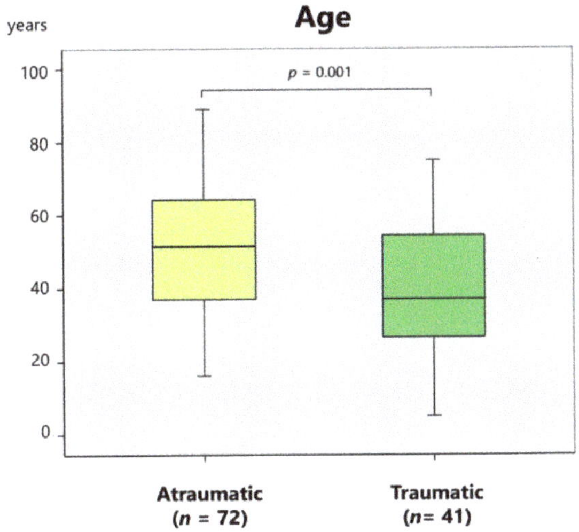

Figure 4. Comparison of the mean age of patients with atraumatic and traumatic etiologies.

3.3. Treatments and Sequelae

Table S2 presents the treatment outcomes, complications, follow-up periods, and sequelae for all patients. A summary of the treatment methods used in these patients is provided in Table 3. Local anesthesia, sedation, and general anesthesia were administered to 18 (7.9%), 51 (22.3%), and 189 (82.5%) patients, respectively (Table S2). Continuous traction with splints or wires was attempted in 29 patients (12.7%), 17 of whom (7.4%) achieved success without requiring an open procedure (Table 3). Additionally, closed manual reduction was performed in 183 patients (79.9%), of whom 28 (12.2%) showed successful outcomes (Table 3). Of these, 22, 5, and 1 were performed under general anesthesia, local anesthesia, and sedation, respectively.

Table 3. Summary of treatments for long-standing TMJ dislocation.

Treatment, (*n* [%])	**Closed reduction**, *n* = 49 (21.4%) Manual reduction, *n* = 28 (12.2%); with instruments, *n* = 3 (1.3%), continuous traction, *n* = 17 (7.4%), 3–40 days
	Open reduction; *n* = 175 (76.4%) Hook placement at the mandibular notch, *n* = 43 (18.8%), condylectomy, *n* = 25 (10.9%), eminoplasty, *n* = 20 (8.7%), eminectomy, *n* = 19 (8.3%), angular traction, *n* = 10 (4.4%), meniscectomy, *n* = 10 (4.4%), orthognathic surgery, *n* = 10 (4.4%), excision of fibrous tissue, *n* = 7 (3.1%), lateral pterygoid myotomy, *n* = 6 (2.6%), condylotomy, *n* = 5 (2.2%), total TMJ prosthesis, *n* = 3 (1.3%), coronoidectomy, *n* = 3 (1.3%), coronoidotomy, *n* = 3 (1.3%), levering condyle, *n* = 3 (1.3%), other, *n* = 10 (4.4%), NR, *n* = 19 (8.3%)
	Incision Preauricular, *n* = 107 (46.7%), submandibular, *n* = 24 (10.5%), zygomatic arch, *n* = 15 (6.6%), intraoral, *n* = 13 (5.7%), Al-Kayat Bramery, *n* = 4 (1.7%), Bockenheimer–Axhausen, *n* = 3 (1.3%), other, *n* = 5 (2.2%)

N, no; TMJ, temporomandibular joint; NR, not reported.

Closed and open reductions were possible in 49 (21.4%) and 175 (76.4%) patients, respectively (Tables 3 and S1). Surgical procedures included hook placement at the mandibular notch (18.8%), condylectomy (10.9%), eminoplasty (8.7%), eminectomy (8.3%), angular traction (4.4%), meniscectomy (4.4%), orthognathic surgery (4.4%), excision of fibrous tissue (3.1%), lateral pterygoid myotomy (2.6%), condylotomy (2.2%), total TMJ prosthesis (1.3%), coronoidectomy (1.3%), coronoidotomy (1.3%), and levering condyle (1.3%) (Table 3, Figure 5).

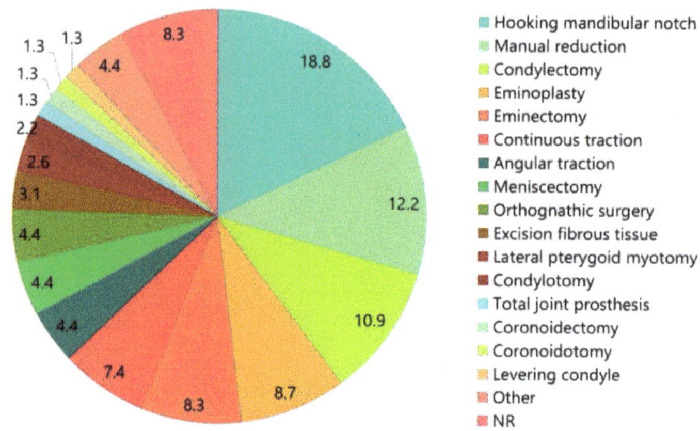

Figure 5. Treatments of patients with long-standing temporomandibular joint dislocation. NR, not reported.

Regarding the approach used during the surgical procedure, a preauricular incision (46.7%) was the most frequent, followed by submandibular (10.5%) and zygomatic arch incisions (Table 3).

A total of 77 patients (66.4%) experienced no complications (Table 4). Post-reduction intermaxillary fixation was performed in 122 patients (53.3%) with an average duration of 17.5 days (Table 4). The average follow-up period was 11.8 months, ranging from 2 weeks to 96 months [99]; however, follow-up data were unavailable for 82 patients (35.8%). At follow-up, the maximal mouth opening was 36.2 mm (Table 4). The sequelae included redislocation (1.7%), deviation (1.3%), and condylar absorption (0.9%). No sequelae were observed in 55.9% of the patients, and data were not reported for 69 patients (30.1%; Table 4).

Table 4. Summary of follow-up and sequelae in patients with long-standing TMJ dislocation.

Treatment complication, (n [%])	Facial nerve paralysis, $n = 8$ (3.5%); redislocation, $n = 3$ (1.3%); others, $n = 3$ (1.3%); N, $n = 77$ (33.6%); NR, $n = 17$ (7.4%)
Fixation (days), (n [%], mean ± SD)	Y, $n = 122$ (53.3%), 17.5 ± 15; N, $n = 20$ (8.7%); NR, $n = 76$ (33.2%)
Follow-up (months), (mean ± SD, n [%], range)	11.8 ± 13, $n = 147$ (64.2%), 0.25–96; NR, $n = 82$ (35.8%)
Maximal mouth opening at follow-up (mm), (mean ± SD, n [%], range)	36.2 ± 6.8, $n = 90$ (39.3%), 22–51, 35; NR, $n = 23$ (10%)
Sequelae, (n [%])	Redislocation; $n = 4$ (1.7%), deviation; $n = 3$ (1.3%), condylar absorption; $n = 2$ (0.9%), other; $n = 9$ (3.9%); N, $n = 128$ (55.9%); NR, $n = 69$ (30.1%)

SD, standard deviation; Y, yes; N, no; TMJ, temporomandibular joint; NR, not reported.

Closed reduction was possible in more than 40% of cases within a 3-month duration; nonetheless, open reduction was required in more than 80% of cases after 4 months or more (Figure 6).

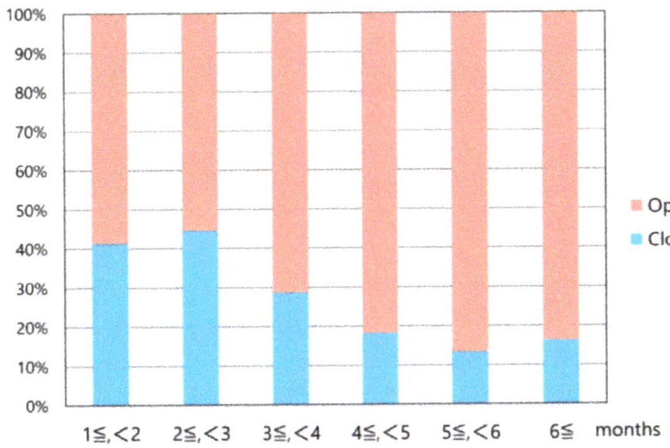

Figure 6. Ratio of closed and open reduction according to duration after dislocation.

The mean age of the patients who underwent closed and open reduction was 55.4 and 51.0 years, respectively, with no significant difference (p = 0.163, unpaired t-test). However, the time from dislocation to reduction was significantly shorter in patients treated with closed reduction than in those who required open reduction (4.9 ± 7.3 vs. 14.8 ± 40.4 months, respectively; p = 0.001, Mann–Whitney U test) (Figure 7).

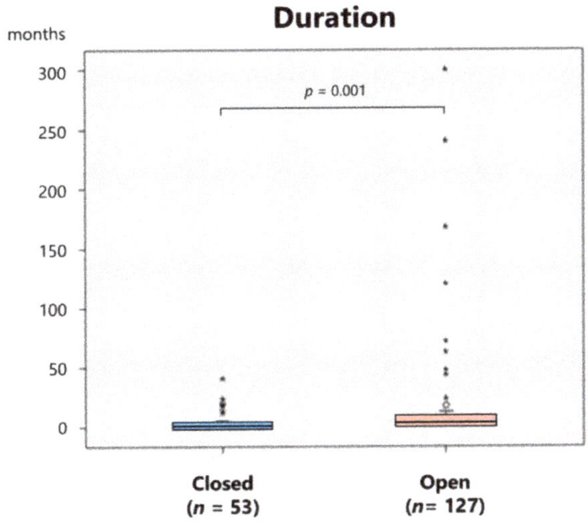

Figure 7. Duration of closed and open reduction in patients with long-standing temporomandibular joint dislocation.

Binomial logistic regression analysis was conducted to evaluate whether age, sex, or duration of dislocation could serve as predictors for determining the appropriate treatment approach (closed versus open procedures); however, no statistically significant factors were identified.

4. Discussion

This is the first extensive review of documented reports on long-standing TMJ dislocations. The clinical courses of 229 patients with long-standing TMJ dislocation that remained unreduced for more than one month were analyzed in this review. Although the early diagnosis and treatment of TMJ dislocation remain primary priorities, treatment is often delayed due to various factors. In cases involving dementia, mental retardation, or unconsciousness, the patients themselves cannot recognize the dislocation; therefore, medical and dental professionals must detect and diagnose it as early as possible. In cases of long-standing dislocation, treatment should proceed systematically, beginning with manual reduction before considering surgical options. However, there is no consensus regarding treatment policies or algorithms, which remains a significant challenge for future research.

4.1. Etiology of Long-Standing TMJ Dislocation

Reasons for TMJ dislocations remaining untreated for more than one month included patients being unaware of the dislocation due to dementia, impaired consciousness, or intellectual disability; edentulous patients not wearing dentures, making occlusal changes less apparent; postponement of TMJ dislocation treatment due to more serious life-threatening conditions; and patients not seeking medical attention, remaining undiagnosed, or being misdiagnosed (Table S1). This review revealed that the most prevalent etiologies of long-standing dislocations were yawning (14.4%), surgery (8.3%), neurological disease (6.6%), and unknown causes (10%) (Figure 2). In contrast, the common etiologies of superior condylar dislocation included motor vehicle accidents (50%), falls (20.7%), bicycle accidents (16.4%), and assault (3.4%) [11]. Compared with superior dislocations, the rate of traumatic etiology is notably lower. Long-standing TMJ dislocations can occur during routine movements such as yawning, and many cases have unknown or unspecified causes. These may result from minimal mouth opening beyond the normal range and often go undetected. Consequently, dislocations tend to recur during daily movements without trauma. If dislocation remains unrecognized due to dementia, mental retardation, psychiatric or neurological diseases, or unconsciousness, it can readily progress to a long-standing condition. In this study, patients with a traumatic etiology ($n = 41$) were significantly younger than those with an atraumatic etiology ($n = 72$) (39.2 years vs. 51.3 years) (Figure 4). The diagnosis and treatment of dislocations are often delayed in cases involving coexisting life-threatening injuries or conditions. Treatment decisions and prognoses may be influenced by factors such as the patient's age, neurological involvement, and etiology.

Pseudoarticulation (nearthrosis) rarely develops in patients with long-standing dislocations when the dislocations persist for extended periods. Although lateral excursion is difficult to achieve, patients maintain a certain degree of function. To date, six cases of pseudoarticulation associated with long-standing TMJ dislocations have been reported [44,72,92,99,107,114].

Medical and dental professionals as well as caregivers should remain vigilant about dislocations in patients who cannot independently recognize abnormalities. Fortunately, recent advances in botulinum toxin therapy have eliminated the need for the surgical treatment of habitual TMJ dislocation when botulinum toxin is administered to the lateral pterygoid muscle following manual reduction [6,125]. If TMJ dislocation is promptly detected and treated, long-standing dislocation can be prevented, surgical treatment for TMJ dislocation will become largely unnecessary, and significant surgical intervention can be avoided [6].

4.2. Diagnosis of Long-Standing TMJ Dislocation

Generally, diagnosis is straightforward and based on clinical signs. The symptoms of bilateral TMJ dislocation include anterior mandibular protrusion, facial elongation, loss of both nasolabial folds, and preauricular depression with anterolateral prominence. Difficulty closing the mouth leads to drooling, impaired speech and pronunciation, and compromised chewing and swallowing. In unilateral dislocation, all symptoms manifest on one side, with mandibular deviation to the unaffected side and a crossbite. Radiography is the primary diagnostic imaging modality. MRI and CT may provide valuable diagnostic information when surgical procedures for the TMJ are necessary.

In most cases, early anterior TMJ dislocations can be reduced manually with relative ease [2]. However, if left untreated for more than one month, the likelihood of successful manual reduction decreases substantially, and the probability of requiring surgical procedures increases (Figure 5). Therefore, the early detection, diagnosis, and treatment of TMJ dislocations are crucial. However, many medical professionals are unfamiliar with TMJ dislocations. This review revealed that numerous cases progressed to chronicity due to missed diagnoses or misdiagnoses (Figure 2). When mouth closure or swallowing becomes difficult, and mouth breathing becomes necessary, the risk of aspiration pneumonia increases. Various neurological diseases cause involuntary contraction of the masticatory muscles, particularly the lateral pterygoid muscle [6,126–128]. Aspiration pneumonia is the most common cause of death in many neurological diseases, and untreated TMJ dislocation may contribute significantly to mortality. Oral surgeons and dentists with TMJ expertise should educate physicians, nurses, and other medical professionals about TMJ dislocations.

4.3. Treatment of Long-Standing TMJ Dislocation

Early diagnosis and treatment are essential for managing TMJ dislocation; however, when the dislocation becomes long-standing, treatment should progress gradually from non-invasive to invasive methods. Manual reduction (using analgesics, muscle relaxants, and local anesthesia as needed), manual reduction under sedation or general anesthesia, and continuous elastic traction using the lever technique should be attempted initially. Continuous traction using splints or wires was attempted in 12.7% of the cases; however, success was achieved without open procedures in only 7.4% of the cases (Table 3). Closed manual reduction was successful in 12.2% of patients (Table 3). Closed reduction was achievable in more than 40% of cases within 3 months of dislocation; however, open reduction was required in more than 80% of cases after 4 months or longer (Figure 6). Furthermore, the duration since dislocation in cases where closed reduction was achievable was significantly shorter than that in cases requiring open reduction (4.9 vs. 14.8 months) (Figure 6).

There are reports of closed reduction even in cases of prolonged dislocation. Caminiti and Weinberg [72] reported on the successful manual reduction of a unilateral TMJ dislocation under general anesthesia that persisted for 2 years. Ogawa et al. [97] successfully performed conservative reduction through lever action using a resin splint in a case of long-standing dislocation that persisted for 3 years and 5 months. Therefore, closed reduction appears feasible even in cases of extra-long-standing dislocations persisting beyond 6 months. However, when reduction using conservative methods is impossible, surgical procedures must be considered. Here, surgical procedures included hook placement at the mandibular notch (18.8%), condylectomy (10.9%), eminoplasty (8.7%), eminectomy (8.3%), angular traction (4.4%), meniscectomy (4.4%), orthognathic surgery (4.4%), excision of fibrous tissue (3.1%), lateral pterygoid myotomy (2.6%), condylotomy (2.2%), total TMJ prosthesis (1.3%), coronoidectomy (1.3%), coronoidotomy (1.3%), and condylar levering (1.3%) (Table 3, Figure 4). The Fink method involves the placement of a hook at the mandibular notch. A strong steel hook is inserted over the mandibular notch, and force is applied in the downward and backward directions to reduce the displaced condyle. McGraw first introduced this method in 1899 [129].

When manual reduction is not possible due to bony adhesions, alternatives such as condylectomy, condylotomy, or craniotomy should be considered. Gottlieb recommended condylectomy as a surgical procedure for long-standing TMJ dislocation because this technique is often necessary to prevent ankylosis [22]. Mazzoni first used this method to treat long-standing TMJ dislocations in 1877 [129].

Although eminectomy or eminoplasty has been applied primarily for habitual TMJ dislocation [130–132], both eminectomy [52,55,58,59,67,72,98,99,101,106,108,110,116,119] and eminoplasty [66,68,69,85,111,117] have also been utilized for long-standing dislocations.

Mandibulotomy enables the independent movement of each condyle, thereby eliminating resistance on the contralateral side [82,90,105]. Although no such cases have been reported, if reduction remains unsuccessful using this technique due to severe fibrous or bony adhesions around the TMJ, an approach to the TMJ may become necessary. The mandibular swing procedure utilizing midline mandibulotomy has been successfully used to access oral and oropharyngeal tumors. The advantage of midline mandibulotomy is the prevention of surgical exposure of the bilateral TMJs, facial scarring, and nerve injuries. Potential complications include lingual hematoma, damage to proximal root apices, malocclusion, and nonunion [90]. Reports are limited, and appropriate case selection requires careful consideration.

Orthognathic surgery is considered appropriate when closed reduction proves impossible, more than 6 months have elapsed since dislocation, and oral function remains maintained to a certain degree with the condyle in a dislocated position [20,36,44,67,81,103,114,124].

TMJ prostheses are gaining popularity and were applied in five cases across four reports included in this review [51,92,113,114]. According to a recent systematic review, TMJ prostheses are recommended only for patients presenting with severe ongoing pain, bony or fibrous ankylosis, or osteomyelitis following primary closed or open reduction of mandibular condyle fractures [133].

Although lateral pterygoid muscle myotomy has been used for recurrent or long-standing dislocations in several reports [12,73,107,116,134–136], botulinum toxin therapy may render myotomy largely unnecessary [11,126].

After successful reduction, intermaxillary fixation is required to preserve occlusion and avoid recurrence. Intermaxillary fixation was applied post-reduction in 122 patients (53.3%) for a mean duration of 17.5 days (Table 4). Redislocation has been reported by several researchers [36,58,74,87,108].

4.4. Limitations and Future Directions

Follow-up data were not available for 35.8% of patients. The mean follow-up period was only 11.8 months. Future research requires sufficient longitudinal follow-up to determine postoperative sequelae. Further investigations, including a larger case series, are necessary to properly analyze the significant factors affecting outcomes. No significant factors were identified through binary logistic analysis, no general treatment policy existed, and treatment was implemented at the discretion of the attending physician. The author proposes an algorithm for managing and treating long-standing TMJ dislocations (Figure 8) based on the results of this review, previously suggested algorithms [84,90,99], and personal experience. Nonetheless, the rarity of this condition means that a consensus and robust evidence are lacking. Patient stratification and the corresponding selection of treatment methods are important when proposing an algorithm. However, previous studies have rarely described these aspects. To date, several clinicians have proposed various algorithms [84,90,99]. This review examined algorithms based on numerous studies including methods that have recently been applied and presented the most appropriate approach. However, this algorithm needs to be further developed and revised in the future to incorporate the opinions of experienced TMJ specialists, oral surgeons, and plastic surgeons based on the latest research results. Diagnostic delays can significantly influence the choice between closed and open reduction. Early diagnosis is crucial to facilitate less-invasive procedures and reduce the risk of long-term sequelae. As such, establishing and optimizing a standardized management approach for chronic dislocations is a pressing need in the medical field.

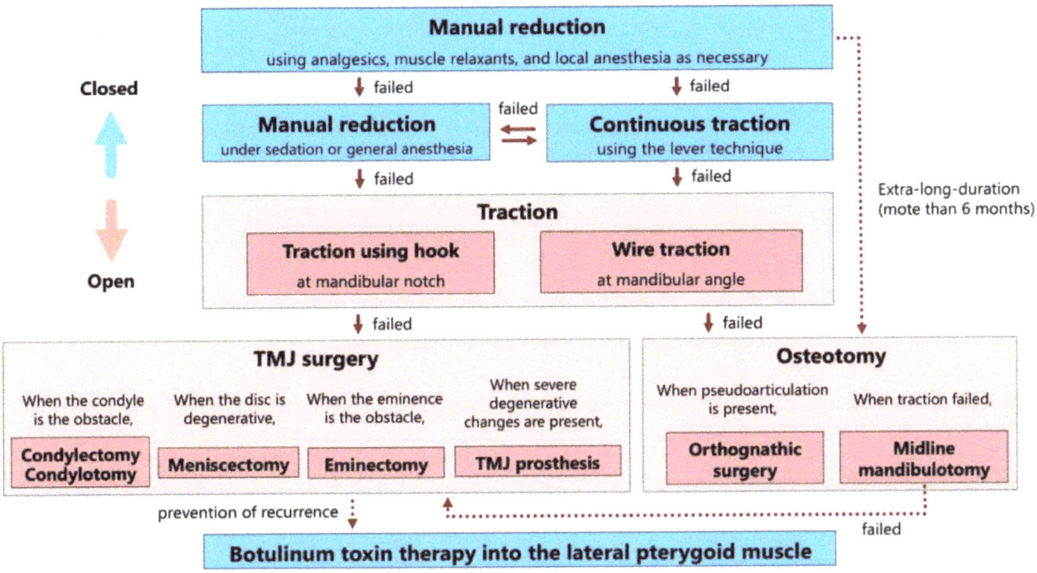

Figure 8. A proposed treatment algorithm for long-standing temporomandibular joint dislocation.

5. Conclusions

Early diagnosis and treatment of TMJ dislocation are essential to significantly reduce progression to chronic dislocation and avoid surgical intervention. Therefore, TMJ specialists should educate medical professionals about TMJ dislocations to increase awareness. For long-standing TMJ dislocations, the treatment approach should advance from conservative to more invasive methods in progressive stages.

Supplementary Materials: The following information can be downloaded from https://www.mdpi.com/article/10.3390/medicina61091505/s1, Table S1. Demographic data and patient symptoms. Table S2. Treatment and follow-up data for all patients.

Funding: This work was supported by JSPS KAKENHI (Grant Number JP22K10091).

Institutional Review Board Statement: Not applicable.

Informed Consent Statement: Not applicable.

Data Availability Statement: Not applicable.

Acknowledgments: The author thanks Kumiko Yasui (Library of Kyoto Medical Center) for collecting the literature.

Conflicts of Interest: The author declares no conflicts of interest.

Abbreviations

The following abbreviations are used in this manuscript:

BC	Before Christ
CT	Computed tomography
MRI	Magnetic resonance imaging
TMJ	Temporomandibular joint

References

1. Neff, A.; Hell, B.; Kolk, A.; Pautke, C.; Schneider, M.; Prechel, U. *S3 Leitlinie Kiefergelenkluxation*; AWMF Registernummer 007–063; Arbeitsgemeinschaft der Wissenschaftlichen medizinischen Fachgesellschaften e V.: Berlin, Germany, 2016.
2. Neff, A.; McLeod, N.; Spijkervet, F.; Riechmann, M.; Vieth, U.; Kolk, A.; Sidebottom, A.J.; Bonte, B.; Speculand, B.; Saridin, C.; et al. The ESTMJS (European Society of Temporomandibular Joint Surgeons) consensus and evidence-based recommendations on management of condylar dislocation. *J. Clin. Med.* **2021**, *10*, 5068. [CrossRef]
3. Akinbami, B.O. Evaluation of the mechanism and principles of management of temporomandibular joint dislocation. Systematic review of literature and a proposed new classification of temporomandibular joint dislocation. *Head Face Med.* **2011**, *7*, 10. [CrossRef]
4. Adams, F. The genuine works of Hippocrates. In *Translated from the Greek with a Preliminary Discourse and Annotations*; William Wood and Company: New York, NY, USA, 1886; Volume 2, p. 107. Available online: https://www.google.co.jp/books/edition/The_Genuine_Works_of_Hippocrates/6BAWAAAAYAAJ?hl=ja&gbpv=1&dq=The+genuine+works+of+HIPPOCRATES,+Vol+2&printsec=frontcover (accessed on 1 July 2025).
5. Daelen, B.; Thorwirth, V.; Koch, A. Neurogene Kiefergelenkluxation Definition und Therapie mit Botulinumtoxin. *Nervenarzt* **1997**, *68*, 346–350. [CrossRef] [PubMed]
6. Yoshida, K. Botulinum neurotoxin injection for the treatment of recurrent temporomandibular joint dislocation with and without neurogenic muscular hyperactivity. *Toxins* **2018**, *10*, 174. [CrossRef] [PubMed]
7. Shorey, C.W.; Campbell, J.H. Dislocation of the temporomandibular joint. *Oral Surg. Oral Med. Oral Pathol. Oral Radiol. Endodontology* **2000**, *89*, 662–668. [CrossRef]
8. Iizuka, T.; Hidaka, Y.; Murakami, K.-I.; Nishida, M. Chronic recurrent anterior luxation of the mandible: A review of 12 patients treated by the LeClerc procedure. *Int. J. Oral Maxillofac. Surg.* **1988**, *17*, 170–172. [CrossRef] [PubMed]
9. Undt, G.; Kermer, C.; Piehslinger, E.; Rasse, M. Treatment of recurrent mandibular dislocation, part I: Leclerc blocking procedure. *Int. J. Oral Maxillofac. Surg.* **1997**, *26*, 92–97. [CrossRef]
10. Yoshida, K. Etiology of pneumoparotid: A systematic review. *J. Clin. Med.* **2022**, *12*, 144. [CrossRef]
11. Yoshida, K. Superior dislocation of the mandibular condyle into the middle cranial fossa: A comprehensive review of the literature. *J. Clin. Med.* **2023**, *12*, 3781. [CrossRef]
12. Kramer. Zur Behandlung der irreponiblen Unterkieferverrenkung. *Centralblatt Chir.* **1901**, *28*, 269.
13. Hildebrand, O. Zur blutigen Reposition veralteter Kieferluxationen. *Arch. Klin. Chir.* **1902**, *66*, 352.
14. Willcutts, M.D. Treatment of an irreducible dislocated lower jaw of 98 days' duration. *U. S. Nav. Med. Bull.* **1927**, *25*, 331–336.
15. Miyakoda, T. Surgical reduction of chronic dislocation of the mandibular joint. *Jpn. Surg. Soc.* **1931**, *32*, 1369–1370.
16. Schwartz, M. Unreduced unilateral dislocation of the jaw. *J. Bone Jt. Surg.* **1940**, *22*, 176–181.
17. Reiß, M. Operative Reposition veralterer doppel-seitiger Unterkieferluxationen. *Zahnärztl. Rundsch.* **1940**, *49*, 1235–1240, 1282–1285, 1309–1311.
18. Watanabe, I.; Hagino, T. A case of chronic bilateral mandibular anterior dislocation successfully reduced by open reduction. *Med. Biol.* **1942**, *1*, 581–583.
19. Müller, G.M. Long-standing dislocation of mandible. *Br. Med. J.* **1946**, *1*, 572. [CrossRef]
20. Jones, J.C.B. Treatment of unreduced bilateral forward dislocation of the temporomandibular joint. *Br. Dent. J.* **1949**, *86*, 275–278.
21. Watanabe, Y.; Otake, O. Unreduced dislocation of the mandibular joint following eclampsia. *Oral Surg. Oral Med. Oral Pathol.* **1950**, *3*, 1010. [CrossRef]
22. Gottlieb, O. Long-standing dislocation of the jaw. *J. Oral Surg.* **1952**, *10*, 25–32.
23. Matsumae, G.; Ito, I. A Case of nonsurgical reduction of chronic anterior dislocation of the mandible. *J. Jpn. Stomatol. Soc.* **1952**, *1*, 91–92.
24. Campbell, J.; White, T.C.; Anderson, H. A case of bi-lateral dislocation of the mandible of nine months duration. *Dent. Rec.* **1952**, *72*, 230–239.
25. Curson, I. Long-standing bilateral dislocation of the temporomandibular joints. *Br. Dent. J.* **1959**, *107*, 351–353.
26. Whinery, J.G. Bilateral condylar neck dissection for long-standing dislocation of the mandible. *J. Oral Surg. Anesth. Hosp. Dent. Serv.* **1961**, *19*, 432–435. [PubMed]
27. Berg, A. Ein Fall einer veralteten, doppelseitigen Unterkieferrenkung. *Zschr. Stomat.* **1962**, *24*, 876.
28. Litzow, T.J.; Royer, R.Q. Treatment of long-standing dislocation of the mandible. *Proc. Staff Meet. Mayo Clin.* **1962**, *37*, 399–403.
29. Glahn, M. Malposition of the mandibular condyle. *Br. J. Oral Surg.* **1964**, *2*, 33–36. [CrossRef]

30. Hogan, N.; Nally, F. Prolonged bilateral temporomandibular joint dislocation. *Ir. Dent. Rev.* **1964**, *10*, 40–42.
31. Fordyce, G.L. Long-standing bilateral dislocation of the jaw. *Br. J. Oral Surg.* **1965**, *3*, 222–225. [CrossRef]
32. Hayward, J.R. Prolonged dislocation of the mandible. *J. Oral Surg.* **1965**, *23*, 585–594.
33. Topazian, R.G.; Costich, E.R. Management of protracted dislocation of the mandible. *J. Trauma* **1967**, *7*, 257–264. [CrossRef]
34. Kameyama, T.; Miura, T.; Moji, K. A case of chronic dislocation of the temporomandibular joint. *Jpn. J. Oral Maxillofac. Surg.* **1968**, *14*, 17–20. [CrossRef]
35. Yoshida, Y.; Terai, H.; Nakashiro, T. Surgical reduction of chronic anterior dislocation of the temporomandibular joint. *J. Jpn. Stomatol. Soc.* **1970**, *19*, 234–240. [CrossRef]
36. Rowe, P.F.; Caldwell, J.B. Correction of permanent temporomandibular joint dislocation. *J. Oral Surg.* **1970**, *28*, 222–226.
37. Ohto, A.; Shimura, K.; Suzuki, K.; Amanai, S. A case of chronic dislocation of the temporomandibular joint. *J. Kanagawa Odontol. Soc.* **1970**, *4*, 83.
38. Okano, M.; Henomatsu, K.; Yoda, K.; Kawai, S. A case of open reduction of chronic temporomandibular joint dislocation. *Jpn. J. Oral Maxillofac. Surg.* **1971**, *17*, 356.
39. Sujaku, C.; Kameyama, T.; Hosino, N. A case of long-standing forward dislocation of the mandible. *Jpn. J. Oral Maxillofac. Surg.* **1972**, *18*, 593–597. [CrossRef]
40. Horii, M.; Murata, A.; Ikeda, S.; Kashiwagi, A.; Ishii, Y. A case of obsolute luxation of jaw joint for 6 years. *Kitano Hosp. J. Med.* **1973**, *18*, 88–90.
41. Rawls, H.C.; Bruni, A.; Hamilton, M.K. Surgical correction of the permanently dislocated mandible. *J. Oral Surg.* **1973**, *31*, 385–388.
42. Gorman, J.M. Condylotomy for bilateral dislocation. *Br. J. Oral Surg.* **1974**, *12*, 96–98. [CrossRef] [PubMed]
43. Hashimoto, K.; Kawachi, S.; Murase, H.; Akashi, Y.; Masuda, M.; Ohtani, T. Two cases of obsolete bilateral dislocation of the temporomandibular joints. *Jpn. J. Oral Maxillofac. Surg.* **1976**, *22*, 423–428. [CrossRef]
44. Adekeye, E.O.; Shamia, R.I.; Cove, P. Inverted L-shaped ramus osteotomy for prolonged bilateral dislocation of the temporomandibular joint. *Oral Surg. Oral Med. Oral Pathol.* **1976**, *41*, 568–577. [CrossRef]
45. Sanders, B.; Schneider, J.; Given, J. Prolonged dislocation of the mandibular condyle. *J. Oral Surg.* **1979**, *37*, 346–348. [PubMed]
46. Littler, B.O. The role of local anaesthesia in the reduction of long-standing dislocation of the temporomandibular joint. *Br. J. Oral Surg.* **1980**, *18*, 81–85. [CrossRef] [PubMed]
47. Kawamura, H.; Takano, N.; Abe, Y.; Kikuchi, M.; Fujita, Y.; Hayashi, S. A case of chronic bilateral dislocation of the temporomandibular joint treated by nonsurgical reduction. *Jpn. J. Oral Maxillofac. Surg.* **1980**, *29*, 341–346. [CrossRef]
48. Mizuno, A.; Fujita, S.; Shimada, T.; Sekiyama, S. Long-standing luxation of the mandible, report of a case and review of the Japanese literature. *Int. J. Oral Surg.* **1980**, *9*, 225–230. [CrossRef]
49. Prabhakara, B.S. Conservative treatment of bilateral persistent anterior dislocation of the mandible. *J. Oral Surg.* **1980**, *38*, 51–52.
50. Stakesby Lewis, J.E. A simple technique for reduction of long-standing dislocation of the mandible. *Br. J. Oral Surg.* **1981**, *19*, 52–56. [CrossRef]
51. Blank, D.M.; Stein, A.C.; Gold, B.D.; Berger, J. Treatment of protracted bilateral mandibular dislocation with proplast-Vitallium prostheses. *Oral Surg. Oral Med. Oral Pathol.* **1982**, *53*, 335–339. [CrossRef] [PubMed]
52. Tipps, S.P.; Landis, C.F. Prolonged bilateral mandibular dislocation. *J. Oral Maxillofac. Surg.* **1982**, *40*, 524–527. [CrossRef]
53. Parekh, P.K.; Bhatia, I.K. Condylectomies for prolonged bilateral temporomandibular dislocation. *Arch. Orthop. Trauma Surg.* **1983**, *102*, 123–125. [CrossRef]
54. Takahashi, T.; Tamura, H.; Ioku, N. Two cases of obsolete dislocation of the temporomandibular joint. *Jpn. J. Oral Maxillofac. Surg.* **1984**, *30*, 1708–1715. [CrossRef]
55. Kudo, K.; Baba, R.; Chen, C.-H.; Komai, T.; Fujioka, Y.; Kanamori, T. Restricting operation of anterior movement for obsolete dislocation of temporomandibular joint: A case report. *Jpn. J. Oral Maxillofac. Surg.* **1985**, *31*, 337–340. [CrossRef]
56. El-Attar, A.; Ord, R.A. Longstanding mandibular dislocations: Report of a case, review of the literature. *Br. Dent. J.* **1986**, *160*, 91. [CrossRef]
57. Wijmenga, J.P.; Boering, G.; Blankestijn, J. Protracted dislocation of the temporomandibular joint. *Int. J. Oral Maxillofac. Surg.* **1986**, *15*, 380–388. [CrossRef]
58. Hammersley, N. Chronic bilateral dislocation of the temporomandibular joint. *Br. J. Oral Maxillofac. Surg.* **1986**, *24*, 367–375. [CrossRef]
59. Suzuki, S.; Mizuno, A.; Torii, S.; Kamiya, H.; Katayama, T.; Yokoi, C.; Shikimori, M.; Motegi, K. Eminectomy for long-standing bilateral forward dislocation of the temporomandibular joint: Report of two cases. *Jpn. J. Oral Maxillofac. Surg.* **1987**, *33*, 386–393. [CrossRef]
60. Kowaka, S.; Hosoda, M.; Segami, N.; Hata, T.; Hanafusa, H.; Fujimura, K.; Fukuda, M. A case of long-standing bilateral dislocation of the mandibular condyle. *Jpn. J. Oral Maxillofac. Surg.* **1987**, *33*, 2131–2135. [CrossRef]
61. Obara, S.; Oka, M.; Harada, T.; Yoshimura, Y. A case of long-standing dislocation of the temporomandibular joint with severe complications. *Jpn. J. Oral Maxillofac. Surg.* **1988**, *34*, 716–721. [CrossRef]

62. Chin, R.S.; Gropp, H.; Beirne, O.R. Long-standing mandibular dislocation: Report of a case. *J. Oral Maxillofac. Surg.* **1988**, 4 693–696. [CrossRef]
63. Tanimoto, Y.; Morizane, T.; Hadano, T.; Yoshiga, K.; Takada, K. The chronic bilateral anterior dislocation of the temporomandibula joint (TMJ): Report of a case. *J. Jpn. Soc. TMJ* **1991**, *3*, 69–74. [CrossRef]
64. Ishihara, A.; Mizuno, K.; Kamiya, Y.; Ito, A.; Imai, T.; Adachi, M.; Yamashita, T.; Fukaya, M. Reduction of obsolete dislocation o temporomandibular joint: Report of a case. *Jpn. J. Oral Maxillofac. Surg.* **1992**, *38*, 500–501. [CrossRef]
65. Ishimaru, T.; Hayatsu, Y.; Ohsawa, S.; Shinozaki, F. A case of prolonged mandibular dislocation of the patient medicated wit antipsychotic drugs. *J. Jpn. Stomatol. Soc.* **1992**, *41*, 504–510. [CrossRef]
66. Ogawa, T.; Mori, M.; Sawatari, S.; Yamamoto, G.; Yamaguchi, Y.; Yoshitake, K. A case of open reduction for long-standing anterio luxation of the temporomandibular joint. *Jpn. J. Oral Maxillofac. Surg.* **1992**, *38*, 1927–1928. [CrossRef]
67. Smith, W.P.; Johnson, P.A. Sagittal split mandibular osteotomy for irreducible dislocation of the temporomandibular joint. A cas report. *Int. J. Oral Maxillofac. Surg.* **1994**, *23*, 16–18. [CrossRef] [PubMed]
68. Kawakami, T.; Tsuzuki, M.; Shohara, E.; Takayama, K.; Morimoto, Y.; Sugimura, M. Surgical treatment by Dautrey procedure fo long-standing anterior luxation of the temporomandibular joints. *J. Jpn. Soc. TMJ* **1995**, *7*, 51–56. [CrossRef]
69. Kato, M.; Isobe, M.; Kamiya, Y.; Ohtani, T. Two cases of obsolete dislocation of the temporomandibular joint with cerebrovascula disease. *J. Jpn. Soc. Dent. Medically Compromised Patient* **1996**, *5*, 30–35. [CrossRef]
70. Iwatsubo, R.; Hosaka, H.; Goto, K.; Murayama, T. Treatment of temporomandibular joint luxation in patients with complications– Case report. *J. Jpn. Soc. Dent. Medically Compromised Patient* **1996**, *4*, 65–73. [CrossRef]
71. Kurita, K.; Mukaida, Y.; Ogi, N.; Toyama, M. Closed reduction of chronic bilateral temporomandibular joint dislocation. *A cas report. Int. J. Oral Maxillofac. Surg.* **1996**, *25*, 422–423. [CrossRef]
72. Caminiti, M.F.; Weinberg, S. Chronic mandibular dislocation: The role of non-surgical and surgical treatment. *J. Can. Dent. Assoc* **1998**, *64*, 484–491.
73. Hoard, M.A.; Tadje, J.P.; Gampper, T.J.; Edlich, R.F. Traumatic chronic TMJ dislocation: Report of an unusual case and discussior of management. *J. Craniomaxillofac. Trauma* **1998**, *4*, 44–47.
74. Mizutani, H.; Hattori, H.; Senga, K.; Seko, K.; Asahina, T.; Kaneko, R.; Shinoda, M.; Ueda, M. Eight cases with chronic mandibula dislocation. *J. Jpn. Soc. TMJ* **2000**, *12*, 52–56.
75. Murakami, K.; Kondo, T.; Irisa, K.; Takahashi, K.; Kishida, T.; Itoh, T. Cases of spectroscopic machinic arthroplasty under genera anesthesia for Chen's old-style mandibular joint dislocation of Parkinson's disease and multiple cerebral infarction patients *J. Jpn. Soc. Dent. Medically Compromised Patient* **2002**, *11*, 41–46. [CrossRef]
76. Takenaka, A.; Fujita, H.; Sasaki, H.; Tanabe, S.; Matsuda, S.; Yoshimura, Y. A case of old anterior temporomandibular join dislocation treated by lysis and lavage using arthroscopic technique and manual reduction. *J. Jpn. Soc. TMJ* **2003**, *15*, 29–32.
77. Aquilina, P.; Vickers, R.; McKellar, G. Reduction of a chronic bilateral temporomandibular joint dislocation with intermaxillary fixation and botulinum toxin A. *Br. J. Oral Maxillofac. Surg.* **2004**, *42*, 272–273. [CrossRef]
78. Ohno, K.; Sumitomo, S.; Mouri, K.; Kuwajima, K.; Takai, Y. Chronic dislocation of temporo-mandibular joint reset by closed reduction with intra-articular pumping technique. *J. Jpn. Soc. TMJ* **2005**, *17*, 215–217. [CrossRef]
79. Kobayakawa, M.; Kamei, K.; Sato, T.; Nakamura, M.; Ito, K.; Kobayashi, K. A case of bilateral chronic dislocation of the temporomandibular joint reduced by removal of fibrous adhesive lesions after eminectomy. *Jpn. J. Oral Maxillofac. Surg.* **2005**, *51*, 212–215. [CrossRef]
80. Terakado, N.; Shintani, S.; Nakahara, Y.; Yano, J.; Hino, S.; Hamakawa, H. Conservative treatment of prolonged bilateral mandibular dislocation with the help of an intermaxillary fixation screw. *Br. J. Oral Maxillofac. Surg.* **2006**, *44*, 62–63. [CrossRef]
81. Debnath, S.C.; Kotrashetti, S.M.; Halli, R.; Baliga, S. Bilateral vertical-oblique osteotomy of ramus (external approach) for treatment of a long-standing dislocation of the temporomandibular joint: A case report. *Oral Surg. Oral Med. Oral Pathol. Oral Radiol. Endod.* **2006**, *101*, e79–e82. [CrossRef] [PubMed]
82. Lee, S.H.; Son, S.I.; Park, J.H.; Park, I.S.; Nam, J.H. Reduction of prolonged bilateral temporomandibular joint dislocation by midline mandibulotomy. *Int. J. Oral Maxillofac. Surg.* **2006**, *35*, 1054–1056. [CrossRef]
83. Yao, M.; Nakayama, S.; Yoshihama, Y.; Mese, H.; Sasaki, A. Conservative reduction of obsolete dislocation of the temporo-mandibular joint –A case report: Innovation for a patient with severe marginal periodontitis. *J. Jpn. Soc. TMJ* **2007**, *19*, 171–176. [CrossRef]
84. Rattan, V.; Rai, S. Management of long-standing anteromedial temporomandibular joint dislocation. *Asian J. Oral Maxillofac. Surg.* **2007**, *19*, 155–159. [CrossRef]
85. Nakashima, M.; Yano, H.; Akita, S.; Tokunaga, K.; Anraku, K.; Tanaka, K.; Hirano, A. Traumatic unilateral temporomandibular joint dislocation overlooked for more than two decades. *J. Craniofacial Surg.* **2007**, *18*, 1466–1470. [CrossRef]
86. Kale, T.P.; Kotrashetti, S.M.; Janardhan, S.; Urolagin, S.B. Long standing TMJ dislocation: Closed reduction –A case report and technical note. *J. Int. Oral Health* **2010**, *2*, 59–67.

87. Huang, I.Y.; Chen, C.M.; Kao, Y.H.; Chen, C.M.; Wu, C.W. Management of long-standing mandibular dislocation. *Int. J. Oral Maxillofac. Surg.* **2011**, *40*, 810–814. [CrossRef]
88. Shakya, S.; Ongole, R.; Sumanth, K.N.; Denny, C.E. Chronic bilateral dislocation of temporomandibular joint. *Kathmandu Univ. Med. J. KUMJ* **2010**, *8*, 251–256. [CrossRef] [PubMed]
89. Kim, C.-H.; Kim, D.-H. Chronic dislocation of temporomandibular joint persisting for 6 months: A case report. *J. Korean Assoc. Oral Maxillofac. Surg.* **2012**, *38*, 305–309. [CrossRef]
90. Rattan, V.; Rai, A.; Sethi, A. Midline mandibulotomy for reduction of long-standing temporomandibular joint dislocation. *Craniomaxillofac. Trauma Reconstr.* **2013**, *6*, 127–132. [CrossRef]
91. Yoshida, M.; Shibayama, N.; Kondo, E.; Ogami, J.; Takekawa, M.; Matsuda, M. A case of chronic mandibular dislocation treated by conservative reduction. *Jpn. J. Oral Maxillofac. Surg.* **2013**, *59*, 18–22. [CrossRef]
92. Baur, D.A.; Jannuzzi, J.R.; Mercan, U.; Quereshy, F.A. Treatment of long term anterior dislocation of the TMJ. *Int. J. Oral Maxillofac. Surg.* **2013**, *42*, 1030–1033. [CrossRef] [PubMed]
93. Elmorsy, K.A. Management of long-standing temporomandibular joint dislocation. *Egypt. J. Oral Maxillofac. Surg.* **2014**, *5*, 39–44. [CrossRef]
94. Hayashi, K.; Onda, T.; Ogane, S.; Yakushiji, T.; Ohata, H.; Takano, N.; Shibahara, T. A case of long standing dislocation of bilateral temporomandibular joints of the elderly. *J. Gerodont.* **2014**, *28*, 284–288. [CrossRef]
95. Saikia, D. Long standing temporomandibular joint dislocation: A case report. *IOSR J. Dent. Med. Sci.* **2014**, *13*, 3–8. [CrossRef]
96. Pradhan, L.; Jaisani, M.R.; Sagtani, A.; Win, A. Conservative management of chronic TMJ dislocation: An old technique revived. *J. Maxillofac. Oral Surg.* **2015**, *14* (Suppl. S1), 267–270. [CrossRef] [PubMed]
97. Ogawa, M.; Kanbe, T.; Kano, A.; Kubota, F.; Makiguchi, T.; Miyazaki, H.; Yokoo, S. Conservative reduction by lever action of chronic bilateral mandibular condyle dislocation. *Cranio* **2015**, *33*, 142–147. [CrossRef]
98. Arzul, L.; Henoux, M.; Marion, F.; Corre, P. Luxation chronique bilatérale des articulations temporo-mandibulaires et syndrome de Meig. *Rev. Stomatol. Chir. Maxillofac. Chir. Orale* **2015**, *116*, 106–110. [CrossRef]
99. Marqués-Mateo, M.; Puche-Torres, M.; Iglesias-Gimilio, M.E. Temporomandibular chronic dislocation: The long-standing condition. *Med. Oral Patol. Oral Cir. Bucal.* **2016**, *21*, e776–e783. [CrossRef]
100. Jeyaraj, P.; Chakranarayan, A. A conservative surgical approach in the management of longstanding chronic protracted temporomandibular joint dislocation: A case report and review of literature. *J. Maxillofac. Oral Surg.* **2016**, *15* (Suppl. S2), 361–370. [CrossRef]
101. Güngörmüş, M.; Yavuz, M.S.; Ömezli, M.M.; Akkaş, İ. Long-term temporomandibular joint dislocation treated with bilateral eminectomy and chin-cap; Case report. *Turk. Klin. J. Dent. Sci. Cases* **2016**, *2*, 75–79. [CrossRef]
102. Negishi, S.; Shibasaki, M. A case of long-standing bilateral temporomandibular joint dislocation treated by intraoral condylectomy. *Jpn. J. Oral Maxillofac. Surg.* **2017**, *63*, 304–309. [CrossRef]
103. Malik, K.; Debnath, S.C.; Adhyapok, A.K.; Hazarika, K. Long-standing temporomandibular joint dislocation: A rare experience. *Saudi J. Oral Sci.* **2017**, *4*, 112–116. [CrossRef]
104. Shaban, S.D.; Sohal, K.S.; Moshy, J.R. A novel technique for surgical reduction of long-standing temporomandibular joint dislocation. *Int. J. Head Neck Surg.* **2017**, *8*, 107–111. [CrossRef]
105. Dhiman, N.K.; Pandey, A.; Vishwakarma, A.K.; Verma, V.; Singh, S. Management of long standing TMJ dislocation: Report of three cases. *J. Adv. Med. Dent. Sci. Res.* **2018**, *6*, 55–58. [CrossRef]
106. Chin, S.Y.; Berahim, N.B.; Andan, K.B.; Ramasamy, S.N. Delayed management of unrecognized bilateral temporomandibular joint dislocation: A case report. *Craniomaxillofac. Trauma Reconstr.* **2018**, *11*, 145–149. [CrossRef]
107. Gholami, M.; Shirzadeh, A.; Khalife, H. Chronic long-standing temporomandibular joint dislocation: Report of three cases and review of literature. *J. Maxillofac. Oral Surg.* **2018**, *17*, 502–507. [CrossRef] [PubMed]
108. Segami, N.; Nishimura, T.; Miyaki, K.; Adachi, H. Tethering technique using bone screws and wire for chronic mandibular dislocation: A preliminary study of refractory cases. *Int. J. Oral Maxillofac. Surg.* **2018**, *47*, 1065–1069. [CrossRef] [PubMed]
109. Balaji, S.M.; Balaji, P. Surgical management of chronic temporomandibular joint dislocations. *Indian J. Dent. Res.* **2018**, *29*, 455–458. [CrossRef]
110. Güven, O. Nearthrosis in true long-standing temporomandibular joint dislocation; a report on pathogenesis and clinical features with review of literature. *J. Cranio-Maxillofac. Surg.* **2019**, *47*, 945–950. [CrossRef]
111. Cuevas Queipo de Llano, A.; Monje Gil, F.; Gonzalez García, R.; Villanueva Alcojol, L.; Gonzalez Ballester, D. Long-term dislocation of the mandible: Is there an algorithm to success? intraoperative decision and review of literature. *J. Maxillofac. Oral Surg.* **2020**, *19*, 12–16. [CrossRef] [PubMed]
112. Karakida, K.; Takahashi, M.; Hamada, Y.; Aoki, J.; Hoshimoto, Y. A case of long-standing temporomandibular joint dislocation: Restoration of oral function following condylectomy. *Tokai J. Exp. Clin. Med.* **2020**, *45*, 152–155.
113. Sarlabous, M.; Psutka, D.J. Total joint replacement after condylar destruction secondary to long-standing dislocation of the temporomandibular joint. *J. Craniofacial Surg.* **2020**, *31*, 989–995. [CrossRef]

114. Bavia, P.F.; Ganjawalla, K.; Keith, D.A. Long-standing unilateral temporomandibular joint (TMJ) dislocation with pseudo-articulation with the base of the skull. *Oral Maxillofac. Surg. Cases* **2020**, *6*, 100205. [CrossRef]
115. Uetsuki, R.; Ono, S.; Tada, M.; Okuda, S.; Takechi, M. Long-standing temporomandibular joint dislocation treated by intraoral condylectomy: A case report and review of the literature. *J. Med. Case Rep.* **2022**, *16*, 245. [CrossRef]
116. Nikunj, A.; Khan, N.; Rajkhokar, D.; Mishra, B.; Rajurkar, S. Deg-induced oromandibular dystonia presenting as chronic temporomandibular joint dislocation: A rare case report. *Cureus* **2022**, *14*, e23478. [CrossRef]
117. Anehosur, V.; Mehra, A.; Kumar, N. Management of chronic long standing condyle dislocation. *Int. Surg. J.* **2023**, *10*, 114–120 [CrossRef]
118. Ekram, S.; Tigga, C.; Prajapati, V.K.; Prakash, O. Elastic traction treatment for the management of chronic dislocation of bilateral condyle—A report of 2 case. *Dent. J. Indira Gandhi Inst. Med. Sci.* **2022**, *1*, 73–75. [CrossRef]
119. Navaneetham, R.; Navaneetham, A.; Pugazhendi, S.K.; Nara, G.; Umarani, P.J. Chronic protracted dislocation of temporomandibular joint in a trauma patient—A case report. *Ann. Maxillofac. Surg.* **2023**, *13*, 130–132. [CrossRef]
120. Gupta, G.; Gupta, D.K.; Gupta, N.; Chandra, N.; Sankhla, D. Conservative management of a 3 months long standing bilateral temporomandibular joint dislocation: A case report. *J. Oral Med. Oral Surg. Oral Pathol. Oral Radiol.* **2023**, *9*, 222–225. [CrossRef]
121. Ogundipe, O.K.; Ugwu, E.I.; Ajayi, O.S.; Ojo, O.O. Reduction of manually irreducible TMJ dislocation with forceps traction: Case report in a 60-year-old woman. *Niger. Dent. J.* **2023**, *31*, 1–7. [CrossRef]
122. Zou, J.; Wang, L.; Acharya, K.; Hou, X.; Li, L.; Li, Y.; Hu, X.; Xing, X. The experience of chronic protracted mandibular dislocation treatment: Manual vs. surgical reduction. *BMC Oral Health* **2024**, *24*, 1127. [CrossRef]
123. Tanaka, T.; Momozaki, N.; Honda, E.; Matsuno, A. Delayed diagnosis of temporomandibular joint dislocation in severe stroke patients. *Cureus* **2024**, *16*, e68896. [CrossRef]
124. Yanagisawa, Y.; Nogami, S.; Iwama, R.; Otake, Y.; Sato, S.; Yamauchi, K. A case of chronic bilateral temporomandibular joint dislocation treated via a bilateral intraoral vertical ramus osteotomy. *Jpn. J. Oral Maxillofac. Surg.* **2024**, *70*, 379–384. [CrossRef]
125. Yoshida, K. How doi inject botulinum toxin into the lateral and medial pterygoid muscles? *Mov. Disord. Clin. Pract.* **2017**, *4*, 285. [CrossRef]
126. Yoshida, K. Botulinum toxin therapy for oromandibular dystonia and other movement disorders in the stomatognathic system. *Toxins* **2022**, *14*, 282. [CrossRef]
127. O'Connor, M.; Rooney, M.D.; Nienaber, C.P. Neuroleptic-induced dislocation of the jaw. *Br. J. Psychiatry* **1992**, *161*, 281–282. [CrossRef]
128. Ibrahim, Z.Y.; Brooks, E.F. Neuroleptic-induced bilateral temporomandibular joint dislocation. *Am. J. Psychiatry* **1996**, *153*, 2–3. [CrossRef]
129. McGraw, T.A. A new method of reducing old dislocations of the lower jaw. *Med. Record* **1899**, *56*, 511.
130. Leclerc, G.; Girard, G. Un nouveau procédé de butée dans le traitement chirurgical de la luxation récidivante de la mâchoire inférieure. *Mém. Acad. Chir.* **1943**, *69*, 457–459.
131. Myrhaug, H. A new method of operation for habitual dislocation of the mandible. Review of former methods of treatment. *Acta Odontol. Scand.* **1951**, *9*, 247–260. [CrossRef]
132. Dautrey, J. Reflexions sur la chirurgie de l'articulation temporo-mandibulaire. *Acta Stomatol. Belg.* **1975**, *72*, 577–581.
133. Niezen, E.T.; van Minnen, B.; Bos, R.R.M.; Dijkstra, P.U. Temporomandibular joint prosthesis as treatment option for mandibular condyle fractures: A systematic review and meta-analysis. *Int. J. Oral Maxillofac. Surg.* **2023**, *52*, 88–97. [CrossRef] [PubMed]
134. Laskin, D.M. Myotomy for the management of recurrent and protracted mandibular dislocations. *Trans. Int. Conf. Oral Surg.* **1973**, *4*, 264–268.
135. Miller, G.A.; Murphy, E.J. External pterygoid myotomy for recurrent mandibular dislocation. *Oral Surg. Oral Med. Oral Pathol.* **1976**, *42*, 705–714. [CrossRef] [PubMed]
136. Sindet-Petersen, S. Intraoral myotomy of the lateral pterygoid muscle for the treatment of recurrent dislocation of the mandibular condyle. *J. Oral Maxillofac. Surg.* **1988**, *46*, 445–449. [CrossRef] [PubMed]

medicina

MDPI

Review

Alveolar Rhabdomyosarcoma of Nasopharynx and Paranasal Sinuses in Children Diagnosis and Treatment—Review of the Literature and Case Report

Cristian Mârțu [1], Ștefan Dragoș Tîrnovanu [2,3], Ioana Mârțu [4,*], Dan Ferariu [5], Dan Mârțu [1], Alexandra Jităreanu [6] and Luminița Rădulescu [1]

1 ENT Clinic Department, "Grigore T. Popa" University of Medicine and Pharmacy Iasi, Universitatii Street 16, 700115 Iasi, Romania; martu.cristian@umfiasi.ro (C.M.); dvmartu@yahoo.com (D.M.); luminita.radulescu@umfiasi.ro (L.R.)
2 Department of Orthopedics and Traumatology, Faculty of Medicine, "Grigore T. Popa" University of Medicine and Pharmacy, 700115 Iasi, Romania; stefan-dragos.tirnovanu@umfiasi.ro
3 Department of Orthopaedics and Traumatology, "Sf. Spiridon" Emergency Universitary Hospital, 700115 Iasi, Romania
4 Department of Oral Implantology, Removable Dentures and Technology, "Grigore T. Popa" University of Medicine and Pharmacy Iasi, Universitatii Street 16, 700115 Iasi, Romania
5 Department of Pathology, Regional Institute of Oncology, 700483 Iasi, Romania; d_ferariu@yahoo.com
6 Department of Toxicology, Faculty of Pharmacy, "Grigore T. Popa" University of Medicine and Pharmacy, 700115 Iasi, Romania; jitareanu.alexandra@umfiasi.ro
* Correspondence: ioanamartu@gmail.com or ioana.martu@umfiasi.ro

Abstract: Alveolar rhabdomyosarcoma (aRMS) is a rare pediatric malignant tumor with a poor prognosis, particularly when located in the rhinopharynx and sphenoidal floor, which complicates diagnosis and increases the risk of misclassification as benign growths. The specific genotype of aRMS is associated with a worse clinical outcome. In young children, especially those aged 4 to 12 years, rhinopharyngeal masses are often attributed to chronic adenoiditis; however, other benign (e.g., angiofibroma in boys) and malignant tumors may also be present. Initial symptoms frequently include nasal obstruction, mucopurulent nasal discharge, serous otitis media, sinusitis, and epistaxis. Rhabdomyosarcoma is the second most common ENT neoplasm in children, following lymphoma, with an incidence of approximately 6 cases per 1,000,000 annually. This report presents the case of an 8-year-old boy diagnosed with aRMS, accompanied by a literature review. Alveolar rhabdomyosarcoma should be suspected in children presenting with a vegetative tumor in the rhinopharynx or paranasal sinuses. Combined treatment approaches (surgery, radiotherapy, and chemotherapy) should be tailored to tumor characteristics. Neuronavigation-guided functional endoscopic sinus surgery (FESS) is an effective option for achieving complete tumor excision, depending on tumor size and extent. The prognosis remains reserved and is contingent upon accurate evaluation and timely intervention. Rigorous follow-up, including endoscopic and imagistic investigation, is crucial for early detection of recurrences, thereby improving treatment outcomes.

Keywords: alveolar rhabdomyosarcoma; rhinopharynx; paranasal sinuses; pediatric

1. Introduction

Rhabdomyosarcoma (RMS) is a malignant tumor composed of rhabdomyoblasts, which microscopically resemble striated muscle cells [1–3]. First described by Weber in 1854 and cited by Ruymann [4], a more comprehensive characterization of pediatric RMS was provided by Pack in 1952 [5]. Alveolar RMS (aRMS) is a common pediatric soft tissue malignancy linked to a chromosomal translocation that results in the expression of a PAX3/7-FOXO1 fusion protein [6]. However, alternative genetic associations have also been documented [7].

Pediatric neoplasms comprise approximately 5% of all cancers in children and are the second leading cause of mortality in those aged 5–14 years [8], following accidental deaths [9]. Annually, 11,000 new cases are diagnosed in individuals under 20 years of age [8]. Among pediatric neoplasms [10], lymphomas are the most prevalent (59%), followed by RMS (13%), rhinopharyngeal cancer (5%), neuroblastoma (5%), soft tissue sarcoma (4.5%), salivary gland tumors (2.5%), and malignant teratomas [8].

RMS represents the most common soft tissue sarcoma in children, accounting for 4.5% of pediatric cancers [11,12], with an incidence of 6 cases per 1,000,000 annually [11]. The most frequently affected sites are the head and neck, genitourinary tract, and extremities [13]. Most cases are diagnosed by age 10, with a male-to-female ratio of 1.5:1 [8]. Head and neck RMS constitute approximately 40% of all RMS cases, and one-third of the cases involving the cephalic extremity invade the orbit [14]. Rare cases have also been reported of RMS localized to the skin of the nasal pyramid [15,16].

Additional case reports further illustrate the complexity of managing RMS in the sinonasal region. For example, a case documented by Liu et al. reported alveolar RMS metastasizing to the breast, highlighting the aggressive nature of the disease [17]. Another case by Watanapokasin et al. presented an unusual case of bilateral proptosis due to adult-onset alveolar RMS of the ethmoid sinus [18].

2. RMS Etiology

The etiology of RMS remains unclear, although genetic predisposition may be a contributing factor. Genetic anomalies associated with aRMS correlate with poorer clinical outcomes, highlighting the importance of genetic evaluation in guiding treatment strategies [19,20]. Li-Fraumeni syndrome, an autosomal dominant disorder associated with germline p53 mutations, is among the risk factors; affected individuals often have a family history of various carcinomas, particularly premenopausal breast cancer. Other cited risk factors include neurofibromatosis, radiation exposure, and maternal use of substances such as cocaine, marijuana, and alcohol during pregnancy [21].

3. RMS Classification

The World Health Organization (WHO) has recently updated staging and classification guidelines for rhabdomyosarcoma (RMS) [22]. Rhabdomyosarcoma (RMS) staging has been updated to incorporate advances in molecular diagnostics and a refined understanding of tumor biology, enabling more accurate risk stratification and personalized treatment. The WHO classification emphasizes the importance of detecting specific gene fusions, such as PAX3-FOXO1 in ARMS and NCOA2 rearrangements in spindle cell variants, to help differentiate RMS subtypes and predict patient outcomes. Genetic profiling is crucial for assessing the prognosis of RMS. For example, tumors with MYOD1 mutations or PAX-FOXO1 fusions tend to have a worse prognosis, while those with VGLL2 rearrangements in the spindle cell subtype often exhibit better clinical outcomes.

The World Health Organization (WHO) classification of rhabdomyosarcoma (RMS) has evolved to include distinct subtypes with updated genetic insights and clinical relevance [22]. The WHO classification now categorizes RMS into several types based on both histological and molecular features:

1. Embryonal Rhabdomyosarcoma (ERMS): This is the most common subtype, primarily affecting children. ERMS can be present in various forms, including botryoid and

diffuse types. The botryoid variant has a favorable prognosis, especially when it arises in mucosal-lined sites such as the bladder or vagina.

2. Alveolar Rhabdomyosarcoma (ARMS): Characterized by PAX3-FOXO1 or PAX7-FOXO1 gene fusions, ARMS is more aggressive than ERMS and is typically found in older children or adolescents. These tumors often have a worse prognosis due to the presence of these fusion genes, which disrupt normal cellular differentiation.
3. Spindle Cell/Sclerosing Rhabdomyosarcoma: This subtype is rare and is noted for its spindle-shaped cells and sclerotic background. It is most commonly found in the head and neck or extremities, with a predilection for the paratesticular region in pediatric patients.
   Spindle cell RMS can be further categorized based on genetic findings:
   - VGLL2 and NCOA2 rearrangements are typically seen in infantile cases, which tend to have a favorable prognosis.
   - MYOD1 mutations, more common in adolescents and adults, are associated with a poor prognosis.
   - The intraosseous variant, involving TFCP2::NCOA2 fusion genes, is an additional form that can be identified in bone tissues.
4. Pleomorphic Rhabdomyosarcoma: This subtype, mainly seen in adults, is characterized by pleomorphic tumor cells (irregular shapes and sizes). Pleomorphic RMS is associated with a poor prognosis due to its more aggressive clinical behavior [22].

1. Embryonal RMS
   - Description: Characterized by primitive, ovoid, or angulated spindle-shaped cells.
   - Histology: Scattered rhabdomyoblasts (cells showing skeletal muscle differentiation).
   - Variant: A subset may exhibit diffuse anaplasia, which is associated with worse prognosis.
   - Significance: It is the most common subtype in children and has a relatively favorable prognosis.
2. Alveolar RMS
   - Description: Composed of monotonous round cells.
   - Histology: May display a distinct alveolar pattern, resembling small clusters of cells in spaces ("alveoli").
   - Genetics: Often associated with fusion genes, such as PAX3-FOXO1 or PAX7-FOXO1, linked to a more aggressive course.
   - Significance: Typically seen in adolescents and young adults.
3. Spindle Cell RMS of MYOD1-mutated Type
   - Description: Features fascicles of spindle cells with areas of primitive round cells.
   - Histology: Dense sclerosis may be present, creating a pseudoalveolar pattern. Rare rhabdomyoblasts may be observed.
   - Genetics: Associated with MYOD1 mutations, which carry a poor prognosis.
   - Significance: This subtype differs from classic spindle cell RMS due to its molecular profile and aggressive behavior.
4. Osseous Spindle Cell RMS
   - Description: Histology ranges from mixed spindled to epithelioid, with less frequent pure spindled or epithelioid patterns.
   - Significance: This rare subtype highlights the morphological diversity of RMS, which can include areas mimicking bone formation.
5. Fusion-Driven Spindle Cell RMS
   - Description: A heterogeneous group with variable spindle cell morphology.

- Genetics: Defined by specific gene fusions, which influence its clinical and pathological behavior.
- Significance: This emerging category underscores the importance of molecular studies in diagnosing RMS.

6. Spindle Cell RMS, NOS (Not Otherwise Specified)
    - Description: Appears as a non-descript spindle cell sarcoma with rhabdomyoblastic differentiation.
    - Significance: Lack of distinct genetic or histological markers places it in this catch-all category.
7. Pleomorphic RMS
    - Description: Composed of large, pleomorphic rhabdomyoblasts.
    - Histology: Displays high-grade features with significant cellular atypia and pleomorphism.
    - Significance: Predominantly occurs in adults and has a poor prognosis.
8. Epithelioid RMS
    - Description: Features a distinct epithelioid morphology resembling carcinoma or melanoma.
    - Histology: A unique presentation of RMS with cells mimicking epithelial tumors.
    - Significance: Highlights the potential diagnostic challenges due to their resemblance to non-sarcomatous malignancies.
9. RMS Arising in Immature Rhabdomyoblastic Tumors (IRMT)
    - Description: Morphology ranges from epithelioid to rhabdoid or undifferentiated spindle to epithelioid cells.
    - Significance: Reflects RMS transformation in a previously identified precursor tumor type, potentially impacting clinical management.

This classification system captures the morphological diversity of RMS and integrates molecular features, aiding in tailored diagnostic and therapeutic approaches [22].

4. RMS in Differential Diagnoses

Among the various subtypes, alveolar RMS (ARMS) represents a significant clinical challenge due to its aggressive nature and potential for local invasion and metastasis [23,24]. In adults, RMS commonly arises in the deep soft tissues; however, it can originate in atypical sites such as the nasal cavity and paranasal sinuses, presenting unique diagnostic and therapeutic challenges [25,26].

The presentation of the nasal cavity or paranasal sinus RMS can be subtle and may mimic more common pathologies. Symptoms may include nasal obstruction, epistaxis, or facial swelling, which can delay diagnosis [24,26].

The presence of a tumor-like mass in the nasal region necessitates a comprehensive clinical and paraclinical evaluation to ensure optimal treatment outcomes [13]. Differential diagnoses must include various benign tumors such as papilloma, fibromyoma, chondroma, adenoma, glioma, neuroblastoma, and angiofibroma. Rapid growth and imaging studies, particularly CT scans showing invasion of adjacent structures, can help exclude many benign conditions. In pediatric cases, lymphoma is the most common malignant tumor affecting the nasal fossa.

Imaging studies, particularly MRI and CT scans, are crucial for assessing tumor extent and involvement of surrounding structures [17,27].

Computed Tomography (CT) is the initial imaging modality for patients with sinonasal pathology, particularly when evaluating persistent symptoms. It is indispensable for assessing bony structures, such as cortical destruction, remodeling, and sclerosis, associated with sinonasal malignancies. CT imaging is particularly effective for identifying aggressive bone destruction patterns (as in squamous cell carcinoma). In sinonasal lymphomas, CT reveals lobulated, hyperdense masses with variable bony involvement [28].

MRI excels in evaluating soft tissue details and tumor extensions, particularly into the skull base or intracranial structures. With superior contrast resolution, MRI helps differentiate tumor tissues from inflammation or post-obstructive secretions. Techniques like diffusion-weighted imaging (DWI) and apparent diffusion coefficient (ADC) mapping enhance MRI's ability to distinguish between benign and malignant sinonasal conditions. For instance, ADC values can help separate lymphomas and SCC from benign lesions [28].

Together, CT, MRI, and PET/CT offer a comprehensive tumor evaluation. While CT defines bone involvement and MRI highlights soft tissue characteristics, PET/CT assesses tumor metabolism, aiding in diagnosis, staging, and surveillance. This multimodality strategy enhances diagnostic accuracy and informs tailored treatment plans for sinonasal malignancies [29].

MRI plays a complementary role to CT, especially in specific clinical scenarios. It is advantageous for staging sinonasal masses, assessing anosmia, and identifying complications of sinusitis. MRI is particularly beneficial in imaging niche anatomical areas, such as the skull base, nasal vestibule, and olfactory niches, where CT may not provide adequate soft tissue detail [29].

On CT, sinonasal SCC appears as a soft tissue mass with bone destruction. MRI shows T1 iso intensity, T2 hypointensity, and variable enhancement, with larger tumors exhibiting heterogeneous signals due to necrosis or hemorrhage [30]. SCC often invades the skull base and cranial fossae and is best seen on contrast-enhanced, fat-suppressed T1 MRI [31]. Moderate to intense FDG uptake on 18F-FDG PET/CT supports diagnosis and staging [32].

Olfactory neuroblastoma (ONB) typically involves the cribriform plate, often with intracranial extension and a dumbbell shape. CT shows an expansile mass with bone erosion and occasional speckled calcifications or hyperostosis [33]. MRI reveals low T1 and high T2 signals with homogeneous or heterogeneous enhancement. Flow voids indicate high vascularity, and cystic changes may appear at the superior margins [30]. 18F-FDG PET/CT aids in detecting metastases and monitoring but shows no correlation between tumor grade and SUVmax [34].

Sinonasal adenocarcinoma shows isointense signals on T1-weighted MRI (T1WI) and variable T2-weighted MRI (T2WI) signals, depending on cellularity: high in paracellular tumors and intermediate in cellular ones [30]. Unlike SCC, which favors the maxillary antrum and nasal cavity, it typically originates in the ethmoid sinuses. Adenocarcinomas have more defined margins and muscular enhancement than SCCs [35]. 18F-FDG PET/CT is useful for staging and detecting recurrences, helping differentiate tumors from postoperative changes [36].

Primary sinonasal malignant melanoma (SNM) commonly appears as a well-defined polypoid mass on CT with smoothly marginated bony remodeling despite its aggressive nature. Contrast enhancement is variable, and melanin often causes T1 shortening, complicating characterization [30].

Amelanotic SNMs show low signal intensity on T1- and T2-weighted MRI [37]. Intense FDG uptake is typically observed on 18F-FDG PET/CT, especially in cases of recurrence or residual disease [38].

On non-contrast CT, sinonasal lymphomas appear as lobulated, slightly hyperdense masses with bone destruction or remodeling. Calcifications are rare, thin, and linear, typically reflecting sinus wall fragments rather than tumor calcification involvement. Contrast-enhanced CT highlights high cellularity with homogeneous enhancement, while necrosis is uncommon [30].

MRI shows isointense T1 signals with homogeneous enhancement and hypointense T2/STIR signals due to high cellularity. Low ADC values on DWI further reflect this feature [39]. Intense FDG uptake is a characteristic finding in PET imaging [40].

Sinonasal undifferentiated carcinoma (SNUC) typically appears as a large, destructive mass with ill-defined margins, bone destruction, and invasion of adjacent structures. CT imaging reveals irregular borders, aggressive bone destruction, and variable enhancement without calcifications [30]. On MRI, the tumor is isointense to muscle on T1WI and iso- to hyperintense on T2WI, with heterogeneous contrast enhancement [41].

SNUC demonstrates a significantly higher SUVmax on 18F-FDG PET/CT than esthesioneuroblastoma (ENB), reflecting its increased metabolic activity and aggressiveness.

Adenoid cystic carcinoma (ACC) commonly affects the maxillary antrum and nasal cavity, with a hallmark tendency for perineural spread, often involving trigeminal nerve branches in the pterygopalatine fossa. Lower-grade ACCs show homogeneous enhancement and bone remodeling, while higher-grade tumors display necrosis and destruction. MRI typically reveals intermediate T2 signal intensity, with low-grade tumors occasionally mimicking inflammatory tissue due to high T2 signal. Neural foraminal enlargement and abnormal perineural signals are key indicators of perineural invasion [30]. 18F-FDG PET/CT has limited utility due to ACC's low metabolic activity [42].

Chondrosarcoma, the most common sinonasal sarcoma, typically arises in the nasal septum and extends along the ethmoid bone to the skull base and palate [43]. CT shows a lobulated, heterogeneous mass with stippled chondroid calcifications and hypodensity due to the chondroid matrix [Articol Cristi]. MRI reveals a hyperintense T2 signal, hypointense T1 signal, and signal voids from calcifications. Contrast-enhanced imaging highlights a heterogeneous enhancement pattern, with the avascular chondroid matrix remaining unchanged [44].

Osteosarcomas in the sinonasal region may be primary or extend from adjacent areas. CT typically shows bone destruction with a soft tissue mass; sclerosis is seen in up to 75% of cases, though the classic sunburst periosteal reaction is often absent. MRI reveals low T1 and intermediate T2 signals, influenced by the tumor's mineral content, and is effective for assessing intramedullary and extraosseous spread [Articol Cristi]. FDG uptake on PET/CT varies with histological grade, with high-grade sarcomas exhibiting more significant FDG accumulation [45].

Sinonasal rhabdomyosarcoma often involves lymph nodes and metastasizes to the lungs and bones [40]. On CT, it appears homogeneous with bone remodeling and destruction. MRI shows isointense T1 and hyperintense T2 signals with moderate to substantial enhancement [30]. While its imaging features, such as homogeneity and skull involvement, are not specific, a lower ADC value can help differentiate it from squamous cell carcinoma, reflecting the tumor's undifferentiated microstructure [46,47].

Juvenile nasal angiofibroma, a highly vascular malformation in young males (15–25 years), typically presents with epistaxis and unilateral nasal obstruction [44]. CT and MRI reveal posterior maxillary antrum bending, pterygopalatine fossa enlargement with bone erosion, and avid enhancement [48]. MRI shows intermediate T1 and intermediate-high T2 signals, with flow voids confirming their vascular nature [30].

Inverted papilloma is a locally aggressive benign tumor often originating from the lateral nasal wall near the middle meatus, sometimes extending to the maxillary antrum [49]. CT reveals a soft tissue mass, occasionally with intratumoral calcifications and focal hyperostosis at the attachment site. MRI shows a convoluted cerebriform pattern on post-contrast T1WI [50], with hypointense epithelium and hyperintense edematous stroma on T2WI [51].

Coexistent squamous cell carcinoma, present in 5–7% of cases, is suggested by necrosis, bone destruction, or loss of cerebriform enhancement. 18F-FDG PET/CT can aid in identifying malignancy through focal increased FDG uptake [52].

Sinonasal schwannomas are benign, slow-growing nerve sheath tumors, typically appearing as well-circumscribed, ovoid soft tissue masses. Larger lesions may show cystic degeneration. On CT, subtle hyperdense areas reflect Antoni A tissue, while adjacent bone remodeling without destruction is paramount [30]. MRI reveals intermediate T1 and variable T2 signals, with contrast enhancement occasionally displaying a characteristic whorled pattern [53].

Osteoma, the most common benign sinonasal tumor, often occurs in the frontal sinus and is usually an incidental finding. On CT, cortical osteomas appear homogeneously dense, while cancellous osteomas may display heterogeneous density or a "ground-glass" pattern, sometimes resembling fibrous dysplasia. MRI typically shows low-to-intermediate signal intensity with no enhancement of the osseous contents, though fibrous tissue may enhance post-contrast [30]. Diagnosis is often aided by patient history or prior imaging studies.

Fibrous dysplasia is a fibro-osseous disorder commonly affecting craniofacial bones [30]. On CT, it may present as heterogeneous osseous and fibrous tissue or exhibit a classic "ground-glass" appearance [54]. MRI reveals variable signals, typically hypointense on T1 and T2, with intense post-contrast enhancement [55]. On 18F-FDG PET/CT, fibrous tissue may show hypermetabolic activity.

Inflammatory myofibroblastic tumor, a rare sinonasal lesion incidentally diagnosed, often mimics malignant tumors like SCC [56]. CT shows bone erosion with sclerosis, unlike malignant tumors exhibiting erosion and destruction. MRI reveals hypointense signals on T1 and T2, with substantial gadolinium enhancement [57]. Differentiating features in imaging are crucial for diagnosis.

Sinonasal hemangiopericytomas often originate from the nasal septum and turbinates, blending with surrounding structures due to substantial enhancement on contrast imaging [58]. CT may reveal a "soap bubble" or "honeycomb" appearance. MRI shows hypointense T1, hyperintense T2 signals, and avid enhancement, with intratumoral flow voids as a characteristic finding [59].

Histopathological diagnosis is confirmed through biopsy and immunohistochemical analysis, where myoglobin, Myo D1, and myogenin are specific markers for RMS [60].

For instance, Torres-Peña et al. documented two cases of alveolar RMS originating in the nasal cavity with orbital extension, emphasizing the aggressive nature of these tumors in adults and the importance of considering RMS in differential diagnoses [23,61]. Similarly, a review by Ahmed and Tsokos noted that RMS in the sinonasal region presents unique challenges, particularly due to the prevalence of the alveolar subtype and the poor prognosis associated with these tumors [26].

Recent studies have also identified characteristic imaging features of sinonasal RMS [62]. Zeng et al. analyzed MRI findings in eleven cases, noting bone destruction and multifocal sinus involvement [63]. This underscores the importance of advanced imaging techniques in diagnosing RMS.

In terms of differential diagnosis, we should include benign tumors such as papilloma, fibromyoma, chondroma, adenoma, glioma or neuroblastoma, and angiofibroma. The macroscopic aspect of the tumor, rapid growth (within a few months), and imagistic (CT/CBCT), which show the invasion of the neighboring structures, exclude most of the above [64]. Out of the malignant tumors of the nasal fossa in the child, lymphoma is the most common.

Knowing that lymphoma responds to chemotherapy, it can be put up for discussion whether it was necessary to just perform the biopsy without removing the mass to establish the right course of treatment.

5. RMS Treatment Options and Survival Rates

The TNM staging of RMS is crucial before treatment and is determined by tumor size and location, local invasion, lymph node involvement, and metastasis [65]. Metastatic RMS presents significant challenges due to its resistance to standard treatments and its ability to evade the body's natural immune responses, necessitating the exploration of innovative therapeutic strategies [66]. Risk assessment is essential to tailor treatment intensity based on tumor location, presence of residual tumor post-resection, histological type, lymph node involvement, and metastasis [67,68].

For over three decades, the standard treatment protocol for RMS in Europe has consisted of a six-month chemotherapy regimen. The European Pediatric Soft Tissue Sarcoma Study Group (EpSSG) has evaluated whether extending treatment with maintenance chemotherapy could improve outcomes [69].

Management of RMS in the nasal cavity and paranasal sinuses requires a multimodal approach that typically includes surgery, chemotherapy, and radiation therapy. Historically, the role of surgery has been limited due to anatomical challenges and the significant role of systemic therapy. However, recent studies indicate that surgical intervention may improve outcomes, particularly in localized cases [25,26,63].

Surgical removal of the tumor and chemotherapy or a combination of both remains the mainstay treatment. A complete resection is achieved by resecting the tumor along with a 0.5 cm rim of normal tissue around it [70,71].

Kana et al. explored the outcomes of surgical management in patients with sinonasal RMS, highlighting that those who underwent surgical resection had improved distant metastasis-free survival compared to those who did not [25]. Moreover, Nayak et al. reported a rare case of alveolar RMS in the paranasal sinus with cervical metastasis, managed through a combination of surgery and chemoradiotherapy [24].

The role of chemotherapy is paramount, particularly in advanced cases. Chemotherapeutic regimens are often tailored based on histological subtype and clinical staging [17,18]. In children and adolescents, Machavoine et al. emphasized that younger patients and those with certain molecular features had better outcomes, indicating the importance of personalized treatment strategies [27].

Taking into account certain aspects like tumor location, stage, and age of the patient, the treatment of RMS is multimodal and individualized. It can be surgical, radiological, and chemotherapeutic.

Radiotherapy is reserved for patients who develop recurrence following completion of initial treatment. The duration of the chemotherapy is determined by the stage of the disease at the time of presentation [71].

5.1. Surgical Approach

Management of RMS involves a multimodal approach tailored to the individual patient, considering tumor location, stage, and age. Surgical excision is the first step, categorized into four clinical groups based on residual disease:

- group 1—The tumor is completely removed;
- group 2—Microscopic residual tumor tissue, invasive loco-regional ganglia, or both;
- group 3—High residual tumor tissue;
- group 4—Distant metastases.

Surgical treatment of RMS depends on the tumor site—It is advised to completely remove the mass if it is possible without causing lesions to impede the function of surrounding organs or disfiguring the patient [25].

Tumor excision is recommended even if there are metastases.

Under ideal conditions, RMS resection should be made 2 cm from the edge of the tumor. In the case of tumors with head localization and especially in children, this limit cannot be met, and resection is recommended at 0.5 cm from the tumor [21]. The resection margins should be noted and sent for histopathological examination in order to have precise evidence of areas where the tumor was not completely resected. They must be marked with titanium clips for targeted irradiation and possibly for reintervention.

Kainhofer et al. evaluated the prognostic significance of margin status in soft tissue sarcoma (STS) patients undergoing curative surgery [72]. Their findings indicated that margin status is an independent factor influencing local recurrence (LR). Specifically, local control rates were higher in cases with a minimal resection margin of 1 mm or more (classified as R0 by UICC standards) compared to margins less than 1 mm (classified as R0 under the R-classification) [73]. Outcomes were notably better for patients who underwent "complete primary resection" compared to those with "incomplete surgery" [74–76].

While a 5 mm surgical margin is often considered an optimal target, achieving such margins may not be feasible or necessary in all anatomical regions or in pediatric patients [73].

The ability to perform en bloc resections with wide margins is highly dependent on the tumor's location, as well as the patient's age and size. In anatomically challenging areas, such as the head and neck, achieving completely negative microscopic margins remains particularly difficult [77].

The surgical stage, when indicated, plays a vital role in treatment stratification, local control, and outcome [42]. The surgeon is assessing the risk of the treatment, he is monitoring the tumor growth and site aspect, and implicitly he contributes to the outcome of the treatment.

Within head and neck localizations, ARMS generally originates within the inferior orbit. For all head and neck RMS, a biopsy is required for diagnostic confirmation. Resection may be limited by the inability to obtain an adequate margin; therefore, the success of resection is heavily dependent on location and resection possibilities [78].

5.2. Radiotherapy Treatment

The patients with post-op residual macroscopic tumor tissue will undergo postoperative radiotherapy. Radiotherapy alone is not capable of destroying macroscopic lesions, while moderate-dose irradiation reduces the risk of local–regional relapse.

Concerns about the long-term toxicity of radiotherapy in children complicate its acceptance by caregivers. The prognosis for children with residual disease is poor without radiotherapy. Pappo [79] estimates a 20% 5-year survival rate in patients with embryonal RMS of group II–III who relapsed and 3% in patients of group III–IV who have relapsed in cases of alveolar RMS. Unfortunately, radiotherapy is not performed in over 40% of patients with RMS [79].

Irradiation will need to be individualized and optimized considering the tumor site and age. The radiation dose is different from author to author. According to risk factors, the American School divides patients into three groups:

- Group I—36 Gy;
- Group II—41.4 Gy;
- Group III—50.4 Gy after lesion extension [8].

The European School applies lower doses of irradiation depending on tumor histology [8]. In patients with microscopic disease, it is intended that in the future, the optimal dose and volume for the affected area should be standardized according to histology, site, and age [80,81].

Proton radiotherapy has been used with good results in a study between 1987 and 2014 on 55 patients, 35 males and 20 females, with a mean age of 5 years and a 1 to 2-year overall survival of 91.9% [82]. Another possibility is brachytherapy [83].

PET-MRI is used to study metabolic imaging using both 2-deoxy-[18 F]-fluoro-D-glucose [18 F] FDG to specify tumor size and activity [84,85].

Numerous studies have found that FDG-PET is a sensitive and specific tool in the clinical determination of disease extension in childhood sarcomas, especially when combined with CT [78,86,87].

Extension of restricted diffusion in RMS in children and hypermetabolic overlap with restricted MRI/PET diffusion demonstrated their prognostic value, indicating an unfavorable prognosis [61,88].

5.3. Chemotherapy Treatment

Standard medical treatment consists of vincristine-based chemotherapy, actinomycin D, and cyclophosphamide [11].

The duration of chemotherapy and dosing of cyclophosphamide is assessed according to the risk of the disease and the response to the treatment, thus limiting the toxicity of the treatment [71].

New therapeutic agents, as well as molecular therapies, are being tested in high-risk patients [89,90].

For the European Scaffolding Group of soft tissue (EpSSG), the standard treatment for RMS is ifosfamide, vincristine, and actinomycin-D [91,92].

Ifosfamide is preferred to cyclophosphamide because it is associated with lower gonadal toxicity.

In the European treatment guidelines, the following three chemotherapy courses are evaluated [93] as follows:

- Complete response—No measurable tumor;
- Good response—Reducing tumor volume by 2/3 compared to the initial volume;
- Poor response—Reduction of tumor volume >1/3 and <2/3 from the initial volume;
- Objective response—Reduction of tumor volume >1/3 compared to an initial volume;
- Progressive disease—The Volume increases >1/3 or new lesions appear.

The purpose of this assessment is to increase chemotherapy in children whose tumor reduction is below 50% [93]. According to US protocols [11], intensification of chemotherapy, according to the data provided by this guide, does not correlate with prognosis. Higher-than-needed doses of chemotherapy can have adverse effects, some also located in the orofacial region [94].

Studies with other chemotherapeutic agents such as doxorubicin [95], ifosfamide with or without etoposide [95], or topotecan [96] do not improve the progression of patients with medium-grade RMS.

Arndt [89], in a recent article, discusses the experience of 50 years of study of RMS on both sides of the Atlantic:

- It is desirable to decrease or omit the alkylating therapy;
- Doxorubicin does not improve prognosis in those at high risk;
- high dose chemotherapy and stem cells do not improve prognosis in those at high risk;
- In the USA, vincristine, actinomycin, and cyclophosphamide remain an important part of the therapy;
- In Europe, the alkylating agent is ifosfamide;

- High-risk patients with the worst prognosis have not improved their prognosis against the 1972 trial;
- Increasing the dose received to be aggressive and decreasing the risk of relapse should be considered, provided it is not possible to identify a priori children with a high risk of relapse.

5.4. Survival Rates

Several factors can influence the survival rates of patients with RMS, such as age at diagnosis, tumor subtype and size, primary site, disease stage and clinical group, and treatment methods. The advances in therapy regimens over the past years have raised the overall 5-year survival rate in pediatric patients to over 70%. Still, the numbers remain low for high-risk RMS and recurrent disease [97]. Furthermore, the percentages published by the Intergroup Rhabdomyosarcoma Study Group (IRSG) based on clinical trials can differ from those from population-based cancer registries due to restrictive inclusion criteria [98].

As previously mentioned, the primary treatment modality is complete surgical resection of the tumor. The IRSG/COG (Intergroup Rhabdomyosarcoma Study Group/Children's Oncology Group) stated that operability was the most significant factor affecting patient survival, with completely resected localized tumors associated with a survival rate of 87% [99].

Tumors less than 5 cm, with no evidence of regional lymph node involvement or distant metastases, have a better prognosis [100]. For a tumor 10 cm in diameter, the survival rate is reduced. Because most RMS lesions are not spherical but irregular in shape, there was a debate regarding the informative value of tumor size vs. tumor volume evaluation for a patient's prognosis. Ferrari et al. addressed this issue and concluded that assessing tumor size from one or three dimensions provided a similar prognostic value [101].

Adjuvant chemotherapy and radiotherapy can be recommended to enhance outcomes. Yang et al. designed a prognostic nomogram based on the records of 1679 RMS pediatric patients to predict patient outcomes. They observed that surgery has significantly increased the survival rate ($p < 0.001$), and radiotherapy was also significantly associated with a better prognosis, but to a much lesser extent [98]. The advanced radiotherapy techniques available (protons, brachytherapy, and rotational intensity-modulated radiotherapy) have contributed to significant improvements in outcomes, as reported by the European Paediatric Soft Tissue Sarcoma Group (EpSSG). However, there are still cases where this approach is ineffective [102].

6. Our Experience—Case Report

CR, an 8-year-old male from a rural area, presents with predominantly left nasal obstruction, purulent rhinorrhea, recurrent epistaxis, and headache. He is under endocrinology surveillance for a chronic adrenogenital syndrome, treated with prednisone (4 mg/day). Symptoms began in 2017, leading to hospitalization in January 2018 at the Pediatric Hospital in Iasi. During hospitalization, antibiotic therapy (Xifia 5 mL every 12 h), mucolytics, and intravenous calcium were initiated. Due to persistent symptoms, a CT scan was performed, and an ENT consultation was sought. Correlating the ENT clinical examination with symptomatology and CT findings, the patient was referred to the ENT department of the Clinical Rehabilitation Hospital for further evaluation and surgical intervention.

Clinical examination revealed a mass in the left nasal fossa that completely obstructed the cavity. The tumor appeared violet, was covered in purulent secretions, and exhibited adherence with bleeding upon palpation. The right nasal fossa contained muco-purulent secretions but no mucosal abnormalities, with a posterior view of the mass occupying the entire opening. Nasal and sinus endoscopy highlights the same issues: a violet mass covered with secretions and puss blocking the left nasal fossa, without invasion in the nasal fossa structures (septum, floor, or lateral wall), and without ulcerations on the mucosal surfaces. Access to the rinopharynx is difficult and reveals a mass that completely obstructs the choane with apparent origin from the superior wall of the rinopharynx. The overlying mucosa with smooth, without ulcerations, but with multiple pink-reddish fleshy polyp-like hypertrophy.

CT imaging revealed a soft tissue mass measuring 72 mm × 42 mm × 22 mm with reduced contrast enhancement, extending from the left nasal fossa into the nasopharynx, posterior wall, and ethmoid cells on the left side, as well as into the left maxillary sinus and posterior part of the right nasal fossa, ultimately occupying the sphenoid sinus. The nasal septum appeared discontinuous in the posterior third. A latero-cervical ultrasound excluded lymph node involvement. CBC results were normal, while coagulation tests indicated minor alterations.

To obtain a biopsy of the lesion, surgical excision of the bulk of the tumor occupying the nasal fossa and nasopharynx was necessary to detect and reach the insertion point. A biopsy sample was sent for extemporaneous examination. While awaiting the result, the paranasal sinuses were accessed, and maxillary antrostomy, ethmoidectomy, sphenoidectomy, and excision of the abnormal-looking tissue from the inferior part of the sphenoid floor were performed. The posterior part of the nasal septum was found to be soft, likely due to compression from the tumor. However, no visible mucosal involvement was observed, possibly because the posterior bony part had thinned under pressure.

The extemporaneous examination suggested a high-grade non-Hodgkin lymphoma (B.A.P. 27855/9. January 2018).

The surgical interventions were deemed necessary for several reasons: obtaining a biopsy close to the insertion point required intubation of the patient; regardless of the biopsy findings, surgical management of the polisinusitis was essential; and excision of the abnormal tissue provided benefits for both immediate and long-term patient outcomes.

All excised tissue was sent for histopathological exam. Further immunohistochemical analysis was conducted to confirm and differentiate the tumor subtype from other morphologically similar malignancies (Figure 1). Although the initial findings suggested non-Hodgkin lymphoma, subsequent tests ruled it out and established the definitive diagnosis of high-grade alveolar rhabdomyosarcoma (RMS) (ICD-O 8920/3).

Chemotherapy was initiated, and following nine rounds, a post-therapeutic MRI indicated minimal inflammatory lesions in the left maxillary sinus mucosa and several ethmoid cells bilaterally.

Post-chemotherapeutic rhinosinusal endoscopy only reveals the presence of mucus in the maxillary sinus and discrete diffuse edema of the nasal mucosa without any local tumor recurrence. Follow-up evaluations were conducted annually, with the most recent assessment in 2024 (6 years after treatment) showing no evidence of tumor recurrence in the rhinopharynx and paranasal sinuses. Endoscopic examination revealed no scarring, stenosis, or mucosal retention (Figure 2). PET CT at 5 years showed no signs of disease persistence.

In this case, the necessity for tumor ablation is underscored by several factors. The tumor caused nasal obstruction and blocked the sinuses that were already suffering, and for the biopsy to be conclusive under conditions of such a large and brittle mass, it was necessary to remove the tumor from its insertion site.

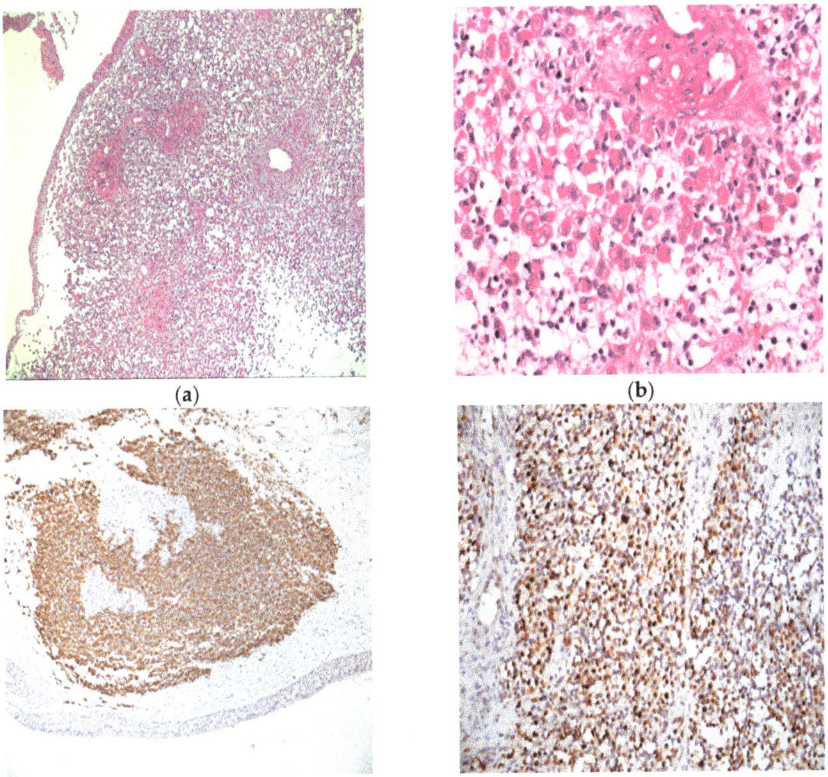

(a) (b) (c) (d)

Figure 1. Histopathology aspect with different colors and magnification (**a**) RMS, HE, ×100, overview, rhabdomyoblastic proliferation with solid pattern, mucosa on a slope (**b**) RMS alveolar, HE, ×400, detail rhabdomyoblast; (**c**) Desmin, ×100, positive diffuse in the tumor; (**d**) Myogenin, ×200, diffuse positive in most cells (nuclear marker).

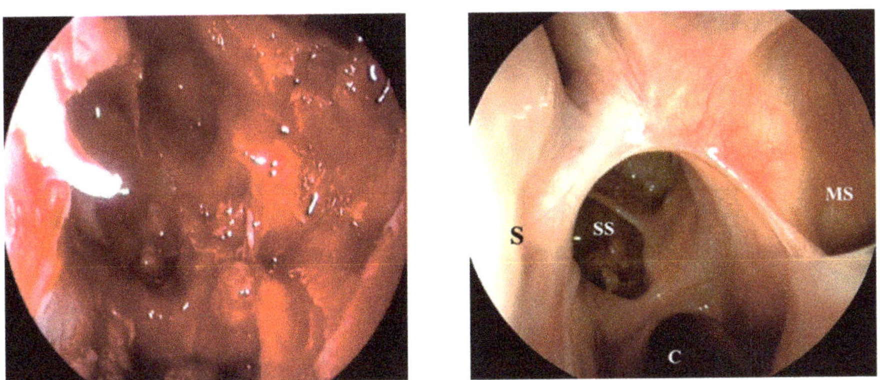

(a) (b)

Figure 2. Endoscopic view at the moment of surgery and at the 6 years follow-up. (**a**) Intraoperative endoscopic image of left nasal fossae and sphenoid sinus; (**b**) follow-up visit at 6 years show cavum (C), septum (S), sphenoid sinus (SS), and maxillary sinus (MS).

The initial result of the histopathological exam was lymphoma, due to which chemotherapy would have been recommended.

Further histochemical examination of the tumor established the diagnosis of RMS.

In the case we presented, the treatment consisted of three rounds of vincristine, actinomycin-D, and cyclophosphamide.

Endoscopic evaluation one month after completing three rounds of chemotherapy could be considered positive regarding the fact that there were no macroscopic signs of tumor recurrence.

However, given that an alveolar RMS has a worse prognosis compared to the embryonal one, radiation therapy is recommended with reassessment after a month. A 3-month basis endoscopic examination and MRI for further follow-up is advised.

The prognosis for this patient remains reserved due to tumor size (tumors larger than 5 cm with a poor prognosis) and histopathological type (alveolar RMS). Recent follow-up has shown disease-free outcomes at 6 years of check-up.

Diagnosis is determined by anatomopathological examination and will be followed by radical surgery, radio, and chemotherapy

7. Conclusions

Alveolar RMS is a rare tumor encountered in the pediatric population. High suspicion is needed in diagnosing this condition in the early stages.

RMS in children should be taken into account whenever a patient is referred for a vegetative tumor in the rhinopharynx or nasal fossa.

Prognosis is reserved and depends on correct evaluation and early treatment. Rigorous follow-up is mandatory and will discover reoccurrences earlier allowing better treatment prognosis.

RMS presents significant challenges in pediatric management, necessitating a coordinated approach involving surgical intervention, radiotherapy, and chemotherapy. Individualized treatment plans are essential to optimize outcomes while minimizing long-term toxicity. Ongoing surveillance through imaging and endoscopic evaluation is crucial for early detection of recurrence, given the complex nature of this malignancy.

Author Contributions: Conceptualization, D.M. and C.M.; methodology, Ș.D.T.; software, A.J.; validation, D.M., L.R. and C.M.; formal analysis, Ș.D.T.; investigation, D.F.; resources, C.M.; data curation, L.R.; writing—original draft preparation, I.M.; writing—review and editing, I.M.; visualization, C.M.; supervision, A.J.; project administration, Ș.D.T. All authors have read and agreed to the published version of the manuscript.

Funding: This research received no external funding.

Institutional Review Board Statement: Ethical approval is deemed unnecessary by The Clinical Rehabilitation Hospital Board as this is a single rare case faced during clinical practice.

Informed Consent Statement: Written informed consent was obtained from the patient's parents for publication of this case report and any accompanying images.

Conflicts of Interest: The authors declare no conflicts of interest.

References

1. Huang, Y.-L.; Tseng, C.-F.; Yang, L.-K.; Tsai, C.-H. Rhabdomyosarcoma of the Adult Nasopharynx A Case Report. *J. Intern. Med. Taiwan* **2005**, *16*, 146–150.
2. Ricker, C.A.; Woods, A.D.; Simonson, W.; Lathara, M.; Srinivasa, G.; Rudzinski, E.R.; Mansoor, A.; Irwin, R.G.; Keller, C.; Berlow, N.E. Refractory alveolar rhabdomyosarcoma in an 11-year-old male. *Cold Spring Harb. Mol. Case Stud.* **2021**, *7*, a005983. [CrossRef]

3. Hettmer, S.; Linardic, C.M.; Kelsey, A.; Rudzinski, E.R.; Vokuhl, C.; Selfe, J.; Ruhen, O.; Shern, J.F.; Khan, J.; Kovach, A.R.; et al. Molecular testing of rhabdomyosarcoma in clinical trials to improve risk stratification and outcome: A consensus view from European paediatric Soft tissue sarcoma Study Group, Children's Oncology Group and Cooperative Weichteilsarkom-Studiengruppe. *Eur. J. Cancer* **2022**, *172*, 367–386. [CrossRef]
4. Ruymann, F.B. Rhabdomyosarcoma in children and adolescents: A review. *Hematol./Oncol. Clin. N. Am.* **1987**, *1*, 621–654. [CrossRef]
5. Pack, G.T.; Eberhart, W.F. Rhabdomyosarcoma of skeletal muscle; report of 100 cases. *Surgery* **1952**, *32*, 1023. [PubMed]
6. Cleary, M.M.; Mansoor, A.; Settelmeyer, T.; Ijiri, Y.; Ladner, K.J.; Svalina, M.N.; Rubin, B.P.; Guttridge, D.C.; Keller, C. NFkappaB signaling in alveolar rhabdomyosarcoma. *Dis. Models Mech.* **2017**, *10*, 1109–1115. [CrossRef]
7. Ohkawa, T.; Nishimura, A.; Kosaki, K.; Aoki-Nogami, Y.; Tomizawa, D.; Kashimada, K.; Morio, T.; Kato, M.; Mizutani, S.; Takagi, M. PAX3/7-FOXO1 fusion-negative alveolar rhabdomyosarcoma in Schuurs-Hoeijmakers syndrome. *J. Hum. Genet.* **2022**, *67*, 51–54. [CrossRef]
8. Rosen, E.J.; Deskin, R.W. Pediatric Head and Neck Malignancies. In *Grand Rounds Presentation*; UTMB Department of Otolaryngology: Chamonix, France, 2003.
9. Choudhary, P.; Sharma, S.; Singh, A.; Agarwal, S.; Singhal, P.; Singh, Y. Primary Alveolar Rhabdomyosarcoma of the Thyroid: A Case Report. *Indian J. Otolaryngol. Head Neck Surg.* **2024**, *76*, 3676–3678. [CrossRef]
10. Bassi, A.; Zamma Gallarati, B.; Sardi, I.; Guidi, M.; Caporalini, C.; Pelosi, P.; de Martino, M. Alveolar rhabdomyosarcoma in a 6-month-old boy. *Arch. Dis. Child.* **2018**, *103*, 95. [CrossRef]
11. Dasgupta, R.; Fuch, J.; Rodeberg, D. Rhabdomyosarcoma, Review. *Semin. Pediatr. Surg.* **2016**, *25*, 276–283. [CrossRef]
12. Hu, Y.; He, Z.; Liu, S.; Ying, W.; Chen, Y.; Zhao, M.; He, M.; Wu, X.; Tang, Y.; Gu, W.; et al. Patient-derived rhabdomyosarcoma cells recapitulate the genetic and transcriptomic landscapes of primary tumors. *iScience* **2024**, *27*, 110862. [CrossRef] [PubMed]
13. Jawad, N.; McHugh, K. The clinical and radiologic features of paediatric rhabdomyosarcoma. *Pediatr. Radiol.* **2019**, *49*, 1516–1523. [CrossRef] [PubMed]
14. Healy, J.N.; Borg, M.F. Paediatric nasopharyngeal rhabdomyosarcoma: A case series and literature review. *J. Med. Imaging Radiat. Oncol.* **2010**, *54*, 388–394. [CrossRef] [PubMed]
15. Chen, J.; Zhang, F.; Wang, L.; Sun, D.; Chen, X. Alveolar Rhabdomyosarcoma of the Nasal Dorsum of a Pediatric Patient: A Case Report. *Ear Nose Throat J.* 2023, *online ahead of print*. [CrossRef]
16. Larson, J.H.; Rutledge, R.; Hunnell, L.; Choi, D.K.; Kellogg, R.G.; Naran, S. Nasal Embryonal Rhabdomyosarcoma in the Pediatric Population: Literature Review and Report of Midline Presentation. *Plast. Reconstr. Surg. Glob. Open* **2021**, *9*, e3534. [CrossRef]
17. Liu, H.; Zhao, W.; Huang, M.; Zhou, X.; Gong, Y.; Lu, Y. Alveolar rhabdomyosarcoma of nasopharynx and paranasal sinuses with metastasis to breast in a middle-aged woman: A case report and literature review. *Int. J. Clin. Exp. Pathol.* **2015**, *8*, 15316–15321.
18. Watanapokasin, N.; Phattraprayoon, N.; Limsiri, T.; Tungyingyong, P.; Ungtrakul, T. Bilateral Proptosis as an Unusual Presentation of Adult-Onset Alveolar-Type Rhabdomyosarcoma of Ethmoid Sinus: A Case Report. *Case Rep. Oncol.* **2022**, *15*, 783–791. [CrossRef]
19. Okuno, K.; Kawaba, D.; Maejima, A.; Kakee, S.; Namba, N. A high-risk alveolar rhabdomyosarcoma case with Duchenne muscular dystrophy. *Pediatr. Int.* **2022**, *64*, e14754. [CrossRef]
20. Tarakanova, A.V.; Sharlay, A.S.; Konovalov, D.M. Alveolar rhabdomyosarcoma: Novel surrogate markers associated with oncogenic translocation. *Arkhiv Patol.* **2023**, *85*, 10–15. [CrossRef]
21. Rodeberg, D.A.; Paidas, C.N.; Lobe, T.L.; Brown, K.; Andrassy, R.J.; Crist, W.M.; Wiener, E.S. Surgical Principles for Children/Adolescents With Newly Diagnosed Rhabdomyosarcoma: A Report from the Soft Tissue Sarcoma Committee of the Children's Oncology Group. *Sarcoma* **2002**, *6*, 111–122. [CrossRef]
22. Dehner, C.A.; Rudzinski, E.R.; Davis, J.L. Rhabdomyosarcoma: Updates on classification and the necessity of molecular testing beyond immunohistochemistry. *Hum. Pathol.* **2024**, *147*, 72–81. [CrossRef] [PubMed]
23. Torres-Peña, J.L.; Castrillo, A.I.R.; Mencía-Gutiérrez, E.; Gutiérrez-Díaz, E.; Rodríguez-Peralto, J.L.; Bengoa-González, Á. Nasal Cavity or Alveolar Paranasal Sinus Rhabdomyosarcoma with Orbital Extension in Adults: 2 Cases. *Plast. Reconstr. Surg. Glob. Open* **2015**, *8*, e414. [CrossRef] [PubMed]
24. Nayak, D.R.; Balakrishnan, R.; Shahab, A.S.; Rao, L. Alveolar rhabdomyosarcoma of paranasal sinus with cervical metastasis-a case report. *Indian J. Otolaryngol. Head Neck Surg.* **2000**, *52*, 162–165. [CrossRef] [PubMed]
25. Kana, L.A.; Smith, J.D.; Bellile, E.L.; Chugh, R.; McKean, E.L. Surgical Management of Rhabdomyosarcoma of the Nasal Cavity and Paranasal Sinuses: Analysis of Operative Indications, Settings, and Outcomes. *J. Neurol. Surg. B Skull Base* **2021**, *83*, 350–358. [CrossRef]
26. Ahmed, A.A.; Tsokos, M. Sinonasal rhabdomyosarcoma in children and young adults. *Int. J. Surg. Pathol.* **2007**, *15*, 160–165. [CrossRef]

27. Machavoine, R.; Helfre, S.; Bernier, V.; Bolle, S.; Leseur, J.; Corradini, N.; Rome, A.; Defachelles, A.-S.; Deneuve, S.; Bernard, S.; et al. Locoregional Control and Survival in Children, Adolescents, and Young Adults with Localized Head and Neck Alveolar Rhabdomyosarcoma—The French Experience. *Front. Pediatr.* **2022**, *9*, 783754. [CrossRef]
28. Ozturk, K.; Gawande, R.; Gencturk, M.; Boegel, K.; Caicedo-Granados, E.; Cayci, Z. Imaging features of sinonasal tumors on positron emission tomography and magnetic resonance imaging including diffusion weighted imaging: A pictorial review. *Clin. Imaging* **2018**, *51*, 217–228. [CrossRef]
29. Pulickal, G.G.; Navaratnam, A.V.; Nguyen, T.; Dragan, A.D.; Dziedzic, M.; Lingam, R.K.; Pulickal, G.G.; Navaratnam, A.V.; Nguyen, T.; Dragan, A.D.; et al. Imaging Sinonasal disease with MRI: Providing insight over and above CT. *Eur. J. Radiol.* **2018**, *102*, 157–168. [CrossRef]
30. Tiwari, R.; Hardillo, J.A.; Mehta, D.; Slotman, B.; Tobi, H.; Croonenburg, E.; van der Waal, I.; Snow, G.B. Squamous cell carcinoma of maxillary sinus. *Head Neck* **2000**, *22*, 164–169. [CrossRef]
31. Hermans, R.; De Vuysere, S.; Marchal, G. Squamous cell carcinoma of the sinonasal cavities. *Semin. Ultrasound CT MR* **1999**, *20*, 150–161. [CrossRef]
32. Paidpally, V.; Chirindel, A.; Lam, S.; Agrawal, N.; Quon, H.; Subramaniam, R.M. FDG-PET/CT imaging biomarkers in head and neck squamous cell carcinoma. *Imaging Med.* **2012**, *4*, 633–647. [CrossRef] [PubMed]
33. Dulguerov, P.; Allal, A.S.; Calcaterra, T.C. Esthesioneuroblastoma: A meta-analysis and review. *Lancet Oncol.* **2001**, *2*, 683–690. [CrossRef] [PubMed]
34. Broski, S.M.; Hunt, C.H.; Johnson, G.B.; Subramaniam, R.M.; Peller, P.J. The added value of ^{18}F-FDG PET/CT for evaluation of patients with esthesioneuroblastoma. *J. Nucl. Med.* **2012**, *53*, 1200–1206. [CrossRef] [PubMed]
35. Raghavan, P.; Phillips, C.D. Magnetic resonance imaging of sinonasal malignancies. *Top. Magn. Reson. Imaging* **2007**, *18*, 259–267. [CrossRef] [PubMed]
36. Maroldi, R.; Ravanelli, M.; Farina, D.; Facchetti, L.; Bertagna, F.; Lombardi, D.; Nicolai, P. Posttreatment evaluation of paranasal sinuses after treatment of sinonasal neoplasms. *Neuroimaging Clin. N. Am.* **2015**, *25*, 667–685. [CrossRef]
37. Yoshioka, H.; Kamada, T.; Kandatsu, S.; Koga, M.; Yoshikawa, K.; Matsuoka, Y.; Mizoe, J.; Itai, Y.; Tsujii, H. MRI of mucosal malignant melanoma of the head and neck. *J. Comput. Assist. Tomogr.* **1998**, *22*, 492–497. [CrossRef]
38. Haerle, S.K.; Soyka, M.B.; Fischer, D.R.; Murer, K.; Strobel, K.; Huber, G.F.; Holzmann, D. The value of ^{18}F-FDG-PET/CT imaging for sinonasal malignant melanoma. *Eur. Arch. Otorhinolaryngol.* **2011**, *269*, 127–133. [CrossRef]
39. Ichikawa, Y.; Sumi, M.; Sasaki, M.; Sumi, T.; Nakamura, T. Efficacy of diffusion-weighted imaging for the differentiation between lymphomas and carcinomas of the nasopharynx and oropharynx: Correlations of apparent diffusion coefficients and histologic features. *Am. J. Neuroradiol.* **2011**, *33*, 761–766. [CrossRef]
40. Tempescul, A.; Querellou, S.; Ianotto, J.-C.; Boisramé, S.; Valette, G.; Berthou, C. ^{18}F-FDG PET/CT in primary non-Hodgkin's lymphoma of the sinonasal tract. *Ann. Hematol.* **2010**, *89*, 635–637. [CrossRef]
41. Rischin, D.; Coleman, A. Sinonasal malignancies of neuroendocrine origin. *Hematol./Oncol. Clin. N. Am.* **2008**, *22*, 1297–1316. [CrossRef]
42. Gil, Z.; Even-Sapir, E.; Margalit, N.; Fliss, D.M. Integrated PET/CT system for staging and surveillance of skull base tumors. *Head Neck* **2007**, *29*, 537–545. [CrossRef] [PubMed]
43. Banks, K.P.; Ly, J.Q.; Thompson, L.D.; Michaelson, P.G.; Davis, S.W. Mesenchymal chondrosarcoma of sinonasal cavity: A case report and brief literature review. *Eur. J. Radiol. Extra* **2004**, *49*, 47–51. [CrossRef]
44. Eller, R.; Sillers, M. Common fibro-osseous lesions of the paranasal sinuses. *Otolaryngol. Clin. N. Am.* **2006**, *39*, 585–600. [CrossRef] [PubMed]
45. Kubo, T.; Furuta, T.; Johan, M.P.; Ochi, M. Prognostic significance of ^{18}F-FDG PET at diagnosis in patients with soft tissue sarcoma and bone sarcoma; systematic review and meta-analysis. *Eur. J. Cancer* **2016**, *58*, 104–111. [CrossRef]
46. Kim, J.H.; Yoon, D.Y.; Baek, S.; Park, M.W.; Kwon, K.H.; Rho, Y.S. CT, MRI, and FDG PET/CT findings of sinonasal sarcoma: Differentiation from squamous cell carcinoma. *J. Korean Radiol.* **2016**, *75*, 17–25. [CrossRef]
47. Wang, X.; Song, L.; Chong, V.; Wang, Y.; Li, J.; Xian, J. Multiparametric MRI findings of sinonasal rhabdomyosarcoma in adults with comparison to carcinoma. *J. Magn. Reson. Imaging* **2017**, *45*, 998–1004. [CrossRef]
48. Chan, K.H.; Gao, D.; Fernandez, P.G.; Kingdom, T.T.; Kumpe, D.A. Juvenile nasopharyngeal angiofibroma. *Laryngoscope* **2013**, *124*, 672–677. [CrossRef]
49. Lee, D.K.; Chung, S.K.; Dhong, H.J.; Kim, H.Y.; Kim, H.J.; Bok, K.H. Focal hyperostosis on CT of sinonasal inverted papilloma as a predictor of tumor origin. *Am. J. Neuroradiol.* **2007**, *28*, 618–621.
50. Jeon, T.Y.; Kim, H.-J.; Chung, S.-K.; Dhong, H.-J.; Kim, H.Y.; Yim, Y.J.; Kim, S.T.; Jeon, P.; Kim, K.H. Sinonasal inverted papilloma: Value of convoluted cerebriform pattern on MR imaging. *Am. J. Neuroradiol.* **2008**, *29*, 1556–1560. [CrossRef]
51. Ojiri, H.; Ujita, M.; Tada, S.; Fukuda, K. Potentially distinctive features of sinonasal inverted papilloma on MR imaging. *Am. J. Roentgenol.* **2000**, *175*, 465–468. [CrossRef]

52. Shojaku, H.; Fujisaka, M.; Yasumura, S.; Ishida, M.; Tsubota, M.; Nishida, H.; Watanabe, Y.; Kawano, M.; Shimizu, M.; Fukuoka, J. Positron emission tomography for predicting malignancy of sinonasal inverted papilloma. *Clin. Nucl. Med.* **2007**, *32*, 275–278. [CrossRef] [PubMed]
53. Yang, B.; Wang, Y.; Wang, S.; Dong, J. Magnetic resonance imaging features of schwannoma of the sinonasal tract. *J. Comput. Assist. Tomogr.* **2015**, *39*, 860–865. [CrossRef] [PubMed]
54. Maroldi, R.; Ravanelli, M.; Borghesi, A.; Farina, D. Paranasal sinus imaging. *Eur. J. Radiol.* **2008**, *66*, 372–386. [CrossRef]
55. Fitzpatrick, K.A.; Taljanovic, M.S.; Speer, D.P.; Graham, A.R.; Jacobson, J.A.; Barnes, G.R.; Hunter, T.B. Imaging findings of fibrous dysplasia with histopathologic and intraoperative correlation. *Am. J. Roentgenol.* **2004**, *182*, 1389–1398. [CrossRef] [PubMed]
56. Werner, R.L.; Castle, J.T. Inflammatory myofibroblastic tumor of the nasal cavity. *Head Neck Pathol.* **2015**, *10*, 336–339. [CrossRef]
57. Yan, Z.; Wang, Y.; Zhang, Z. Inflammatory myofibroblastic tumor: An entity of CT and MR imaging to differentiate from malignant tumors of the sinonasal cavity. *J. Comput. Assist. Tomogr.* **2014**, *38*, 14–19. [CrossRef]
58. Duval, M.; Hwang, E.; Kilty, S.J. Systematic review of treatment and prognosis of sinonasal hemangiopericytoma. *Head Neck* **2012**, *35*, 1205–1210. [CrossRef]
59. Hennessey, P.T.; Reh, D.D. Benign sinonasal neoplasms. *Am. J. Rhinol. Allergy* **2013**, *27*, 31–34. [CrossRef]
60. Fyrmpas, G.; Wurm, J.; Athanassiadou, F.; Papageorgiou, T.; Beck, J.-D.; Iro, H. Constantinidis Management of pediatric sinonasal rhabdomyosarcoma. *J. Laryngol. Otol.* **2009**, *123*, 990–996. [CrossRef]
61. Hiroshima, Y.; Otomi, Y.; Shinya, T.; Otsuka, H.; Harada, M. ^{11}C-Methionine PET/CT and ^{18}F-FDG PET/CT in the Evaluation of Adult Alveolar Rhabdomyosarcoma. *Mol. Imaging Radionucl. Ther.* **2023**, *32*, 62–64. [CrossRef]
62. Liu, J.H.; Qi, M.; Huang, W.H.; Sha, Y.; Zhang, F. The magnetic resonance characteristics of sinonasal rhabdomyosarcoma in adults: Analysis of 27 cases and comparison with pathological subtypes. *BMC Med. Imaging.* **2023**, *23*, 98. [CrossRef] [PubMed]
63. Zeng, J.; Liu, L.; Li, J.; Huang, Q.; Pi, L.; Jin, K. MRI features of different types of sinonasal rhabdomyosarcomas: A series of eleven cases. *Dentomaxillofacial Radiol.* **2021**, *50*, 20210030. [CrossRef] [PubMed]
64. Beltran, C.; Lukose, R.; Gangadharan, B.; Bani-Hashemi, A.; Faddegon, B.A. Image quality & dosimetric property of an investigational imaging beam line MV-CBCT. *J. Appl. Clin. Med. Phys.* **2009**, *10*, 3023–3036.
65. Cripe, T.P.; Coppes, M.J. Pediatric Rhabdomyosarcoma Treatment & Management. 2018. Available online: https://emedicine.medscape.com/article/988803-treatment?form=fpf (accessed on 15 October 2024).
66. Heim, C.; Moser, L.M.; Kreyenberg, H.; Bonig, H.B.; Tonn, T.; Wels, W.S.; Gradhand, E.; Ullrich, E.; Meister, M.T.; Koerkamp, M.G.; et al. ErbB2 (HER2)-CAR-NK-92 cells for enhanced immunotherapy of metastatic fusion-driven alveolar rhabdomyosarcoma. *Front. Immunol.* **2023**, *14*, 1228894. [CrossRef] [PubMed]
67. Dorado García, H.; Pusch, F.; Bei, Y.; von Stebut, J.; Ibáñez, G.; Guillan, K.; Imami, K.; Gürgen, D.; Rolff, J.; Helmsauer, K.; et al. Therapeutic targeting of ATR in alveolar rhabdomyosarcoma. *Nat. Commun.* **2022**, *13*, 4297. [CrossRef]
68. Filbin, M.; Monje, M. Developmental origins and emerging therapeutic opportunities for childhood cancer. *Nat. Med.* **2019**, *25*, 367–376. [CrossRef]
69. Bisogno, G.; De Salvo, G.L.; Bergeron, C.; Melcón, S.G.; Merks, J.H.; Kelsey, A.; Martelli, H.; Minard-Colin, V.; Orbach, D.; Glosli, H.; et al. Vinorelbine and continuous low-dose cyclophosphamide as maintenance chemotherapy in patients with high-risk rhabdomyosarcoma (RMS 2005): A multicentre, open-label, randomised, phase 3 trial. *Lancet Oncol.* **2019**, *20*, 1566–1575. [CrossRef]
70. Rajinder, S.; Rohaizam, J.; Irfan, M. Alveolar-type rhabdomyosarcoma of nasal cavity and paranasal sinus in adult with pulmonary metastasis: A case report. *Egypt. J. Ear Nose Throat Allied Sci.* **2016**, *17*, 177–179. [CrossRef]
71. Moretti, G.; Guimarães, R.; Oliveira, K.M.; Sanjar, F.; Voegels, R.L. Rhabdomyosarcoma of the head and neck: 24 cases and literature review. *Braz. J. Otorhinolaryngol.* **2010**, *76*, 533–537. [CrossRef]
72. Kainhofer, V.; Smolle, M.; Szkandera, J.; Liegl-Atzwanger, B.; Maurer-Ertl, W.; Gerger, A.; Riedl, J.; Leithner, A. The width of resection margins influences local recurrence in soft tissue sarcoma patients. *Eur. J. Surg. Oncol.* **2016**, *42*, 899–906. [CrossRef]
73. Sparber-Sauer, M.; Ferrari, A.; Spunt, S.L.; Vokuhl, C.; Casey, D.; Lautz, T.B.; Meyer, W.H.; Walterhouse, D.O.; Pajtler, K.W.; Alaggio, R.; et al. The significance of margins in pediatric Non-Rhabdomyosarcoma soft tissue sarcomas: Consensus on surgical margin definition harmonization from the INternational Soft Tissue SaRcoma ConsorTium (INSTRuCT). *Cancer Med.* **2023**, *12*, 11719–11730. [CrossRef] [PubMed]
74. Ferrari, A.; Casanova, M.; Collini, P.; Meazza, C.; Luksch, R.; Massimino, M.; Cefalo, G.; Terenziani, M.; Spreafico, F.; Catania, S.; et al. Adult-type soft tissue sarcomas in pediatric-age patients: Experience at the Istituto Nazionale Tumori in Milan. *J. Clin. Oncol.* **2005**, *23*, 4021–4030. [CrossRef] [PubMed]
75. Spunt, S.L.; Million, L.; Chi, Y.-Y.; Anderson, J.; Tian, J.; Hibbitts, E.; Coffin, C.; McCarville, M.B.; Randall, R.L.; Parham, D.M.; et al. A risk-based treatment strategy for non-rhabdomyosarcoma soft-tissue sarcomas in patients younger than 30 years (ARST0332): A Children's Oncology Group prospective study. *Lancet Oncol.* **2020**, *21*, 145–161. [CrossRef] [PubMed]

76. Ferrari, A.; van Noesel, M.M.; Brennan, B.; Zanetti, I.; Corradini, N.; Casanova, M.; Berlanga, P.; Merks, J.H.M.; Alaggio, R. Schifflers, S.; et al. Paediatric non-rhabdomyosarcoma soft tissue sarcomas: The prospective NRSTS 2005 study by the European Pediatric Soft Tissue Sarcoma Study Group (EpSSG). *Lancet Child Adolesc. Health* **2021**, *5*, 546–558. [CrossRef]
77. Liu, Z.; Zhu, F.; Cao, W.; Sun, J.; Zhang, C.; He, Y. Surgical treatment of pediatric rhabdomyosarcoma in the parameningeal nonparameningeal region. *J. Craniomaxillofacial Surg.* **2020**, *48*, 75–82. [CrossRef]
78. Dasgupta, R.; Rodeberg, D.A. Update on rhabdomyosarcoma. *Semin. Pediatr. Surg.* **2012**, *21*, 68–78. [CrossRef]
79. Pappo, A.S.; Anderson, J.R.; Crist, W.M.; Wharam, M.D.; Breitfeld, P.P.; Hawkins, D.; Raney, R.B.; Womer, R.B.; Parham, D.M. Qualman, S.J.; et al. Survival after relapse in children and adolescents with rhabdomyosarcoma: A report from the Intergroup Rhabdomyosarcoma Study Group. *J. Clin. Oncol.* **1999**, *17*, 3487–3493. [CrossRef]
80. Million, L.; Anderson, J.; Breneman, J.; Hawkins, D.S.; Laurie, F.; Michalski, J.; Rodeberg, D.; Wharam, M.; Wolden, S.; Donaldson S.S.; et al. Influence of noncompliance with radiation therapy protocol guidelines and operative bed recurrences for children with rhabdomyosarcoma and microscopic residual disease: A report from the children's oncology group. *Int. J. Radiat. Oncol. Biol. Phys.* **2011**, *80*, 333–338. [CrossRef]
81. Merchant, T.E. Proton beam therapy in pediatric oncology. *Cancer J.* **2009**, *15*, 298–305. [CrossRef]
82. Mizumoto, M.; Murayama, S.; Akimoto, T.; Demizu, Y.; Fukushima, T.; Ishida, Y.; Oshiro, Y.; Numajiri, H.; Fuji, H.; Okumura, T. et al. Preliminary results of proton radiotherapy for pediatric rhabdomyosarcoma: A multi-institutional study in Japan. *Cancer Med.* **2018**, *7*, 1870–1874. [CrossRef]
83. Dávila Fajardo, R.; Scarzello, G.; Gaze, M.N.; Boterberg, T.; Cameron, A.; Fuchs, J.; Guérin, F.; Hoskin, P.; Krasin, M.J.; Kroon, P. et al. Brachytherapy for rhabdomyosarcoma: Survey of international clinical practice and development of guidelines. *Radiother Oncol.* **2024**, *195*, 110273. [CrossRef] [PubMed]
84. Yokouchi, M.; Terahara, M.; Nagano, S.; Arishima, Y.; Zemmyo, M.; Yoshioka, T.; Tanimoto, A.; Komiya, S. Clinical implications of determination of safe surgical margins by using a combination of CT and ^{18}FDG-positron emission tomography in soft tissue sarcoma. *BMC Musculoskelet. Disord.* **2011**, *12*, 166. [CrossRef] [PubMed]
85. O'Sullivan, F.; Wolsztynski, E.; O'Sullivan, J.; Richards, T.; Conrad, E.U.; Eary, J.F. A statistical modeling approach to the analysis of spatial patterns of FDG-PET uptake in human sarcoma. *IEEE Trans. Med. Imaging* **2011**, *30*, 2059–2071. [CrossRef]
86. Kumar, R.; Shandal, V.; Shamim, S.A.; Halanaik, D.; Malhotra, A. Clinical applications of PET and PET/CT in pediatric malignancies. *Expert Rev. Anticancer Ther.* **2010**, *10*, 755–768. [CrossRef] [PubMed]
87. Mody, R.J.; Bui, C.; Hutchinson, R.J.; Yanik, G.A.; Castle, V.P.; Frey, K.A.; Shulkin, B.L. FDG-PET imaging of childhood sarcomas *Pediatr. Blood Cancer* **2010**, *54*, 222–227. [CrossRef]
88. Pourmehdi Lahiji, A.; Jackson, T.; Nejadnik, H.; von Eyben, R.; Rubin, D.; Spunt, S.L.; Quon, A.; Daldrup-Link, H. Association of Tumor [^{18}F]FDG Activity and Diffusion Restriction with Clinical Outcomes of Rhabdomyosarcomas. *Mol. Imaging Biol.* **2019**, *21*, 591–598. [CrossRef]
89. Arndt, C.A.; Bisogno, G.; Koscielniak, E. Fifty years of rhabdomyosarcoma studies on both sides of the pond and lessons learned. *Cancer Treat. Rev.* **2018**, *68*, 94–101. [CrossRef]
90. Hawkins, D.S.; Gupta, A.A.; Rudzinski, E.R. What is new in the biology and treatment of pediatric rhabdomyosarcoma? *Curr. Opin. Pediatr.* **2014**, *26*, 50–56. [CrossRef]
91. Dantonello, T.M.; Int-Veen, C.; Harms, D.; Leuschner, I.; Schmidt, B.F.; Herbst, M.; Juergens, H.; Scheel-Walter, H.-G.; Bielack, S.S.; Klingebiel, T.; et al. Cooperative trial CWS-91 for localized soft tissue sarcoma in children, adolescents, and young adults. *J. Clin. Oncol.* **2009**, *27*, 1446–1455. [CrossRef]
92. Oberlin, O.; Rey, A.; de Toledo, J.S.; Martelli, H.; Jenney, M.E.; Scopinaro, M.; Bergeron, C.; Merks, J.H.; Bouvet, N.; Ellershaw, C.; et al. Randomized comparison of intensified six-drug versus standard three-drug chemotherapy for high-risk nonmetastatic rhabdomyosarcoma and other chemotherapy-sensitive childhood soft tissue sarcomas: Long-term results from the International Society of Pediatric Oncology MMT95 study. *J. Clin. Oncol.* **2012**, *30*, 2457–2465.
93. Dantonello, T.M.; Stark, M.; Timmermann, B.; Fuchs, J.; Selle, B.; Linderkamp, C.; Handgretinger, R.; Hagen, R.; Feuchtgruber, S.; Kube, S.; et al. Tumour volume reduction after neoadjuvant chemotherapy impacts outcome in localised embryonal rhabdomyosarcoma. *Pediatr. Blood Cancer* **2015**, *62*, 16–23. [CrossRef] [PubMed]
94. Nitescu, D.C.K.; Constantin, M.; Martu, S. Evaluation of Cumulative Effects of Chemotherapy and Bevacizumab (Avastin) in Oncological Patients with Periodontal Disease. *Rev. Chim.* **2017**, *68*, 549–552. [CrossRef]
95. Crist, W.; Gehan, E.A.; Ragab, A.H.; Dickman, P.S.; Donaldson, S.S.; Fryer, C.; Hammond, D.; Hays, D.M.; Herrmann, J.; Heyn, R. The Third Intergroup Rhabdomyosarcoma Study. *J. Clin. Oncol.* **1995**, *13*, 610–630. [CrossRef] [PubMed]
96. Arndt, C.A.S.; Stoner, J.A.; Hawkins, D.S.; Rodeberg, D.A.; Hayes-Jordan, A.A.; Paidas, C.N.; Parham, D.M.; Teot, L.A.; Wharam, M.D.; Breneman, J.C.; et al. Vincristine, actinomycin, and cyclophosphamide compared with vincristine, actinomycin, and cyclophosphamide alternating with vincristine, topotecan, and cyclophosphamide for intermediate-risk rhabdomyosarcoma: Children's oncology group study D9803. *J. Clin. Oncol.* **2009**, *27*, 5182–5188. [CrossRef]

97. Zarrabi, A.; Perrin, D.; Kavoosi, M.; Sommer, M.; Sezen, S.; Mehrbod, P.; Bhushan, B.; Machaj, F.; Rosik, J.; Kawalec, P.; et al. Rhabdomyosarcoma: Current Therapy, Challenges, and Future Approaches to Treatment Strategies. *Cancers* **2023**, *15*, 5269. [CrossRef]
98. Yang, L.; Takimoto, T.; Fujimoto, J. Prognostic model for predicting overall survival in children and adolescents with rhabdomyosarcoma. *BMC Cancer* **2014**, *14*, 654. [CrossRef]
99. Choi, P.J.; Iwanaga, J.; Tubbs, R.S.; Yilmaz, E. Surgical Interventions for Advanced Parameningeal Rhabdomyosarcoma of Children and Adolescents. *Cureus* **2018**, *10*, e2045. [CrossRef]
100. Jacobson, J.; Jamieson, J.; Mushunje, S.; Harrison, D. Management and outcomes of children with rhabdomyosarcoma in a low-to-middle-income country: A first report from Chris Hani Baragwanath Academic Hospital, South Africa. *J. Pediatr. Surg. Open* **2024**, *6*, 100139. [CrossRef]
101. Ferrari, A.; Miceli, R.; Meazza, C.; Casanova, M.; Favini, F.; Morosi, C.; Trecate, G.; Marchianò, A.; Luksch, R.; Cefalo, G.; et al. Comparison of the prognostic value of assessing tumor diameter versus tumor volume at diagnosis or in response to initial chemotherapy in rhabdomyosarcoma. *J. Clin. Oncol.* **2010**, *28*, 1322–1328. [CrossRef]
102. Mandeville, H.C. Radiotherapy in the Management of Childhood Rhabdomyosarcoma. *Clin. Oncol.* **2019**, *31*, 462–470. [CrossRef]

medicina

MDPI

Case Report

Fibrous Dysplasia of the Ethmoid Bone Diagnosed in a 10-Year-Old Patient

Zofia Resler [1], Monika Morawska-Kochman [2], Katarzyna Resler [2,*] and Tomasz Zatoński [2]

1 Student Scientific Society of Otolaryngology, Department of Otolaryngology, Head and Neck Surgery, Wroclaw Medical University, 50-556 Wrocław, Poland
2 Department of Otolaryngology, Head and Neck Surgery, Wroclaw Medical University, 50-556 Wrocław, Poland; monika.morawska-kochman@umw.edu.pl (M.M.-K.); tomasz.zatonski@umw.edu.pl (T.Z.)
* Correspondence: katarzyna.resler@umw.edu.pl

Abstract: Fibrous dysplasia is an uncommon bone disorder affecting various parts of the skeleton, often affecting facial and cranial bones. In this case, a 10-year-old patient was diagnosed with fibrous dysplasia of the ethmoid sinus at an early age. The patient has experienced nasal congestion, snores, and worsening nasal patency since 2019. A CT scan revealed an expansive proliferative lesion, likely from the frontal or ethmoid bone, protruding into the nasal cavity, ethmoid sinus, and right orbit. The tumor causes bone defects in the area of the nasal bone, leading to fluid retention in the peripheral parts of the right maxillary sinus. The patient's parents decided not to undergo surgery to remove the diseased tissue and reconstruct the area, as it would be very extensive, risky, and disfiguring. The patient is being treated conservatively with an MRI, with a contrast performed approximately every six months and infusions of bisphosphonates. Despite the lesion's size, the patient does not experience pain characteristic of dysplasia, and functions typically. Fibrous dysplasia of bone is a rare condition that presents with the most visually apparent manifestations, often mistaken for other bone conditions. Advanced diagnostic tools, like CT and MRI, are used to identify conditions affecting the ethmoid sinus more frequently. However, diagnostic errors often occur in imaging studies, leading to confusion. The most common period for clinical manifestations and diagnosis is around 10 years of age. The preferred approach in managing fibrous dysplasia involves symptomatic treatment, which can alleviate airway obstruction, restore normal globe position and visual function, and address physical deformities. Surgical intervention is recommended only for patients with severe functional impairment, progressive deformities, or malignant transformation.

Keywords: fibrous dysplasia; children; bone disease; ethmoid bone; osteitis; craniofacial lesion

1. Introduction

Fibrous dysplasia (FD) is an uncommon bone disorder that can impact various parts of the skeleton, primarily affecting facial and cranial bones, such as the mandible and maxilla [1]. An irregular mix of weak fibrous and osseous tissue replaces the normal bone marrow in the affected bones in fibrous dysplasia. The precise etiology of the disease is currently not fully elucidated [1,2]. However, some studies suggest that fibrous dysplasia is caused by sporadic post-zygotic mutations in the *GNAS* gene located on chromosome 20 [3,4]. The mutation disrupts the intrinsic GTPase activity of *Gsα*, causing receptor activation. This leads to abnormal cyclic adenosine monophosphate (cAMP)-mediated signaling, which results in elevated cAMP levels within mutated cells. Mutated osteoblastic cells overexpress the receptor activator of nuclear factor kappa-B ligand (RANKL) and interleukin-6 (IL-6), which subsequently activate osteoclasts. This activation promotes bone resorption, replacing normal bone with an overproduced, disorganized collagenous matrix, ultimately causing the FD lesion to expand [3,5] (Figure 1). Fibrous dysplasia has a female predilection [6]. This condition has three forms: monostotic (70% of cases), polyostotic (30% of cases), and the most severe form, McCune-Albright syndrome, which is defined as the combination of FD and one or more extra-skeletal features, or the presence of two or more extra-skeletal features, such as skin pigmentation manifestation and premature sexual maturation [7,8]. The monostotic form involves one skeletal site without extra-skeletal manifestations, usually a benign presentation encountered in the second and third decades of life. In contrast, the polyostotic form affects multiple bones without extra-skeletal manifestations [7,9]. It often presents with significant morbidity, thus requiring careful management to alleviate symptoms and prevent complications such as fractures or deformities associated with the condition [10]. Isolated monostotic bone lesions have a wide differential diagnosis and often involve diagnostic uncertainty, usually require histological confirmation. Moreover, in some cases a molecular diagnosis of affected tissues is indicated (Figure 2). Management strategies for fibrous dysplasia typically involve a multidisciplinary approach, including orthopedic intervention, pharmacological treatment for pain relief, and regular monitoring to assess potential complications, such as osteosarcoma, in patients with the polyostotic form of the disease.

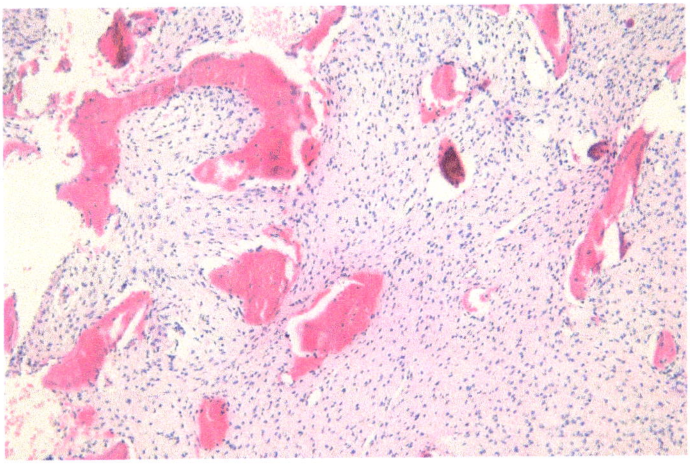

Figure 1. Histopathological findings. Tumor tissue composed of diffuse irregular, circular attenuated bone trabeculae on a background of fibrous tissue (H + E, ×100).

Fibrous dysplasia of the ethmoid sinus is rarely encountered, and diagnosing it at such an early age as in our 10-year-old patient is exceptionally uncommon. This case illustrates the challenges of diagnosing fibrous dysplasia, especially in pediatric patients, where clinical manifestations may overlap with other conditions, leading to potential misdiagnosis or delayed treatment [10].

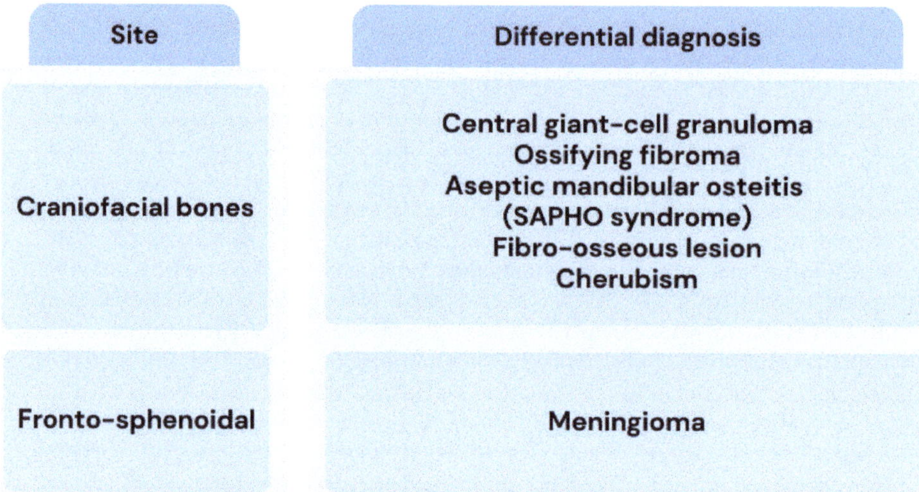

Figure 2. Differential diagnosis of craniofacial fibrous dysplasia [7].

2. Case Description

A 10-year-old patient was admitted to the hospital for a scheduled computer tomography (CT) scan of the craniofacial area due to suspected growth changes in the right nasal cavity. During the interview, the patient testified to experiencing nasal congestion for a long time. Since 2019, her symptoms have worsened. The child breathes through the mouth constantly, snores and has experienced a significant worsening of nasal patency. The patient's mother also reports observing gradual changes in her daughter's facial features on the right side. The patient states that there have been no previous bleeding episodes or pathological discharge from the nasal cavity. Nasal endoscopy revealed proliferative changes in the right nasal cavity, causing obstruction of the right nasal passage and associated external swelling at the base of the nose. No pathological discharge was observed in the nasal cavities. Ocular examination revealed a mild strabismus of the right eye, with round, normally reactive pupils. A contrast-enhanced CT scan of the craniofacial and neck region was performed for a more detailed diagnosis. The examination revealed an expansive proliferative lesion, most likely originating from the frontal or ethmoid bone and protruding into the nasal cavity, ethmoid sinus, and right orbit. The lesion exhibited a peripheral structure consistent with preserved bone structure, with islands, calcifications, and ossifications mainly localized at the lower pole of the tumor. The central part of the lesion was filled with irregular space containing dense fluid. The overall dimensions of the lesion were 35 mm in transverse diameter, 43 mm in anteroposterior diameter, and 52 mm in craniocaudal diameter. The tumor causes the formation of bone defects in the area of the nasal bone. It leads to fluid retention in the peripheral parts of the right maxillary sinus. Additionally, it affects the right nasal conchae and the palate. It causes exophthalmos and the peripheral displacement of the right eyeball. The remaining facial and temporal bones exhibit no structural changes. The anatomical spaces of the face and neck present a picture within normal limits. In the CT scan examination, the image of the lesion was not conclusive (Figure 3). Initially, fibrous dysplasia was considered for differentiation from osteofibrous dysplasia as a possible diagnosis. The patient was subsequently scheduled for a biopsy of the lesion under general anesthesia. After preparing the surgical field under endoscopic visualization, the mucosa was anesthetized and incised, revealing a significant protrusion of the sphenoid bone. The histopathological examination revealed a sample composed of bony trabeculae with typical architecture. The intertrabecular spaces were filled with bone marrow tissue and predominantly vascular fibrous connective tissue (Figure 1). In April 2020, the patient underwent a significant resection of the lesion in a part of the nasal cavity. Unfortunately, the resection did not bring any positive changes. An MRI performed in August 2020 showed a lesion of dimensions similar to those before the biopsy. In the Pediatric Surgery Department, the patient was advised to undergo surgery to remove the diseased tissue and reconstruct the area. However, the patient's parents decided not to proceed with this step because the surgery would be very extensive, risky, and disfiguring, with an uncertain outcome. Removing all of the diseased bone is impossible, which means there is a risk that the lesion could change its dynamics and continue to grow. The girl is being treated conservatively, with an MRI with contrast performed approximately every six months. She is also receiving infusions of bisphosphonates. Unfortunately, this drug has not caused a regression of the lesion but is being administered to limit the progression of the disease. The most recent MRI, performed in January 2024, showed the lesion size as $6.0 \times 4.2 \times 6.2$ cm. Fortunately, the patient does not experience the characteristic pain of dysplasia, although she has limited ability to breathe through her nose but functions normally. The patient remains under regular supervision at the Pediatric Outpatient Otolaryngology Clinic and with an ophthalmologist [11].

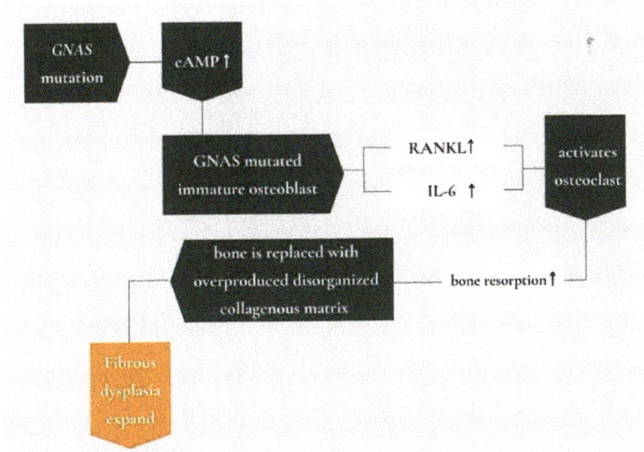

Figure 3. The pattern of cascade of events resulting from GNAS mutations leading to fibrous dysplasia. (↑—rise).

3. Discussion

Diagnostic challenges in identifying fibrous dysplasia of bone arise from the rare location of the lesions in this anatomical region and the considerable variability in CT and MRI imaging, due to the varying proportions of fibrous and bony tissue within the affected bones [7]. The most commonly affected bones are the maxilla (12%) and mandible (12%), while the involvement of the ethmoid, sphenoid, frontal, and temporal bones is less frequent [6]. Due to advanced diagnostic tools, like endoscopy, computed tomography (CT), and magnetic resonance imaging (MRI), conditions affecting the ethmoid sinus are being identified more frequently [12]. Additionally, a complicating factor in diagnosis is the similarity of radiological images to many other bone conditions. Diagnostic errors are common in imaging studies (CT and MRI), where fibrous dysplasia is often mistaken for chondrosarcoma, sinusitis, meningioma, inflammatory polyps, adenoma, aspergilloma, and old fractures [7] (Figure 4). On the other hand, the literature describes the fibrous dysplasia involving craniofacial bones as the most frequently diagnosed form among all locations of fibrous dysplasia, due to its visually apparent manifestations, as observed by Adeyemo in 100% of cases [13]. However, this condition primarily affects the more visible craniofacial bones, such as the maxilla or mandible, where the manifestations are more noticeable. Early diagnosis of fibrous dysplasia in the ethmoid bone is infrequent at this stage, as it presents with nonspecific symptoms [3]. Although sinus involvement frequently has no symptoms, it can manifest as rhinitis, nasal congestion or obstruction, sinusitis, pain, or headache [4]. Furthermore, given that fibrous dysplasia is estimated to occur before 15 years of age, and its main development occurs during adolescence, the most common period for clinical manifestations and diagnosis is around 10 years of age [3].

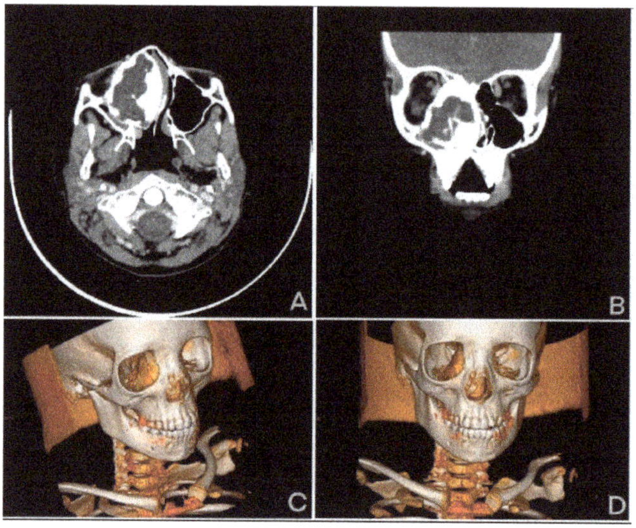

Figure 4. CT image in: (**A**) sagittal projection, (**B**) frontal, (**C**,**D**) 3D image reconstructions.

Due to diagnostic uncertainties following a CT scan examination in our 10-year-old patient, it was concluded that histopathological evaluation is decisive in distinguishing fibrous dysplasia and serves as the basis for the final diagnosis. Localizing lesions within the ethmoid sinus necessitates a higher level of surgical expertise to obtain tissue samples. According to the international literature, an endoscopic biopsy approach was employed in the described scenario. This method offers a less invasive means of accessing areas that traditionally require a more invasive transcranial approach [7].

Currently, there is no established consensus on the treatment of craniofacial FD, and no therapy exists to limit the expansion of the disease [9]. Bisphosphonates are often used; however, they only contribute to pain relief [14,15]. Recent studies indicate that Denosumab (a RANKL inhibitor), may effectively control disease activity, but further research is needed to determine the potential benefits [16,17]. The preferred approach in managing craniofacial fibrous dysplasia involves symptomatic treatment, due to the benign nature of the condition [7]. Lesions in the naso-ethmoid region can result in airway compromise and displacement of the eyeball, leading to substantial deformity and functional impairment. It is advised to undergo an evaluation by an otorhinolaryngologist and a comprehensive ophthalmological assessment. Treatment approaches focus on alleviating airway obstruction, restoring normal globe position, visual function, and addressing physical deformities [3]. The patient should be advised to promptly report any changes in their vision, including loss of color perception and especially any sudden decline in vision, as these are absolute indications for therapeutic optic nerve decompression [18].

Surgical intervention is recommended only for patients with severe functional impairment, progressive deformities, or malignant transformation [7]. Surgical interventions in this region may involve partial or extensive excision with subsequent reconstruction of the skull base and orbits [3]. Conservative surgery may not be sufficient for all cases of craniofacial fibro-osseous lesions. For more extensive lesions, a more radical approach, such as craniofacial resection or total maxillectomy, may be necessary [18]. Radiation therapy is contraindicated due to the risk of malignant transformation. The surgical procedures do not negatively impact the growth rates of healthy tissue, and do not seem to trigger the onset of malignancy [18]. The risk of malignant transformation is estimated to be less than 1% for the monostotic form, and around 4% for the polyostotic form [7]. Patients with moderate to severe disease, particularly those experiencing significant functional disabilities or craniofacial deformities affecting appearance, should be considered for referral to a psychologist. Additionally, a referral to a social worker might also be necessary [7]. It is also advised to evaluate the psychological impact on both the patient and their family using the Craniofacial Experience Index [19].

4. Conclusions

Fibrous dysplasia is an uncommon bone disorder, very rarely occurring in children. Nevertheless, it is very important to consider it during diagnosis. There are both conservative and surgical therapies that can be applied. It is very important to provide the patient with psychological care.

Author Contributions: Conceptualization, methodology K.R. and M.M.-K.; resources, Z.R., K.R. and M.M.-K.; data curation, Z.R. and K.R.; writing—original draft preparation, Z.R., K.R. and M.M.-K.; writing—review and editing, Z.R., K.R., M.M.-K. and T.Z.; visualization, Z.R., K.R. and M.M.-K.; supervision, T.Z. All authors have read and agreed to the published version of the manuscript.

Funding: This research was funded by Wroclaw Medical University SUBZ.C250.24.088.

Institutional Review Board Statement: The study was conducted in accordance with the Declaration of Helsinki and approved by the Bioethics Committee nr 47/2024, 25 January 2024.

Informed Consent Statement: The patient's written consent form for publication was granted.

Data Availability Statement: Data are contained within the article.

Conflicts of Interest: The authors declare no conflicts of interest.

References

1. Buyuklu, F.; Tarhan, E.; Cakmak, O.; Ozgirgin, N.; Arikan, U. Isolated fibrous dysplasia of the sphenoid sinus. *Rhinology* **2005**, *43*, 309–312. [PubMed]
2. Singh, H.; Mohan, C. Fibrous dysplasia of Sphenoid bone. *Indian. J. Otolaryngol. Head. Neck Surg.* **2007**, *59*, 157–159. [CrossRef] [PubMed]
3. Kim, D.Y. Current concepts of craniofacial fibrous dysplasia: Pathophysiology and treatment. *Arch. Craniofacial Surg.* **2023**, *24*, 41–51. [CrossRef] [PubMed]
4. Szymczuk, V.; Taylor, J.; Boyce, A.M. Craniofacial Fibrous Dysplasia: Clinical and Therapeutic Implications. *Curr. Osteoporos. Rep.* **2023**, *21*, 147. [CrossRef] [PubMed]
5. Riminucci, M.; Kuznetsov, S.A.; Cherman, N.; Corsi, A.; Bianco, P.; Gehron Robey, P. Osteoclastogenesis in fibrous dysplasia of bone: In situ and in vitro analysis of IL-6 expression. *Bone* **2003**, *33*, 434–442. [CrossRef] [PubMed]
6. Chandavarkar, V.; Patil, P.M.; Bhargava, D.; Mishra, M.N. A rare case report of craniofacial fibrous dysplasia. *J. Oral. Maxillofac. Pathol.* **2018**, *22*, 406. [CrossRef] [PubMed]
7. Wardas, P.; Piotrowska-Seweryn, A.; Markowski, J.; Ślaska-Kaspera, A.; Golonka, A.; Dorosz, R.; Sokołowski, M. Fibrous dysplasia of sphenoid bone—Diagnostic difficulties. *Pol. Otorhinolaryngol. Rev.* **2015**, *4*, 30–35. [CrossRef]

8. Kuśmierczyk, K.; Owczarek, K.; Michalska, J.; Miłoński, J.; Olszewski, J. Dysplazja włóknista kości klinowej—Trudnośc diagnostyczne. *Onkol. Po Dyplomie* **2017**, *4*, 181.
9. Bouet, B.; Schlund, M.; De Massary, M.; Nicot, R. Craniofacial fibrous dysplasia: Systematic review of facial management. *Stomatol. Oral. Maxillofacial Surg.* **2023**, *124*, 101660. [CrossRef] [PubMed]
10. Rosen, C.; Compston, J.; Lian, J.B. *Primer on the Metabolic Bone Diseases and Disorders of Mineral Metabolism*; John Wiley & Sons Hoboken, NJ, USA, 2009.
11. Javaid, M.K.; Boyce, A.; Appelman-Dijkstra, N.; Ong, J.; Defabianis, P.; Offiah, A.; Arundel, P.; Shaw, N.; Dal Pos, V.; Underhil, A. et al. Best practice management guidelines for fibrous dysplasia/McCune-Albright syndrome: A consensus statement from the FD/MAS international consortium. *Orphanet J. Rare Dis.* **2019**, *14*, 139. [CrossRef] [PubMed]
12. Ng, Y.H.; Sethi, D.S. Isolated sphenoid sinus disease: Differential diagnosis and management. *Curr. Opin. Otolaryngol. Head Neck Surg.* **2011**, *19*, 16–20. [CrossRef] [PubMed]
13. Adeyemo, A.A.; Ogunkeyede, S.A.; Daniel, A.; Lasisi, A.O. Paediatric paranasal sinus fibrous dysplasia. *Trop. Doct.* **2023**, *53* 117–120. [CrossRef] [PubMed]
14. Boyce, A.M.; Kelly, M.H.; Brillante, B.A.; Kushner, H.; Wientroub, S.; Riminucci, M.; Bianco, P.; Robey, P.G.; Collins, M.T. A randomized, double blind, placebo-controlled trial of alendronate treatment for fibrous dysplasia of bone. *J. Clin. Endocrinol. Metab.* **2014**, *99*, 4133–4140. [CrossRef]
15. Wang, Y.; Wang, O.; Jiang, Y.; Li, M.; Xia, W.; Meng, X.; Xing, X. Efficacy and Safety of Bisphosphonate Therapy in Mccune-Albright Syndrome–Related Polyostotic Fibrous Dysplasia: A Single-Center Experience. *Endocr. Pract.* **2019**, *25*, 23–30. [CrossRef]
16. Gun, Z.H.; Arif, A.; Boyce, A.M. Fibrous dysplasia in children and its management. *Curr. Opin. Endocrinol. Diabetes Obes.* **2024** *31*, 60–66. [CrossRef] [PubMed]
17. Pan, K.S.; Boyce, A.M. Denosumab Treatment for Giant Cell Tumors, Aneurysmal Bone Cysts, and Fibrous Dysplasia-Risks and Benefits. *Curr. Osteoporos. Rep.* **2021**, *19*, 141–150. [CrossRef]
18. Panda, N.K.; Parida, P.K.; Sharma, R.; Jain, A.; Bapuraj, J.R. A clinicoradiologic analysis of symptomatic craniofacial fibro-osseous lesions. *Otolaryngol. Head Neck Surg.* **2007**, *136*, 928–933. [CrossRef]
19. Roberts, R.M.; Shute, R. Living with a craniofacial condition: Development of the Craniofacial Experiences Questionnaire (CFEQ) for adolescents and their parents. *Cleft. Palate Craniofacial J.* **2011**, *48*, 727–735. [CrossRef] [PubMed]

medicina

MDPI

Case Report

A Clinical Approach for the Removal of a Large Antral Pseudocyst with Simultaneous Maxillary Sinus Augmentation: A Case Series

Won-Bae Park [1], Jina Shin [2], Seungil Shin [3] and Ji-Youn Hong [3,*]

1 Private Practice in Periodontics and Implant Dentistry, Seoul 02771, Republic of Korea; wbpdds@naver.com
2 Department of Dentistry, Graduate School, Kyung Hee University, Seoul 02447, Republic of Korea; jina_s7528@naver.com
3 Department of Periodontology, College of Dentistry, Kyung Hee University Dental Hospital, Kyung Hee University, Seoul 02447, Republic of Korea; shin.dmd@khu.ac.kr
* Correspondence: periohjy@khu.ac.kr; Tel.: +82-2-958-9380

Abstract: For a large benign lesion within the maxillary sinus, such as an antral pseudocyst, maxillary sinus floor augmentation is more commonly performed using a two-stage approach. This involves first removing the lesion, and then, re-entry following several months of healing. In this case series, we described the "one-bony-window" approach, which is a technical surgical modification of the previous one-stage approach, for simultaneous cyst removal and maxillary sinus floor augmentation. Four patients with large maxillary antral pseudocysts were included. The "one-bony-window" approach involves the preparation of a large window opening of approximately 15 mm × 20 mm at the lateral wall. A mesiodistally extended intentional perforation was made in the upper part of the exposed membrane to enhance the access for instrumentation. The antral pseudocyst was removed in its entirety without being deformed to prevent rupture or leakage of the cystic contents. Subsequent detachment and elevation of the Schneiderian membrane at the sinus floor significantly reduced the perforation site, and bone grafting with implant placement was performed simultaneously. This alleviated the need to surgically repair the perforation. The lateral opening was either uncovered or repositioned using bony window lids. Healing abutments were connected after six months, and the final prosthesis was placed after two months. At the 1-year follow-up, the antral pseudocysts had resolved with no specific recurrence, and the stability of the augmented sinus was maintained with excellent implant survival. Within the limitations of our findings, the "one-bony-window" technique can be suggested for the simultaneous removal of large antral pseudocysts and maxillary sinus floor augmentation with favorable clinical outcomes.

Keywords: antral pseudocyst; dental implant; lateral sinus window; maxillary sinus floor augmentation; Schneiderian membrane

1. Introduction

Maxillary sinus floor augmentation (MSFA) using the lateral window approach involves elevation of the Schneiderian membrane through an access opening in the maxillary sinus lateral wall and creates confined space underneath the elevated membrane filled with grafting materials to increase limited residual ridge height [1,2]. A predictable long-term outcome regarding implant survival in MSFA has been reported [3]. However, risks of intraoperative and postoperative complications may occur related to the lateral window approach, and perforation of the Schneiderian membrane is the most frequent complication during the procedure [4]. Different treatment strategies including post-perforation clot formation, placement of collagen membrane, suturing, and use of platelet-rich fibrin are introduced to manage the membrane perforation [4–6]. Other complications such as wound infection, post-operative sinusitis, and graft failure may also be involved with MSFA, although the incidence is relatively low [4]. In the presence of maxillary sinus pathologies, the potential risks of complications are increased; therefore, an accurate diagnosis and careful clinical and radiographic assessments before surgery are critical [7].

Maxillary sinus cysts are frequently diagnosed on radiographs. These cysts are classified into mucoceles, postoperative maxillary cysts, mucous retention cysts, and pseudocysts, with different clinicopathologic aspects [8]. Mucous retention cysts and antral pseudocysts are among the most common lesions of the maxillary sinus [9]. Mucous retention cysts are fluid-filled masses with thin epithelial linings that result from the obstruction of seromucous glands, and several etiologies including trauma from tooth extraction, dental infection, and allergies are suggested to be involved with the occurrence of the lesions [10]. On the other hand, pseudocysts lack epithelial walls due to diffuse subepithelial accumulation of inflammatory exudate and have been associated with allergies and respiratory and viral infections, although the etiologies are yet to be confirmed [11]. Antral pseudocysts usually appear as faint and dome-shaped radiopaque lesions with homogenous density [12]. It is an asymptomatic benign lesion that does not require treatment under normal circumstances. However, the presence of large antral pseudocysts may increase the risk of ostial obstruction and dysventilation following upward shift of the lesions by sinus lift [13]. Moreover, preoperative sinus pathology may interfere with Schneiderian membrane mobilization and increase the risk of membrane perforation, which can contaminate and infect graft materials with the leakage of cystic fluid or purulent exudate [14,15].

Conventionally, antral cystic lesions are usually treated before MSFA, and Caldwell–Luc surgery was considered the gold standard for complete removal of the lesion from maxillary sinus, which is replaced with new mucosa [16,17]. However, Caldwell–Luc surgery is associated with increased postoperative surgical trauma, patient morbidity, and longer healing periods. Endoscopic sinus surgery can also be considered in the treatment of sinonasal impairments. Endoscopic-assisted MSFA through the lateral maxillary wall allows for a direct and clear visualization of the surgical field without preparation of huge or multiple bone windows, which helps to reduce the risk of membrane perforation during sinus lift [18]. It also allows for a one-stage procedure for MSFA combined with the removal of maxillary sinus pathologies [19]. Despite the advantages, it is not easy to access endoscopic surgery due to the need for special instruments or settings accompanied by medical assistance.

Recently, technical surgical modifications to simultaneously remove antral pseudocysts and perform MSFA using either the one- or two-stage approach have been introduced into dentistry [20–22]. Chiapasco et al. described the formation of an additional small round bony access above the sinus window opening for enucleation of pseudocyst while preserving the integrity of the Schneiderian membrane periosteal layer during the simultaneous approach [20]. Yu et al. prepared a bony window (a smaller rounded opening) to first remove the pseudocyst, and then, created a larger bony window surrounding the former to elevate the sinus membrane [21,22]. Previous studies have utilized a smaller size of bony window during the first surgical step to remove a cyst following the aspiration of mucous fluid, which may be advantageous in minimizing damage to the sinus mucosa by limiting the membrane perforation. However, small windows make it difficult to access instruments and remove large cysts without rupture. Leakage of inflammatory exudate from disintegrated lesion can increase the risk of graft contamination when one-stage MSFA is planned simultaneously with the cyst removal.

In this case series, we describe the "one-bony-window" approach, which is a technical surgical modification of the previous one-stage approach, for simultaneous cyst removal and MSFA in four patients. It includes the creation of a large-sized lateral window opening and mesiodistally long intentional incision on the upper part of the Schneiderian membrane to facilitate cyst removal without deformation or leakage from the rupture. The purpose of this article is to present a one-bony-window approach for favorable clinical outcomes in the removal of a large antral pseudocyst and one-stage MSFA.

2. Case Presentation

This case series includes four patients who visited a private practice in periodontics and implant dentistry. All the patients presented with a limited residual bone height in the posterior maxilla that would benefit from sinus lifting. Moreover, a large antral pseudocyst was present in each patient. To simultaneously remove the antral cyst and perform MSFA, we modified the lateral window opening technique to develop the "one-bony-window approach". Briefly, a mucoperiosteal flap with vertical incisions in the posterior maxilla was fully reflected and an oval-shaped lateral access window opening, measuring approximately 15 mm × 20 mm, was prepared. After exposing the Schneiderian membrane of the lateral wall, a long horizontal incision was made in the upper part of the membrane using a #15 Bard-Parker blade. The antral pseudocyst was removed through the incised hole within the membrane using a Pincette or tissue plier. Subsequently, membrane elevation of the sinus floor, which should not be performed prior to cyst removal, was carried out carefully to avoid membrane perforation and to secure the space for bone graft materials. The incised membrane in the upper part was left without additional repair. The graft materials for MSFA were deposited into the confined space beneath the membrane elevation, and dental implants were placed simultaneously. The lateral opening was either repositioned with the bony window removed or left uncovered. Finally, the mucoperiosteal flap was sutured to facilitate primary closure.

2.1. Case 1

A 67-year-old male smoker was scheduled for dental implant placement in the maxillary right posterior edentulous ridge. The residual bone height was limited to within 3 mm, due to the alveolar ridge resorption and a pneumatized sinus floor (Figure 1a). A preoperative CBCT (sagittal and coronal views) showed a large dome-shaped antral cyst (20.5 mm × 27.8 mm) in the right maxillary sinus, which occupied half of the sinus cavity (Figure 1b,c). After mucoperiosteal flap reflection, a single bony lateral window was prepared using a rotary round bur, and the bony lid was removed (Figure 1d). Part of the mucous membrane was incised by intentionally perforating the upper Schneiderian membrane, exposing a yellowish cystic wall (Figure 1e). Using a pair of tissue pliers, the antral pseudocyst was removed through the perforated membrane. The original shape of the cyst was preserved and there was no rupture of the cystic wall or outflow of cystic fluid (Figure 1f). A large perforation was observed (Figure 1g), and the remaining membrane attached to the sinus floor was carefully separated using sinus elevation instruments (Genoss, Suwon, Republic of Korea). By elevating the membrane of the sinus floor, the size of the perforated area was greatly reduced. This reduction is due to the perforated area moving further to the buccal side, with a reduction in tension applied to the mucous membrane and mucosal folding (Figure 1h). The sinus floor was augmented with xenografts (OsteonTM Xeno; Genoss, Suwon, Republic of Korea). Additional repair of the perforated membrane was not necessary (Figure 1i). Two Ø 4.8 mm × 10 mm SLA (sandblasts, large grit, acid-etched) implants (Implantium, Dentium, Suwon, Republic of Korea) were simultaneously placed and submerged (Figure 1j). Postoperatively, systemic antibiotics (ciprofloxacin 500 mg; Ildong Pharmaceutical Co., Seoul, Republic of Korea) and nonsteroidal anti-inflammatory drugs (etodolac; Yuhan Pharmaceutical Co., Seoul, Republic of Korea) were prescribed for 7 days. To avoid increasing pressure within the sinus, the patient was advised not to blow his nose. Histological examination of the resected specimen demonstrated an inflamed maxillary sinus lining surrounding an inner fibrous connective tissue, which was diagnosed as an antral pseudocyst (Figure 1k). The patient had transient nasal bleeding, facial swelling, and hematoma, but healing was uneventful (Figure 1l). Surgical re-entry and abutment connection were performed after six months (Figure 1m,n). Regenerated hard tissue covering the lateral window site was observed. Prosthetic loading was performed 2 months after healing (Figure 1o). At the 1-year follow-up, a dome-shaped augmentation of the graft volume surrounding the implant fixtures was observed in the panoramic view (Figure 1p). Additionally, resolved cystic lesions adjacent to the well-defined grafted borders were observed on sagittal and coronal CBCT images (Figure 1q,r).

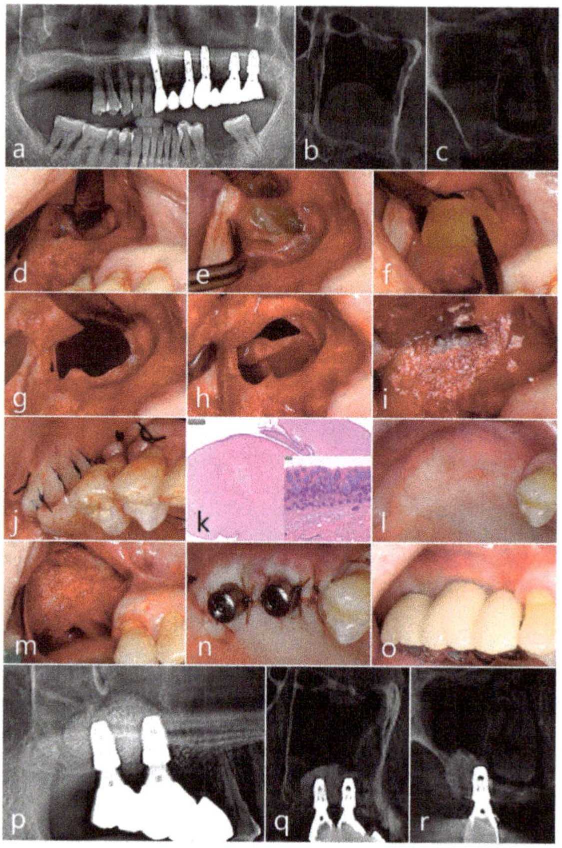

Figure 1. Case 1. Preoperative radiographs. A dome-shaped antral pseudocyst in the right maxillary sinus is shown in the panoramic (**a**), sagittal (**b**), and coronal (**c**) CBCT images. The "one-bony-window" technique including preparation of an elliptical lateral sinus access opening (**d**), intentional perforation at the upper part of the exposed Schneiderian membrane (**e**), removal of the antral pseudocyst with a large mucosal perforation site (**f**,**g**), detachment and elevation of sinus floor membrane with significant reduction in the perforation size (**h**), sinus floor augmentation with graft materials and implant placements (**i**), and flap closure (**j**). Histological features of the antral pseudocyst specimens (**k**). The clinical appearance at 6 months of follow-up (**l**). Surgical re-entry and healing abutment connection (**m**,**n**). Post-prosthetic delivery (**o**). Postoperative radiographic features of the augmented sinus floor in the panoramic (**p**), sagittal (**q**), and coronal (**r**) CBCT images, taken 1 year after prosthetic loading.

2.2. *Case 2*

A 72-year-old male non-smoker, who was taking antihypertensive drugs, presented for consultation regarding a faint dome-shaped lesion in the right maxillary sinus (Figure 2a). The panoramic CBCT view demonstrated a well-delineated homogenous lesion, measuring approximately 22.5 mm × 22.7 mm, on the sinus floor (Figure 2b). The lesion was removed using the one-bony-window technique described in Case 1 (Figure 2c,d). However, for this patient, the removed bony window was repositioned at the opening. Synthetic biphasic calcium phosphate (OsteonTM II; Genoss, Suwon, Republic of Korea) was used as a bone graft substitute (Figure 2e). One Ø 4.3 mm × 10 mm and two Ø 4.8 mm × 10 mm SLA-surface implants (Implantium, Dentium, Suwon, Republic of Korea) were placed. The implants were submerged, and the patient received the same prescription and postoperative precautions as in Case 1. The patient experienced postoperative pain, swelling, nasal bleeding, and hematoma. Healing was uneventful. The healing abutment was connected after 6 months, and prosthetic loading was performed 2 months after uncovering the abutments. In the post-surgical panoramic radiographs (Figure 2f) (taken at prosthesis delivery (Figure 2g) and 1 year of loading (Figure 2h), respectively), no specific crestal bone loss around the implants was observed, and the augmented sinus floor showed no significant decrease. In the coronal CBCT images obtained at the first molar site (Figure 2i–l) and second molar site (Figure 2m–p), taken at each procedure corresponding to the panoramic view, no specific leakage of the bone graft material, or recurrence of the antral pseudocyst, was evident.

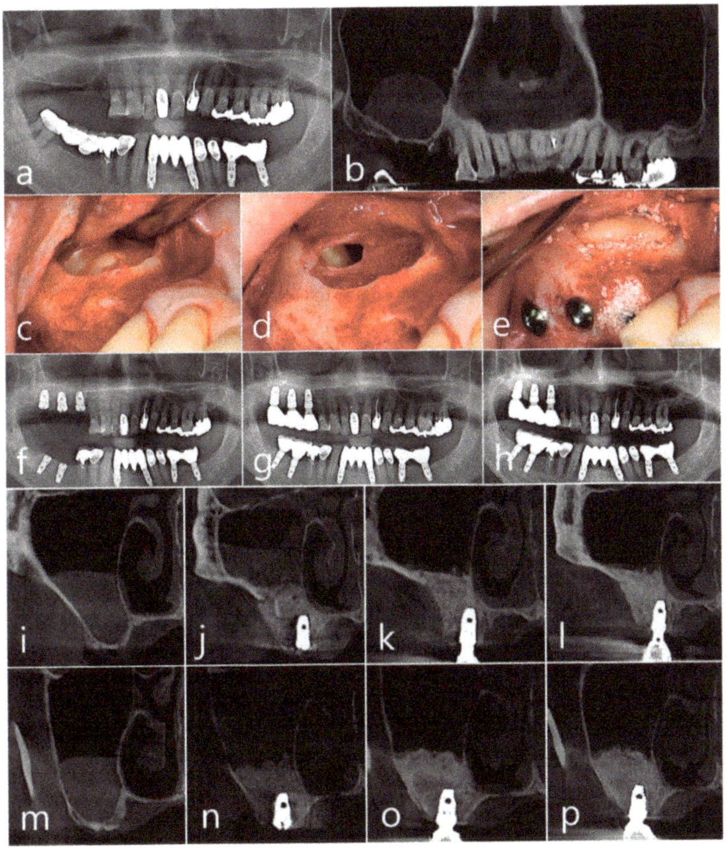

Figure 2. Case 2. Preoperative radiographs. A dome-shaped antral pseudocyst in the right maxillary sinus is shown in the panoramic radiograph (**a**) and CBCT (**b**). The "one-bony-window" technique showing lateral sinus window opening (**c**), intentional perforation at the upper part of the Schneiderian membrane and removal of antral pseudocyst (**d**), and sinus floor membrane elevation following bone grafting with implant placements, with repositioning of bony window (**e**). Panoramic view taken immediately after sinus floor augmentation and implant placement (**f**), after prosthetic delivery (**g**), and after 1 year of loading (**h**). Coronal CBCT images of the right maxillary first molar site before surgery (**i**), immediately after surgery (**j**), after prosthetic delivery (**k**), and after 1 year of loading (**l**). Coronal CBCT images of the right maxillary second molar site in the corresponding periods are described above (**m–p**).

2.3. Case 3

A 79-year-old female non-smoker visited the clinic for implant placement at the left maxillary first molar site. The site had limited residual bone height and a large dome-shaped cystic appearance, measuring 21.2 mm × 30.4 mm, in the left maxillary sinus cavity (Figure 3a,b). After removing the cyst and lifting the sinus floor using the one-bony-window technique (Figure 3c,d), xenograft bone augmentation (OsteonTM Xeno, Genoss, Suwon, Republic of Korea) was performed simultaneously with the placement of one Ø 4.8 mm × 10 mm SLA-surface implant (Implantium, Dentium, Suwon, Republic of Korea). Similar to Case 2, we repositioned the lateral bony window (Figure 3f), and then submerged the implant (Figure 1g). During early healing, a partial wound dehiscence developed at the incision line, and the patient experienced nasal bleeding and hematoma. Subsequently, healing occurred without further complications. The abutments were uncovered 6 months after MSA, and the prosthesis was placed 2 months later (Figure 3h). Preoperative coronal CBCT images showed a large antral pseudocyst (Figure 3i) and traces of graft leakage at the intentionally perforated site after surgery (Figure 3j). However, the leak was limited and did not change the augmented volume significantly. At the 1-year follow-up, recurrence of the antral cyst was not evident (Figure 3k).

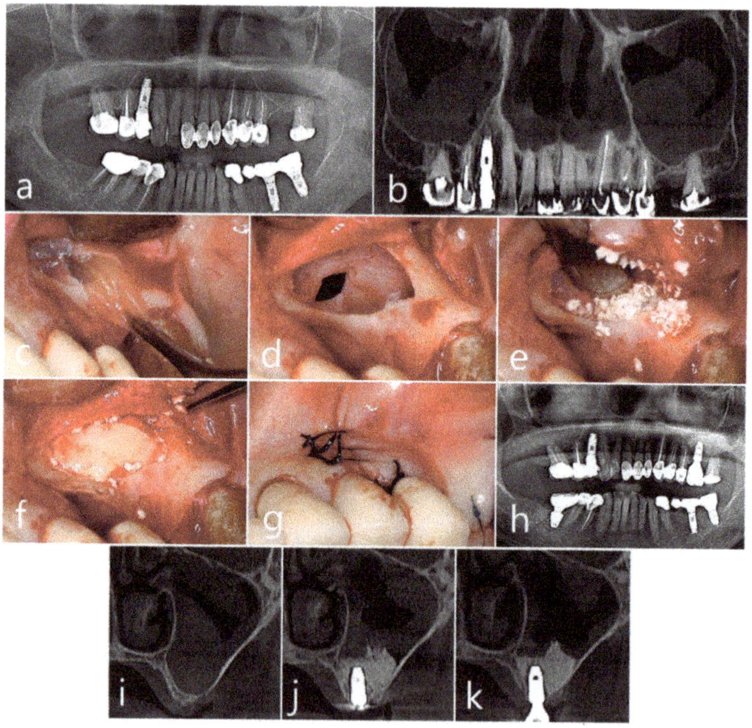

Figure 3. Case 3. Preoperative radiographic features of both maxillary sinuses are shown in the panoramic (**a**) and CBCT (**b**) images. The "one-bony-window" technique in left maxillary sinus showing lateral sinus window opening and removal of antral pseudocyst via intentional perforation site (**c**), sinus floor membrane elevation and reduced size of perforation (**d**), sinus bone grafting with implant placements (**e**), repositioning of bony window (**f**), and primary flap closure (**g**). Panoramic view obtained immediately after sinus augmentation and implant placement (**h**). Coronal CBCT images before surgery (**i**), immediately after surgery (**j**), and after 1 year of loading (**k**).

2.4. Case 4

A 42-year-old male smoker visited the clinic because of severe mobility of the posterior teeth in both the right and left maxilla. Preoperative panoramic radiography and CBCT revealed severe periodontal loss at the root apex of both maxillary molars (Figure 4a). Additionally, a dome-shaped antral pseudocyst, measuring 20.5 mm × 25.3 mm, attached to the sinus floor was observed in the sinus cavities bilaterally (Figure 4b). Replacement with an implant-supported fixed bridge from the first premolar to the second molar of the left maxilla was planned to be carried out first. After extraction of the left maxillary second premolar and first and second molars, MSFA was immediately performed using the one-bony-window technique with an elliptical lateral sinus window. The Schneiderian membrane was exposed without tears. A horizontal incision was made at the top of the window to access the cyst in the sinus, and the antral pseudocyst was removed in its entirety using tissue pliers (Figure 4c). After the detachment and elevation of the Schneiderian membrane from the floor, xenograft bone augmentation (OsteonTM Xeno, Genoss, Suwon, Republic of Korea) and implant placement (Implantium, Dentium, Suwon, Republic of Korea; one Ø 3.8 mm × 10 mm and two Ø 4.3 mm × 10 mm implants) were performed (Figure 4d). The peri-implant defects were grafted, covered with a resorbable collagen membrane (Genoss, Suwon, Republic of Korea) (Figure 4e,f), submerged, and closed with a primary flap (Figure 4g). After surgery, the patient experienced severe facial swelling, hematoma, and pain. The surgical site healed uneventfully (Figure 4h). The abutments were uncovered six months after surgery, which showed regenerated bone at the peri-implant defects (Figure 4i,j). The final prosthesis was placed two months later (Figure 4k). Panoramic radiography and CBCT taken after 1 year of prosthetic loading showed a well-maintained volume of augmented bone, with no cystic lesions observed (Figure 4l–n).

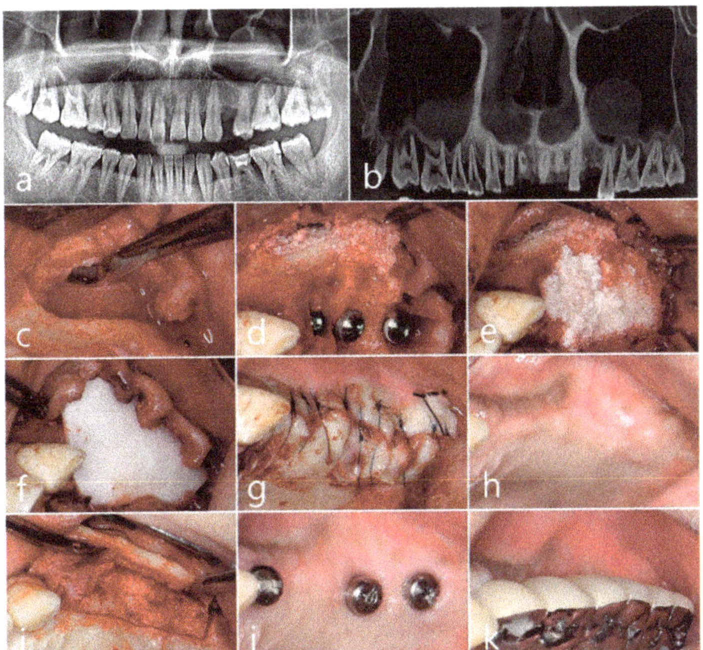

Figure 4. *Cont.*

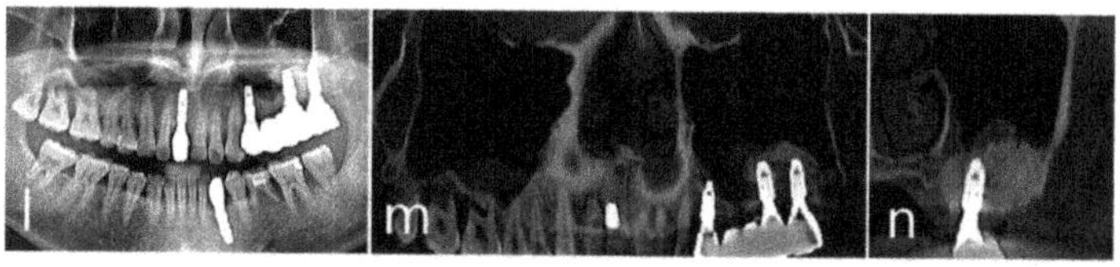

Figure 4. Case 4. Preoperative radiographs. Dome-shaped antral pseudocysts in both maxillary sinuses are shown in the panoramic (**a**) and CBCT (**b**) images. The "one-bony-window" technique including the preparation of an elliptical lateral window opening at the left maxilla and the removal of the antral pseudocyst through intentional perforation (**c**), sinus bone augmentation with implant placement (**d**), additional bone graft for peri-implant bone defects covered by a resorbable collagen membrane (**e**,**f**), and flap closure (**g**). The clinical appearance after 6 months of healing (**h**), at surgical reentry (**i**), connection of healing abutments (**j**), and prosthetic delivery (**k**). Panoramic (**l**) and CBCT (**m**,**n**) images at the 1-year follow-up.

3. Discussion

The one-stage approach using the one-bony-window technique in the presence of a large antral pseudocyst resulted in successful cyst removal and simultaneous MSFA without graft contamination or postoperative sinus infection. Early postoperative complications, such as nasal bleeding, swelling, and hematoma, occurred. Subsequently, healing occurred with no further clinical problems. Cyst recurrence or graft failure was not observed during the follow-up period, and all implants were successfully maintained.

Schneiderian membrane perforation is the most common accidental intraoperative complication during sinus lift [23,24]. Factors, such as thickness and morphology of the Schneiderian membrane, anatomy of the sinus, limited residual ridge height, and sinus pathology, can increase the risk. Sinus pathology may be accompanied by poor membrane vascularity and elasticity and reduced membrane resistance to elevation [15,24]. Membrane perforation in the presence of sinus pathoses may also lead to graft contamination and sinus infection with the leakage of cystic fluid or inflammatory exudate unless the lesion is enucleated ahead of MSFA. Management of the preexisting maxillary lesions should be carefully planned.

The size and location of the lesion may influence the timing of MSFA (either immediately after the removal of antral pseudocysts or after delayed healing for several months) [12,25]. For small pseudocysts, MSFA can be performed without removal or other treatment [26]. However, large antral pseudocysts are likely to block osteomeatal complex patency, which can cause postoperative sinusitis or retention cysts and perforation during sinus lift [19]. Aspiration of cystic fluid can compress the volume and simplify removal. However, treatment confined to mucus aspiration showed recurrence in 30% of maxillary cysts, due to residual connective tissue from the pseudocyst [21,27]. The two-stage approach is relatively problem-free, especially issues related to leakage and graft displacement. However, it requires a postoperative healing period of at least 3 months and additional surgeries thereafter. Difficulties in elevation of the Schneiderian membrane due to scar tissues during the first access may also occur.

In a recent report comparing one- and two-stage interventions for cyst removal and MSFA, both approaches showed comparable histological results and clinical outcomes, including implant survival, marginal bone resorption, and complication rates [22]. Postoperative complications, such as infection, were also infrequent in both groups. However, the one-stage approach was technically more challenging. Previous studies have described the enucleation of an antral pseudocyst through a smaller bony access prepared additionally or prior to an enlarged bony window for sinus membrane elevation [20–22]. The purpose was to avoid excessive damage to the sinus mucosa adjacent to the intentional perforation and to minimize progressive tearing, but the access to the lesion could still be limited. The one-bony-window technique used in the present study involved the preparation of a large bony opening to enucleate the pseudocyst, with a relatively long incised intentional perforation in the upper portion. The wide access facilitates cyst removal without damaging the original shape of the lesion. The risk of graft contamination can also be reduced especially when the cystic wall is vulnerable and likely to rupture even with light manipulation.

In severe cases, Schneiderian membrane perforation may result in mucosal thickening, displacement of graft particles, and postoperative maxillary sinusitis. Some studies have reported an association between membrane perforation and adverse effects, compromising sinus floor augmentation and implant survival [28,29]. On the other hand, several studies have supported the conflicting opinion that membrane perforation is not associated with postoperative infection or implant failure, probably because of improved access for instruments and materials, and repair techniques [23,26,30]. Proper strategies to manage a perforated membrane are suggested to reduce complications [6,24,31]. Currently, intentional perforation during sinus lift is mostly indicated for the removal of implants displaced into the sinus cavity [32] and for treating sinus mucosal thickening or pathology. It is assumed that the procedure may help manage minor pathologic lesions, such as antral pseudocysts.

The proposal to create an intentional long incised perforation in the Schneiderian membrane as required in the one-bony-window technique can be counter-intuitive to clinicians as the efforts to block perforation are pursed. Furthermore, the perforated membrane was not covered by some collagen membrane or sutured. Instead, careful detachment and elevation of the Schneiderian membrane at sinus floor distant from the intentional perforation relieved the tension on the sinus mucosa, reduced the size of the perforation, and moved the position further buccally with mucosal folding. The whole procedure could be easily performed with good visual access through a large-sized window. Interestingly, a previous study by Park et al. reported that a non-repaired perforation of the Schneiderian membrane did not adversely affect the clinical and radiographic outcomes of MSFA [15]. In the study, a Prichard elevator was inserted into the sinus cavity to prevent displacement of bone graft material, and the material was condensed only in the direction of the sinus floor. Successful bone grafting was possible without notable leakage of the bone graft material into the perforated mucosa that had not been repaired, and the leakage of bone graft particles was naturally drained by mucociliary clearance and did not stagnate in the maxillary sinus [33]. In the present cases, although the perforation site was not repaired with an additional collagen membrane and was not completely covered, the collapsed perforation, with its size and buccally displaced location after sinus lift, was compatible with stabilizing the space and minimizing contact with the graft materials.

Implant survival and ossification of sinus bone grafts may be enhanced when the lateral access opening sites are covered with barrier membranes or repositioned using a bony window [34,35]. However, controversial opinions suggest that there are no significant differences in implant treatment outcomes after MSFA, with or without coverage of the lateral windows, although a higher percentage of newly formed bone was detected in the coverage group [36]. Cases in this study were treated with either repositioning of the lateral bony window or a lateral opening without coverage, and the clinical and radiographic outcomes were comparable and consistent.

Despite the favorable outcomes in implant survival, maintenance of augmented bone height, and no recurrence of cystic lesions, the findings are limited in small-sized samples with short-term observation periods. To verify our results, controlled prospective studies with larger sample sizes should be conducted in the future.

4. Conclusions

Despite the limitations present in the case series of four patients with large maxillary antral pseudocysts, the "one-bony-window" technique can be utilized in simultaneous cyst removal and sinus floor augmentation and showed favorable outcomes of implant survival and well-maintained augmented bone height in short-term periods.

Author Contributions: Conceptualization, W.-B.P.; methodology, W.-B.P. and S.S.; validation, W.-B.P.; formal analysis, W.-B.P. and J.-Y.H.; investigation, W.-B.P. and J.S.; data curation, W.-B.P. and J.S.; writing—original draft preparation, W.-B.P.; writing—review and editing, W.-B.P. and J.-Y.H.; visualization, W.-B.P., J.S. and J.-Y.H.; supervision, W.-B.P. and J.-Y.H.; project administration, W.-B.P. and S.S. All authors have read and agreed to the published version of the manuscript.

Funding: This research received no external funding.

Institutional Review Board Statement: Not applicable.

Informed Consent Statement: Informed consent was obtained from all subjects involved in the study. Written informed consent has been obtained from the patients to publish this paper.

Data Availability Statement: Data are contained within the article.

Conflicts of Interest: The authors declare no conflicts of interest.

References

1. Boyne, P.J.; James, R.A. Grafting of the maxillary sinus floor with autogenous marrow and bone. *J. Oral Surg.* **1980**, *38*, 613–616. [PubMed]
2. Tatum, H.J. Maxillary and sinus implant reconstructions. *Dent. Clin. N. Am.* **1986**, *30*, 207–229. [CrossRef] [PubMed]
3. Raghoebar, G.M.; Onclin, P.; Boven, G.C.; Vissink, A.; Meijer, H.J.A. Long-term effectiveness of maxillary sinus floor augmentation: A systematic review and meta-analysis. *J. Clin. Periodontol.* **2019**, *46* (Suppl. S21), 307–318. [CrossRef] [PubMed]
4. Hsu, Y.T.; Rosen, P.S.; Choksi, K.; Shih, M.C.; Ninneman, S.; Lee, C.T. Complications of sinus floor elevation procedure and management strategies: A systematic review. *Clin. Implant Dent. Relat. Res.* **2022**, *24*, 740–765. [CrossRef] [PubMed]
5. Park, W.B.; Kang, K.L.; Han, J.Y. Factors influencing long-term survival rates of implants placed simultaneously with lateral maxillary sinus floor augmentation: A 6- to 20-year retrospective study. *Clin. Oral Implants Res.* **2019**, *30*, 977–988. [CrossRef]
6. Díaz-Olivares, L.A.; Brinkmann, J.C.B.; Martínez-Rodríguez, N.; Martínez-González, J.M.; López-Quiles, J.; Leco-Berrocal, I.; Meniz-García, C. Management of Schneiderian membrane perforations during maxillary sinus floor augmentation with lateral approach in relation to subsequent implant survival rates: A systematic review and meta-analysis. *Int. J. Implant Dent.* **2021**, *7*, 91. [CrossRef]
7. Kim, S.W.; Lee, I.H.; Kim, S.W.; Kim, D.H. Points to consider before the insertion of maxillary implants: The otolaryngologist's perspective. *J. Periodontal Implant. Sci.* **2019**, *49*, 346–354. [CrossRef]
8. Beaumont, C.; Zafiropoulos, G.G.G.; Rohmann, K.; Tatakis, D.N. Prevalence of maxillary sinus disease and abnormalities in patients scheduled for sinus lift procedures. *J. Periodontol.* **2005**, *76*, 461–467. [CrossRef]
9. Meer, S.; Altini, M. Cysts and pseudocysts of the maxillary antrum revisited. *J. South Afr. Dent. Assoc.* **2006**, *61*, 10–13.
10. Anitua, E.; Alkhraisat, M.; Torre, A.; Eguia, A. Are mucous retention cysts and pseudocysts in the maxillary sinus a risk factor for dental implants? A systematic review. *Med. Oral Patol. Oral Cir. Bucal.* **2021**, *26*, e276–e283. [CrossRef]
11. Mardinger, O.; Manor, I.; Mijiritsky, E.; Hirshberg, A. Maxillary sinus augmentation in the presence of antral pseudocyst: A clinical approach. *Oral Surg. Oral Med. Oral Pathol. Oral Radiol. Endod.* **2007**, *103*, 180–184. [CrossRef]
12. Kara, I.M.; Küçük, D.; Polat, S. Experience of maxillary sinus floor augmentation in the presence of antral pseudocysts. *J. Oral Maxillofac. Surg.* **2010**, *68*, 1646–1650. [CrossRef]
13. Kara, M.I.; Kirmali, O.M.I.; Kirmali, O.; Ay, S. Clinical evaluation of lateral and osteotome techniques for sinus floor elevation in the presence of an antral pseudocyst. *Int. J. Oral Maxillofac. Implants* **2012**, *27*, 1205–1212. [PubMed]
14. Pikos, M.A. Maxillary sinus membrane repair: Update on technique for large and complete perforations. *Implant Dent.* **2008**, *17*, 24–31. [CrossRef]
15. Park, W.B.; Han, J.Y.; Kang, P.; Momen-Heravi, F. The clinical and radiographic outcomes of Schneiderian membrane perforation without repair in sinus elevation surgery. *Clin. Implant Dent. Relat. Res.* **2019**, *21*, 931–937. [CrossRef]
16. Datta, R.K.; Viswanatha, B.; Harsha, M.S. Caldwell Luc Surgery: Revisited. *Indian J. Otolaryngol. Head Neck Surg.* **2016**, *68*, 90–93. [CrossRef]
17. Lin, Y.; Hu, X.; Metzmacher, A.R.; Luo, H.; Heberer, S.; Nelson, K. Maxillary sinus augmentation following removal of a maxillary sinus pseudocyst after a shortened healing period. *J. Oral Maxillofac. Surg.* **2010**, *68*, 2856–2860. [CrossRef] [PubMed]
18. Giovannetti, F.; Raponi, I.; Priore, P.; Macciocchi, A.; Barbera, G.; Valentini, V. Minimally-Invasive Endoscopic-Assisted Sinus Augmentation. *J. Craniofac. Surg.* **2019**, *30*, e359–e362. [CrossRef] [PubMed]
19. Abu-Ghanem, S.; Kleinman, S.; Horowitz, G.; Balaban, S.; Reiser, V.; Koren, I. Combined maxillary sinus floor elevation and endonasal endoscopic sinus surgery for coexisting inflammatory sinonasal pathologies: A one-stage double-team procedure. *Clin. Oral Implants Res.* **2015**, *26*, 1476–1481. [CrossRef]
20. Chiapasco, M.; Palombo, D. Sinus grafting and simultaneous removal of large antral pseudocysts of the maxillary sinus with a micro-invasive intraoral access. *Int. J. Oral Maxillofac. Surg.* **2015**, *44*, 1499–1505. [CrossRef]
21. Yu, H.; Qiu, L. Histological and clinical outcomes of lateral sinus floor elevation with simultaneous removal of maxillary sinus pseudocysts. *Clin. Implant Dent. Relat. Res.* **2019**, *21*, 94–100. [CrossRef]

22. Yu, H.; Tang, Y.; He, D.; Qiu, L. Immediately or delayed sinus augmentation after pseudocyst removal: A randomized trial. *Clin. Implant Dent. Relat. Res.* **2023**, *25*, 967–973. [CrossRef] [PubMed]
23. Testori, T.; Weinstein, T.; Taschieri, S.; Wallace, S.S. Risk factors in lateral window sinus elevation surgery. *Periodontol. 2000* **2019**, *81*, 91–123. [CrossRef]
24. Testori, T.; Tavelli, L.; Scaini, R.; Saibene, A.M.; Felisati, G.; Barootchi, S.; Decker, A.M.; Deflorian, M.A.; Rosano, G.; Wallace, S.; et al. How to avoid intraoperative and postoperative complications in maxillary sinus elevation. *Periodontol. 2000* **2023**, *92*, 299–328. [CrossRef] [PubMed]
25. Bhattacharyya, N. Do maxillary sinus retention cysts reflect obstructive sinus phenomena? *Arch. Otolaryngol. Head Neck Surg.* **2000**, *126*, 1369–1371. [CrossRef] [PubMed]
26. Timmenga, N.M.; Raghoebar, G.M.; van Weissenbruch, R.; Vissink, A. Maxillary sinus floor elevation surgery. A clinical, radiographic and endoscopic evaluation. *Clin. Oral Implants Res.* **2003**, *14*, 322–328. [CrossRef] [PubMed]
27. Wang, J.H.; Jang, Y.J.; Lee, B.J. Natural course of retention cysts of the maxillary sinus: Long-term follow-up results. *Laryngoscope* **2007**, *117*, 341–344. [CrossRef] [PubMed]
28. Hernandez-Alfaro, F.; Torradeflot, M.M.; Marti, C. Prevalence and management of Schneiderian membrane perforations during sinus-lift procedures. *Clin. Oral Implants Res.* **2008**, *19*, 91–98. [CrossRef]
29. Tükel, H.C.; Tatli, U. Risk factors and clinical outcomes of sinus membrane perforation during lateral window sinus lifting: Analysis of 120 patients. *Int. J. Oral Maxillofac. Surg.* **2018**, *47*, 1189–1194. [CrossRef]
30. Becker, S.T.; Terheyden, H.; Steinriede, A.; Behrens, E.; Springer, I.; Wiltfang, J. Prospective observation of 41 perforations of the Schneiderian membrane during sinus floor elevation. *Clin. Oral Implants Res.* **2008**, *19*, 1285–1289. [CrossRef]
31. Park, W.B.; Kim, J.K.; Kim, Y.J.; Kang, P.; Lim, H.C.; Han, J.Y. Changes in sinus mucosal thickening in the course of tooth extraction and lateral sinus augmentation with surgical drainage: A cone-beam computed tomographic study. *Clin. Oral Implants Res.* **2023**, *34*, 95–104. [CrossRef] [PubMed]
32. An, J.H.; Park, S.H.; Han, J.J.; Jung, S.; Kook, M.S.; Park, H.J.; Oh, H.K. Treatment of dental implant displacement into the maxillary sinus. *Maxillofac. Plast. Reconstr. Surg.* **2017**, *39*, 35. [CrossRef] [PubMed]
33. Park, W.B.; Cho, N.J.; Kang, P. Tomographic Imaging of Mucociliary Clearance Following Maxillary Sinus Augmentation: A Case Series. *Medicina* **2022**, *58*, 672. [CrossRef]
34. Wang, W.B.; Zhang, J.; Ren, L.; Yang, G. Repositioning of the bone window in lateral sinus floor elevation with simultaneous implant placement: A retrospective radiographic study. *Clin. Oral Implants Res.* **2022**, *33*, 816–833. [CrossRef] [PubMed]
35. Tawil, G.; Tawil, P.; Khairallah, A. Sinus Floor Elevation Using the Lateral Approach and Bone Window Repositioning I: Clinical and Radiographic Results in 102 Consecutively Treated Patients Followed from 1 to 5 Years. *Int. J. Oral Maxillofac. Implants* **2016**, *31*, 827–834. [CrossRef]
36. Starch-Jensen, T.; Deluiz, D.; Duch, K.; Tinoco, E.M.B. Maxillary Sinus Floor Augmentation with or without Barrier Membrane Coverage of the Lateral Window: A Systematic Review and Meta-Analysis. *J. Oral Maxillofac. Res.* **2019**, *10*, e1. [CrossRef]

medicina

MDPI

Case Report

The Temporary Mental Nerve Paresthesia as an Outcome of Dentigerous Cyst Removal during Preparation for Dental Implant Placement: A Case Report

Kamil Nelke [1,2,*], Maciej Janeczek [3], Edyta Pasicka [3,*], Krzysztof Żak [2], Marceli Łukaszewski [4], Radosław Jadach [5] and Maciej Dobrzyński [6]

1 Privat Practice of Maxillo-Facial Surgery and Maxillo-Facial Surgery Ward, EMC Hospital, Pilczycka 144, 54-144 Wrocław, Poland
2 Academy of Applied Sciences, Health Department, Academy of Silesius in Wałbrzych, Zamkowa 4, 58-300 Wałbrzych, Poland
3 Department of Biostructure and Animal Physiology, Wrocław University of Environmental and Life Sciences, Kożuchowska 1, 51-631 Wrocław, Poland; maciej.janeczek@upwr.edu.pl
4 Department of Anaesthesiology and Intensive Care, Sokołowski Hospital, Sokołowskiego 4, 58-309 Wałbrzych, Poland
5 Dental Salon Privat Dental Office, Horbaczewskiego 53a, 54-130 Wrocław, Poland
6 Department of Pediatric Dentistry and Preclinical Dentistry, Wrocław Medical University, Krakowska 26, 50-425 Wrocław, Poland
* Correspondence: kamil.nelke@gmail.com (K.N.); edyta.pasicka@upwr.edu.pl (E.P.)

Abstract: The usage of xenograft material is widely used in almost all oral cavity bone defects for regenerative and reconstructive purposes. The presented xenograft usage in the following care report enabled good bone defect healing and enabled the preservation of affected premolars. It is quite common to use any possible variations of bone materials to ensure bone defect improved healing. In some cases, the scope of surgeries requires the removal of each cyst within close proximity to various nerves and vessels. The inferior alveolar, infraorbital, lingual, and mental nerves are those most commonly adjacent to most operating sites in jaw bones. The usage of some additional materials such as collagen sponges, bone substitutes, resorbable membranes, or other additional materials are useful in each bone defect reconstruction but should be handled with care, as described in the following case. Before planning their usage, it is important to perform each surgery with close cone beam computed tomography imaging, which is very helpful to establish the scope of each lesion and the proximity of vital structures. There are a lot of factors that might influence any possible nerve damage, especially the different nerve anatomical variations. Even factors including the subperiosteal preparation and compression of adjacent tissues might influence later nerve function. When the lesion is expanding through the buccal cortical plate and when soft tissue fluctuation is present, some special care is needed. Similar to the presented case, a limitation in crushing, blowing, or any irritation of nerve fibers improves later postoperative outcomes. When the wound and surrounding tissues are handled with care, a limited possibility of any damage or paresthesia can occur. When the nerve itself is damaged or cut, loss of function can be permanent. Immediately after or even prophylactic prescription 1–2 days before the surgery of Vitamin B with NSAIDs (Non-steroidal anti-inflammatory drugs) (or other additional supplementary medicaments can improve nerve function in time. Possible nerve damage can be divided into many etiological factors. A quite different situation arises when the nerve is pulled in by the cyst growth into the cyst wall. The presented case report describes the outcomes of a cyst removal from the mandibular basis and treatment modalities.

Keywords: mandibular cyst; xenograft; mental nerve; case report; bone reconstruction

1. Introduction

In the oral cavity, the main innervation of jaw bones is related to the second and third branches of the trigeminal nerve (CNV). The mental nerve (MN) is a sensory nerve from the posterior trunk of the mandibular nerve (CNV3). It provides sensation to the front of the chin and the lower lip, the gums of the anterior mandibular teeth, the area of the chin and skin, and the mucous membrane of the inner cheek. Problems with the nerve cause the chin, the area of the mouth angle, and part of the lower lip on the affected side numbness (loss of sensation) [1,2]. This situation is related to the scope of mandibular body anatomy, where, just under the lingula of the mandible, the mandibular foramen is located with the inferior alveolar nerve passing to the canal, and the lingual nerve, which descends more medially to the floor of the mouth contained in the structures above the mylohyoid line until the gonial tubercules at the mandibular symphysis area [3]. On the other hand, in the middle of the mandibular body, between the premolar mandibular teeth, a mental nerve foramen is present. In normal conditions, these nerves arise from the mental foramen located inferiorly between the roots of the mandibular premolars. The location of the foramen has some anatomical variations as well. After leaving the mental foramen, the MN divides into three main branches beneath the depressor anguli oris muscle, where one branch descends directly to the chin skin area and two others ascend in the skin and mucous membrane of the lower lip. Some additional nerve fibers can also be seen. These branches communicate and anastomose freely with the facial nerve (CNVII, marginal mandibular and cervical branches) and some fibers of the buccal nerve (CNV3). Accessory mental foramen (AMF) can also be present, along with various nerve fibers (Figure 1) [1–6].

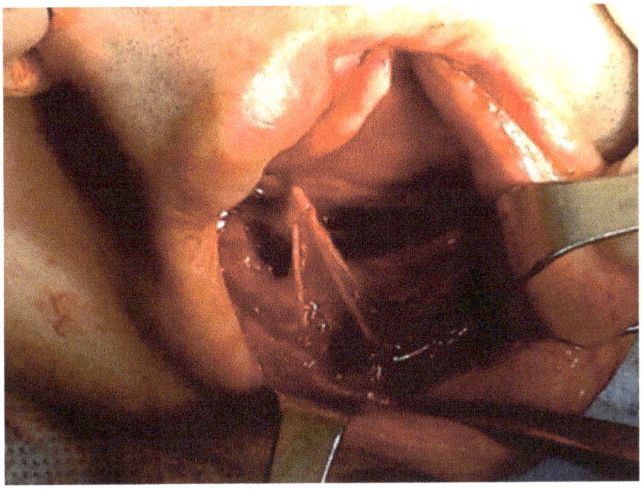

Figure 1. An illustrative figure where the branches of mental nerve are visible during a chin wing osteotomy of the lower border of the mandible during orthognathic surgery.

Possible damage of the mental nerve can be caused by various factors, such as trauma (mandibular fracture); endodontic treatment of mandibular premolars and surgery close to this premolar area (iatrogenic factors (cyst removal)); periapical cyst, abscess, and inflammatory/periapical infections; tumor spread (oral cancer, leukemia, lymphoma (Vincent Sign, tumor spread into the nerve structure)); orthognathic surgery (BSSO-Bilateral Sagittal Split Osteotomy/genioplasty, chin wing approaches); damage to the nerve after abscess drainage; lower lip mucocele removal/labial minor salivary gland retention cyst (nerve fiber damage); local anesthesia administration; compression of the nerve and adjacent tissue pulling; or others [4–10]. These factors might cause transient or permanent paresthesia. Mental nerve paresthesia (MNP) is reported to be a cause of dental treatment (dental implant, trauma, endodontic approaches) in approximately 15–20% of cases. On the other hand, according to the Chai et al. study, because of growing interest in the transoral endoscopic thyroidectomy vestibular approach (TOETVA), many studies indicate that because of the following, in order to minimize MN damage, special anatomical landmarks should be used [8–11].

The type and scope of nerve damage can be described by many classifications. Some injuries to any nerve can be easily described by Seddon's (1942) nerve damage classification, Sunderland's (1951) or Lundborg's (1988), and Mackinnon's (1989). The etiological factors, such as mechanical, chemical, biological, iatrogenic, or other factors, influence the nerve condition and its later degree of regeneration. As reported by Chhabra et al., the Seddon classification is mostly used by electrophysiologists, while the Sunderland grading is more often used by surgeons. Seddon nerve injury is divided into neuropraxia, axonotmesis, and neurotmesis, while the Sunderland classification describes Grades I-V of nerve injuries. Both Grade I and neuropraxia are considered non-degenerative injuries, while the rest are degenerative ones with poorer outcomes [11–14]. The MN scope, and etiology of its damage, influence the type of nerve damage, which can be either transient hypoesthesia, neuropathic pain, trigeminal neuralgia, or partial sensory loss in different anatomical sites. When present, this can be called numb chin syndrome [11–16].

CBCT (cone beam computed tomography) is nowadays a golden standard for the evaluation of any changes in the mandibular and maxillary bones [17]. In cases of cysts and tumors in the bone, not only the shape, size, and diameter of the lesions should be evaluated but also the close proximity of nerves, such as the infraorbital nerve (ION), the lingual nerve (LN), the mental nerve (MN), and the inferior alveolar nerve (IAN) should be closely evaluated. The pathological spread of any lesion in the nerve area might cause some potential nerve damage during any surgery in the jaw bones. Before scheduling any surgical intervention, a good diagnostic approach is mandatory, along with full patient awareness of possible transient or permanent nerve damage. Authors would want to point out their early pharmacological protocol, which can be improved and scheduled even 1–2 days before any major surgery with a close proximity to any nerve structure in the jaw bones.

The following case describes a patient with transient mental nerve injury, who had an instant presurgical pharmacological protocol implemented to affect the possible mental nerve deficiency after the removal of a big radicular cyst in the left mandibular basis as preparation for dental implant procedures.

2. Case Description

A 56-year-old patient was referred for consultation because of a cyst in the left mandibular body that was discovered accidentally during CBCT screening before a dental implant placement. An additional clinical survey chart was scheduled to exclude any other diseases that might influence future outcomes, healing, or complications. Because of the bone defect size, a GBR (guided bone regeneration procedure) was scheduled. The presented case report was written according to CARE (case report guidelines) [17–22].

The cyst had well-defined borders and was situated between two left mandibular premolar roots. The entire left mental nerve (MN) was surrounded by the cyst, while the inferior alveolar nerve was situated just inferiorly from the cyst (Figure 2). The alveolar ridge remained intact. Two teeth, the 34/35, were stable in the bone without any pathological movement. Because of their lack of vital stimulus to cold, an endodontic treatment was planned. Further extraoral examination revealed no changes within the lymph nodes nor other adjacent tissues. The function of the trigeminal nerve was normal. Firstly, some hygienization and scaling were scheduled.

An intraoral examination revealed some swelling near the 34/35 teeth, with slight fluctuation but without crepitation, and a presence of a purulent fistula close to the vestibular surface under the old prosthetic bridge in the area of missing 36 teeth (Figures 3 and 4). The close radiological and clinical evaluation indicated that it was really a granulation tissue with some inflammation. Because this was the first source of an active infection, it was scheduled for an excisional biopsy with curettage (Figure 5).

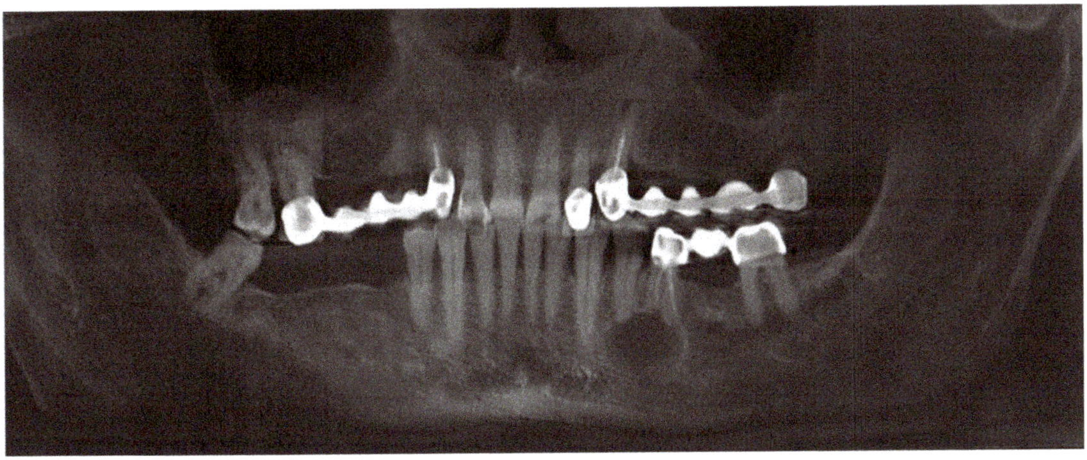

Figure 2. CBCT (cone-beam computed tomography)with clearly visible cyst in the 34/35 area and close proximity of the inferior alveolar nerve.

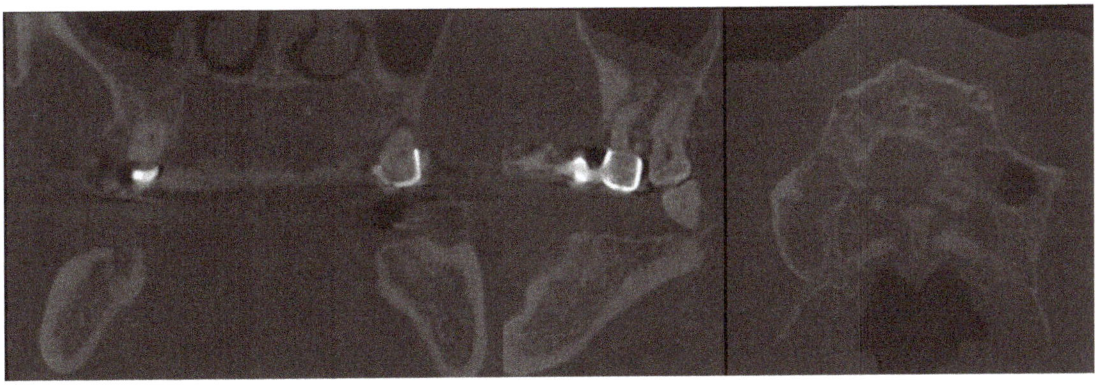

Figure 3. CBCT with visible sources of dental infection. CBCT scans: coronal, sagittal, and axial.

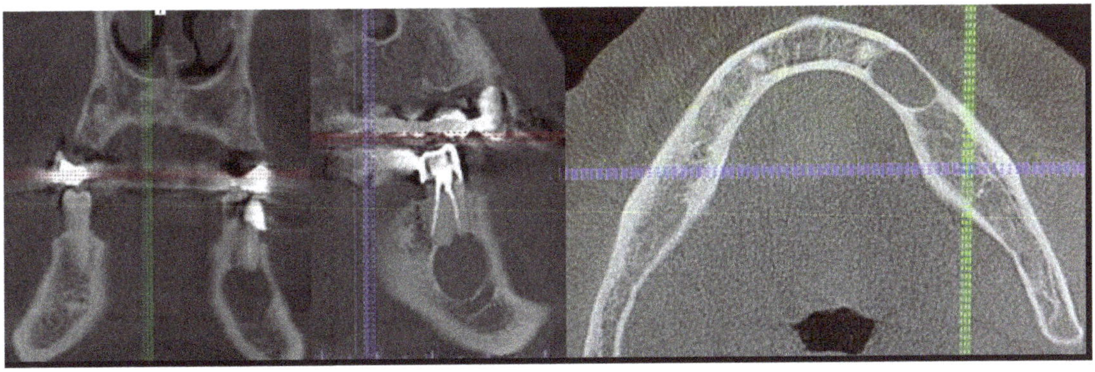

Figure 4. The sagittal, coronal, and axial view of the cystic lesion in the left mandibular basis.

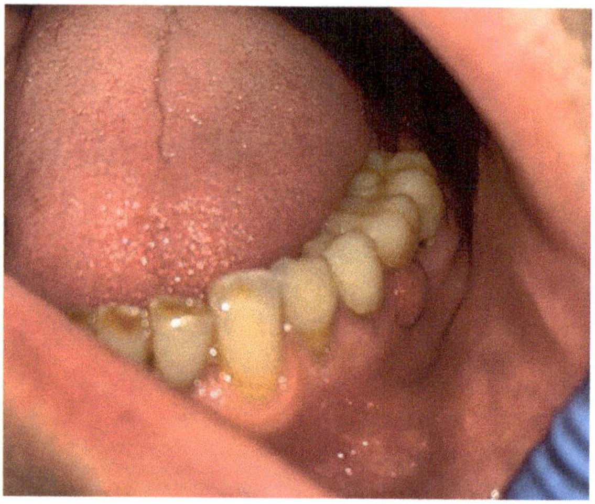

Figure 5. Intraoral photograph with granulation tissues arising from under the dental bridge.

Clinical anamnesis and a clear significant physical examination (PE) revealed additional hypertension and hypothyroidism, which had been under pharmacological control. No other genetic, hereditary, psychosomatic, or other disease or disturbance was noted. Familiar history and past surgical intervention history were unrelated to the current condition. The patient was in an overall good clinical status.

After the preparation of the 34/35 teeth and good endodontic treatment, the granulation tissue was first removed. The histopathological evaluation confirmed the presence of granulation tissues with inflammation. During the same visit, two loosened dental bridges on both sides of the maxilla were removed, along with the 13, 23, and 26/16 teeth because of their poor periodontal status, inflammation periapical lesions, and their pathological mobility in the maxillary arch. After a month, when no signs of infection were noted, the cyst removal was scheduled. Further dental implant treatment was planned after the cyst and other sources of dental inflammations would be removed and tissues would be properly healed (Figures 6 and 7).

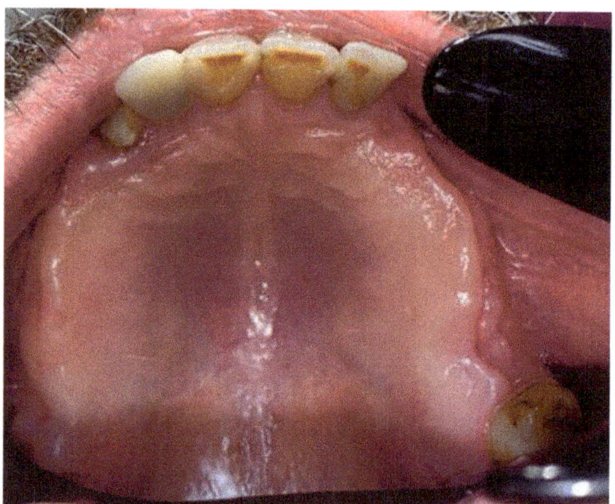

Figure 6. First stages of treatment.

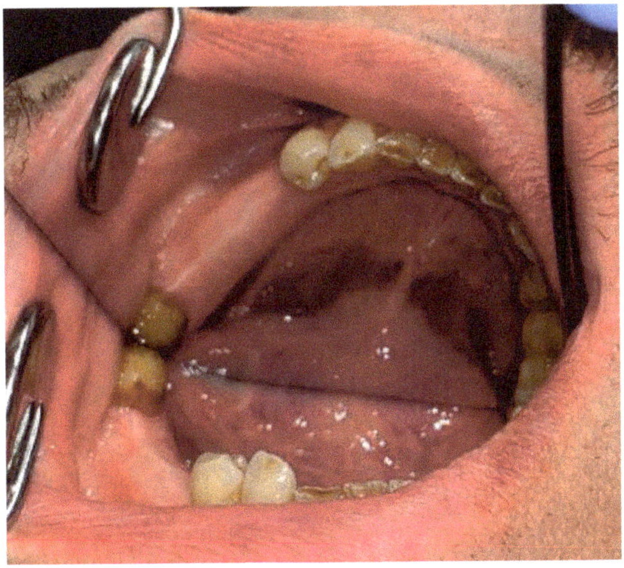

Figure 7. Visible scope of missing teeth scheduled for dental implant placement.

The main surgical approach was scheduled under local anesthesia and consisted of 3ampules (1.7 mL each) of Ubistesin Forte (articaine with epinephrine, 3M, Maplewood, MN, United States). Approximately 60 min before the procedure, the patient took intraoral premedication consisting of 2 g Amotaks (Polfa Tarchomin, Warsaw, Poland), 400 mg Ibuprofen (Polfarmex, Kutno, Poland), and 1 g of Paracetamol (Biofarm, Poznań, Poland). Both the skin and oral cavity were rinsed with Octanisept solution (Schulke, Hamburg, Germany). Surgical draping U-shaped was used (Matopat, TZMO, Toruń, Poland). To ensure good mouth angle and lips lubrication, a sterile Vaseline (Unilever, London, UK) cream was used. The initial incision was made with blade No 15c B (Swann Morton, WR Swann, Owlerton Grn, Hillsborough, Sheffield, UK). A typical horizontal incision approximately 2 mm below the mucogingival fold was used. The horizontal incision was made in the distance between teeth 33–36. The superior part of the flap was not elevated to maintain any contact with the previously treated tissues near 36 area and gingival sulcus surrounding the 34/35 teeth. A Minnesota retractor (Hossa International, Medinstruments, Warsaw, Poland) was used to ensure good visibility. A full-thickness mucoperiosteal flap was elevated inferiorly and in the medial aspect to ensure the subperiosteal elevation until the mental foramen was identified. The Obwegeser Periosteal elevators (Obwegeser 38-630-06-07-38-630-11-07 17.5 cm/6 7/8", KLS Martin, Tuttlingen, Germany) ensured the mental nerve safe retraction with the adjacent mucoperiosteal flap. With the usage of a surgical burr (Lindemann, Aesculap, Tuttlingen, Germany), the thinned buccal cortical plate was removed and the cyst cavity was identified. Surgical curettage and bone debridement were performed. Both tooth apexes of the left mandibular premolar were cut with a surgical burr. Inferiorly, a part of the mandibular canal was visible. Slight bleeding from the IAN canal was secured with BloodSTOP hemostatic dressing (Life Science Plus, Mountain View, San Jose, CA, USA). A total of 1 g xenograft bone (1 g The Graft 0.25–1 mm, Manufacturer Purgo Biologics Inc., Korea) and resorbable collagen membrane (15 $\times$ 20 mm-OsseoGuard Membrane- Zimmer Biomet, Collagen Matrix Inc., Oakland, CA, USA) was used, while the bone substitute was mixed with two iPRF tubes. Centrifuge (Model: MiniFuge, AMD Company, New Delhi, India) was used at 2660 rpm for 12 min. Careful packing on the bone to maintain adequate pressure on the hemostatic dressing helped maintain the bleeding. The MN was repositioned inferiorly with care when the collagen membrane was placed subperiosteally from the superior and inferior aspects of the bone defect. A control CBCT evaluation confirmed a good final surgical outcome (Figure 8). The wound was sutured with 4-0 interrupted vertical mattress sutures (Dafilon, B Braun, Aesculap AG Am Aesculap-Platz, Tuttlingen Germany). The healing period was uneventful; however, the MN temporary MN paresthesia was present for about 6–7 weeks (Figure 9).

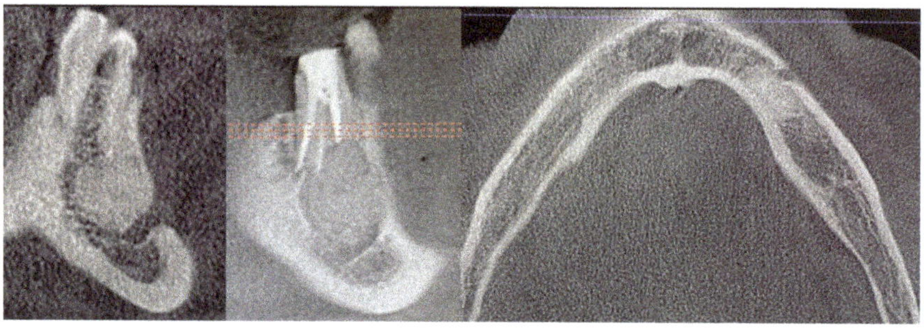

Figure 8. CBCT just after the cyst removal. CBCT presented with the following scans, from the left: coronal, sagittal, and axial. A close proximity to the left mental nerve is seen. Some image disturbances from 3D evaluation are visible.

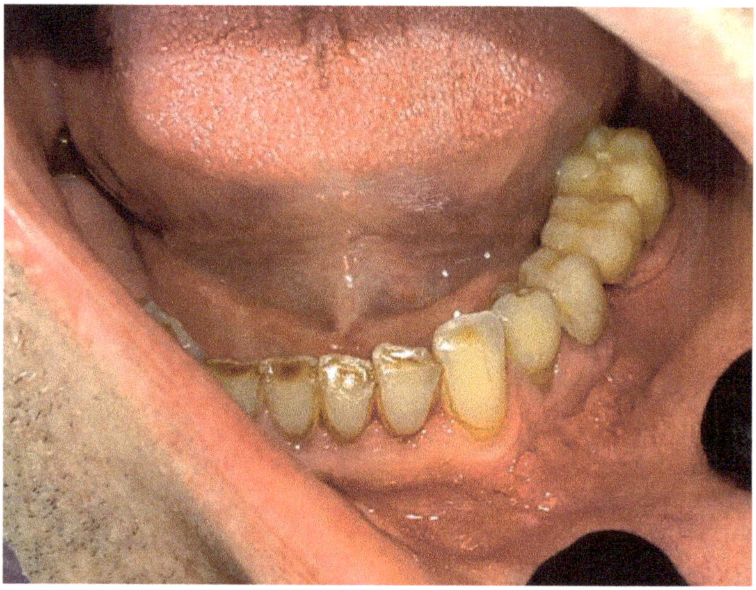

Figure 9. Final view of the operated area after 14 days during suture removal.

The patient continued intraoral antibiotics consisting of Amoxiclav Quick Tab (2 × 1 g—Sandoz Poland, Warsaw, Poland) for seven days and NSAIDs: Ketonal (2 × 0.1 g—Sandoz Poland, Warsaw, Poland) for 3 days, followed by Dexak Sl 0.025 mg three times a day for 5 days (dexketoprofenum, Berlin Chemie Menarini, Berlin, Germany) with Controloc 0.040 mg once a day (pantoprazolum, Takedda Pharma, Tokyo, Japan) for 10 days and local wound care with: 0.1% CHX (chlorhexidine gluconate) (Eludril, Pierre-Fabre Oral care, France) and Alfa Implant Care Mouthwash solution (Atos MM, Warsaw, Poland) was carried away until the 4th week post-operatively. Additional Neurovit 0.32 mg was scheduled two times per day for fifty days in total (1 tabl. Consists of 100 mg wit. B1, 200 mg wit. B6, 0,2 mg wit. B12; 100 tabl.; G.L. Pharma, Gerot-Lannah, Wien, Austria) in the postsurgical period for nerve healing stimulation immediately after the surgery, approximately 4–5 h after the procedure. If the cyst shape, position, and nerve impact is significantly bigger and radiologically relevant, the authors advise to start administration of Vitamin B and NSAIDs 2 days prior to surgery if nerve damage is highly possible. Final outcomes after 1.5 years from surgery are satisfactory with good full oral cavity dental implant rehabilitation procedures (Figures 10 and 11). Further patient prognosis is overall very good and other follow-up appointments have been scheduled.

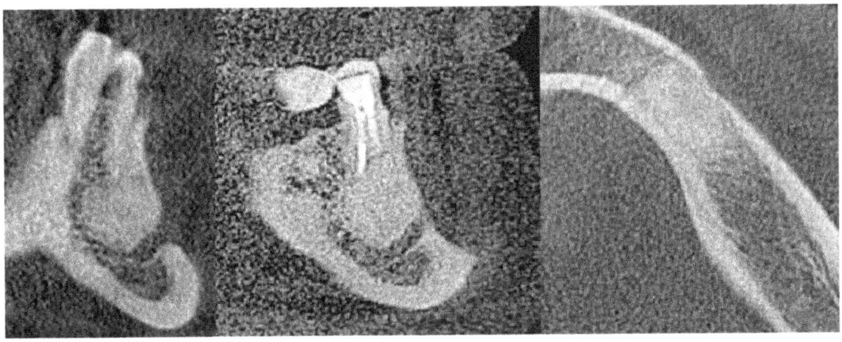

Figure 10. Control CBCT evaluation 1.5 years after a cyst removal. Presented from the left on coronal, sagittal and axial scans. Some image disturbances from 3D evaluation are visible.

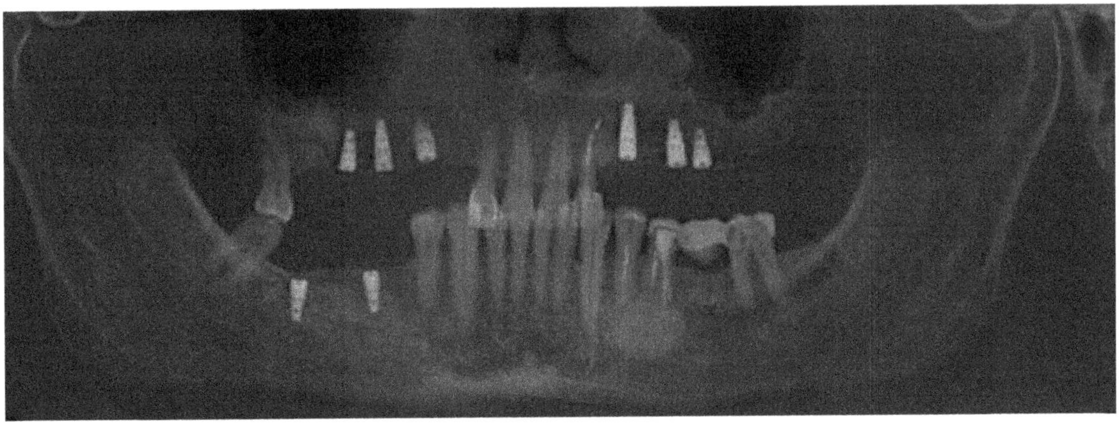

Figure 11. Final result after two years of treatment and dental implant placement.

The MN function in the post-operative period started to improve at the 6th week. Some tingling and stinging was present in the skin of the chin and left mouth angle, while the lip remained numb. The first signs of sensitivity spread in the next 12 weeks and resulted in a total nerve regeneration. Full function was visible at the middle of the 3rd month postoperatively, both in the skin, oral mucosa, lip, mouth angle, and chin area.

3. Discussion

Every cyst removal from the jaw bones requires careful planning and CBCT evaluation. Quite commonly, when additional bone grafting or dental implant procedures will be scheduled simultaneously, the patient should be free of any possible inflammation tissues and one of the various possible dental hygienization protocols should be implemented. Furthermore, when the oral cavity before each surgery is also rinsed with an antiseptic solution, it also improves later outcomes. Any potential inflammation present in the oral cavity influences future dental implant healing [14–18]. Each clinician should carefully plan a step-by-step treatment protocol. This can be achieved by various methods and mostly is related to properly scheduled dental treatment consisting of conservative, periodontal, surgical, and other related procedures to improve the dental status of each patient. It is already known and widely established that any bone surgery in the jaw bones should be scheduled when no active source of inflammation is present in the oral cavity [15–23]. This situation is also quite important, because, if teeth are not free of plaque and bacteria, or even the same can be associated with inappropriately endodontic treated teeth, whose poor dental status might promote inflammation in the operating field and might cause the necessity of secondary surgery close to the operated site and cause even more possible serious damage to the nerve located in such close proximity.

A close anatomical nerve exposure during the procedure reduces its possible damage or palsy. Intraoperative nerve monitoring could be advisable to reduce this damage and to track the MN, especially during TOETVA surgery, while a normal cyst removal from the oral cavity does not require such a method [20–22]. When each nerve is visible and widely exposed, its neuroprotection is more efficient. Factors such as compression, stretching, elevation, and nerve flexion during subperiosteal elevation might lead to MN function deficiencies. When the MN is visible, it is more exposed to any handpiece drills, surgical burrs, and saws; this requires one of the techniques used for its protection. Chhikara et al. described a nerve shield protection technique for different mandibular surgeries [21–23]. Similar methods for protection can be used when a periosteal elevator or a Farabeuf or Minnesota retractor is bone based to secure its stable position and avoid unnecessary lateral movements and inappropriate tissue compression in the MN area [20–25].

Each surgery in the mandibular located between the premolar region should be made with care. Dentigerous cyst enucleation is the most common procedure. A cystectomy procedure sometimes can be combined with bone curettage or can be used as a second approach after a big cyst marsupialization procedure. The scope of many surgical procedures is still widely discussed. Each surgical approach can be related to various factors such as surgeon preferences, the age of the patient, the size of the bone defect that will heal on its own, will require GBR procedures, or can be treated with marsupialization, overall patient good cooperation, the biology of the cyst/tumor, and its histopathological result from a biopsy or other factors [25–27].

Regardless of the type of surgery, each can be burdened by some percentage of possible nerve damage and MN palsy. The discussion on possible oral supplementation for nerve rehabilitation is a topic of many studies. In nerve rehabilitation, a lot of attention is focused on vitamin B12, acetyl-L-carnitine (ALC), adenosine triphosphate/ATP, and others [27–30]. According to Hasegawa et al.'s study on refractory hypoesthesia, the authors highlight that early oral administration of ATP/vitamin B12 should be used in all cases of hypoesthesia. Presented neurosensory deficits tend to improve in time, within 6 months or less. On the other hand, some authors advise some nerve stimulation, physiotherapy, or other agents [27–29]. Moreover, the type of nerve damage influences its healing and future outcome. The Mensink study highlights that chisels and sharp burrs tend to damage more nerve tissues and decrease their healing [30–33]. The novelty of this case presents that early post-operative or even early pre-surgical intervention pharmacological treatment might improve overall nerve healing if the nerve is handled with care during surgery.

In the author's presented case, some key surgical points should be addressed:

1. A close CBCT evaluation before surgery;
2. Elimination of all possible inflammation sources in the oral cavity and pre-surgical hygienization;
3. Good local anesthetic injection into the operation can improve tissue preparation;
4. Local anesthetic injection in the nerve should be avoided;
5. Appropriate visibility to the operated field with retractors and periosteal elevators;
6. Surgical field irrigation with saline for improved visibility;
7. Identification of the nerve in the subperiosteal plane grants more nerve safety;
8. Traction of the adjacent tissues is safer than only nerve traction;

9. MN compression should be limited when retractors are positioned on the bone and not on the MN fibers;
10. When using high-speed drills, good irrigation and visibility should be used;
11. When suturing the wound, any nerve fibers should be identified to avoid their possible damage;
12. Early intraoral vitamin B or other agents should be used;
13. Close patient monitoring after the surgery to avoid any hematoma or purulent formation in the operating area.

Limitations of the following study include the small number of cyst lesion cases located in between premolar tooths and mental nerve foramen. On the other hand, the presented case's strong point could indicate that any similar case of a cyst arising from the jaw bones that is closely related to the inferior alveolar or lingula nerve close proximity can be treated with the same surgical, pharmacological, and subperiosteal elevation technique with good outcomes. Furthermore, a take-away message indicates that CBCT greatly helps each surgeon to avoid unnecessary complications, while a gentle subperiosteal tissue elevation followed by an early postsurgical or a 1–2 day presurgical pharmacological approach also might increase the number of unnecessary complications.

4. Conclusions

Possible nerve damage in different surgery types is related to the type of approaches used, the nerve location within a cyst or a tumor, and the method of nerve preparation and retraction with surgical hooks or subperiosteal elevators. In each situation, it is not only wise to identify the nerve fibers during the radiological examination before the surgery but also to know the surgical field anatomy and be able to identify each nerve fiber and its location during each procedure. If possible damage or injury to the nerve will happen, it is worth informing the patient about possible decreased nerve function after the surgery. Careful nerve retraction and good postoperative care grant more satisfactory outcomes.

Author Contributions: Conceptualization, K.N., M.J. and K.Ż.; methodology, K.N. and R.J.; software, M.J.; validation, K.N., E.P. and M.Ł.; formal analysis, K.N., M.Ł. and R.J.; investigation, K.N.; resources, M.Ł. and K.Ż.; data curation, M.J. and M.D.; writing—original draft preparation, K.N., E.P. and M.D.; writing—review and editing, E.P., K.Ż. and R.J.; visualization, K.N., M.Ł. and R.J.; supervision, M.Ł.; project administration, M.J., M.D., E.P. and K.Ż.; funding acquisition, M.J. and M.D. All authors have read and agreed to the published version of the manuscript.

Funding: This work was financed by a subsidy from Wroclaw Medical University, number SUBZ.B180.23.054.

Institutional Review Board Statement: The study was conducted in accordance with the Declaration of Helsinki and approved by the Bioethics Committee nr 4-BNR-2022. The approval date is 12 October 2022.

Informed Consent Statement: Patient written consent form for publication was granted. Informed consent was obtained from all subjects involved in the study.

Data Availability Statement: Availability of supporting data: the datasets used and/or analyzed during the current study are available from the corresponding author on reasonable request.

Conflicts of Interest: The authors declare no conflict of interest.

References

1. Alsaad, K.; Lee, T.C.; McCartan, B. An anatomical study of the cutaneous branches of the mental nerve. *Int. J. Oral Maxillofac. Surg.* **2003**, *32*, 325–333. [CrossRef]
2. Won, S.Y.; Yang, H.M.; Woo, H.S.; Chang, K.Y.; Youn, K.H.; Kim, H.J.; Hu, K.S. Neuroanastomosis and the innervation territory of the mental nerve. *Clin. Anat.* **2014**, *27*, 598–602. [CrossRef]
3. Bernardi, S.; Angelone, A.M.; Macchiarelli, G. Anatomy in dentistry: From the beginnings to contemporary reality. *Clin. Anat.* **2022**, *35*, 711–722. [CrossRef] [PubMed]

4. Hu, K.S.; Yun, H.S.; Hur, M.S.; Kwon, H.J.; Abe, S.; Kim, H.J. Branching patterns and intraosseous course of the mental nerve. *J. Oral Maxillofac. Surg.* **2007**, *65*, 2288–2294. [CrossRef]
5. Iwanaga, J.; Haikata, Y.; Nakamura, K.; Kusukawa, J.; Watanabe, K.; Tubbs, R.S. An anatomical and histological study of mental nerve branches to the inferior labial glands. *Surg. Radiol. Anat.* **2021**, *43*, 1801–1804. [CrossRef]
6. Kieser, J.; Kuzmanovic, D.; Payne, A.; Dennison, J.; Herbison, P. Patterns of emergence of the human mental nerve. *Arch. Oral Biol.* **2002**, *47*, 743–747. [CrossRef] [PubMed]
7. Sen, O.G.; Kaplan, V. Temporary Mental Nerve Paresthesia Originating from Periapical Infection. *Case Rep. Dent.* **2015**, *2015*, 457645. [CrossRef]
8. Aljarbou, F.; Riyahi, A.M.; Altamimi, A.; Alabdulsalam, A.; Jabhan, N.; Aldosimani, M.; Alamri, H.M. Anatomy of the accessory mental foramen in a Saudi subpopulation: A multicenter CBCT study. *Saudi Dent. J.* **2021**, *33*, 1012–1017. [CrossRef]
9. Patel, N.; Langaliya, A.; Kanodia, S.; Kumbhar, A.; Buch, A.; Shah, A.; Bhatt, H.; Panchal, D.; Shah, S.; Shah, J. Mental Nerve Paraesthesia: A Report of Two Cases Associated with Endodontic Etiology. *Case Rep. Dent.* **2021**, *2021*, 1747519. [CrossRef]
10. Kumar, U.; Kaur, C.K.; Vashisht, R.; Rattan, V. Paresthesia diagnosed using cone-beam computed tomography: A case report. *J. Dent. Anesth. Pain Med.* **2020**, *20*, 95–99. [CrossRef] [PubMed]
11. Chai, Y.J.; Chae, S.; Oh, M.Y.; Kwon, H.; Park, W.S. Transoral Endoscopic Thyroidectomy Vestibular Approach (TOETVA): Surgical Outcomes and Learning Curve. *J. Clin. Med.* **2021**, *10*, 863. [CrossRef]
12. Chhabra, A.; Ahlawat, S.; Belzberg, A.; Andreseik, G. Peripheral nerve injury grading simplified on MR neurography: As referenced to Seddon and Sunderland classifications. *Indian J. Radiol. Imaging* **2014**, *24*, 217–224. [CrossRef] [PubMed]
13. Thakkar, R.S.; Del Grande, F.; Thawait, G.K.; Andreisek, G.; Carrino, J.A.; Chhabra, A. Spectrum of high-resolution MRI findings in diabetic neuropathy. *Am. J. Roentgenol.* **2012**, *199*, 407–412. [CrossRef]
14. Chhabra, A.; Thakkar, R.S.; Andreisek, G.; Chalian, M.; Belzberg, A.J.; Blakeley, J. Anatomic MR imaging and functional diffusion tensor imaging of peripheral nerve tumors and tumorlike conditions. *Am. J. Neuroradiol.* **2013**, *34*, 802–807. [CrossRef] [PubMed]
15. Seddon and Sunderland Classification of Nerve Injury. Available online: https://www.ncbi.nlm.nih.gov/books/NBK557746/figure/article-25766.image.f1/ (accessed on 9 February 2023).
16. Do, T.A.; Le, H.S.; Shen, Y.W.; Huang, H.L.; Fuh, L.J. Risk Factors related to Late Failure of Dental Implant-A Systematic Review of Recent Studies. *Int. J. Environ. Res. Public Health* **2020**, *17*, 3931. [CrossRef] [PubMed]
17. Varvara, G.; Feragalli, B.; Turkyilmaz, I.; D'Alonzo, A.; Rinaldi, F.; Bianchi, S.; Piattelli, M.; Macchiarelli, G.; Bernardi, S. Prevalence and Characteristics of Accessory Mandibular Canals: A Cone-Beam Computed Tomography Study in a European Adult Population. *Diagnostics* **2022**, *12*, 1885. [CrossRef]
18. Fatani, B.; Almutairi, E.S.; Almalky, H.A.; Mubarki, M.I.; Al-Safadi, A. A Comparison of Knowledge and Skills Related to Up-to-Date Implant Techniques Among Prosthodontists, Periodontists, and Oral Surgeons: A Cross-Sectional Study. *Cureus* **2022**, *14*, 30370. [CrossRef]
19. The CARE Guidelines (for CAse REports) Were Developed. Available online: https://www.care-statement.org/checklist (accessed on 16 March 2023).
20. Yao, L.; Xu, X.; Ren, M.; Liu, D.; Ni, Z.; Lin, F. Inflammatory dentigerous cyst of mandibular first premolar associated with endodontically treated primary first molar: A rare case report. *Eur. J. Paediatr. Dent.* **2015**, *16*, 201–204. [PubMed]
21. Golob Deeb, J.; Deeb, G.R.; Schafer, D.R. Odontogenic Keratocyst Is Frequently Misdiagnosed for a Lateral Periodontal Cyst in Premolar and Anterior Tooth-Bearing Areas. *J. Endod.* **2022**, *48*, 337–344. [CrossRef]
22. Wu, Z.; Fang, J.G.; Chen, X.; Hou, L.Z.; Zhong, Q.; Ma, H.Z.; Zhang, Y.; Shen, X.X. Protection of nerve function during transoral endoscopic thyroidectomy by vestibular approach. *Zhonghua Er Bi Yan Hou Tou Jing Wai Ke Za Zhi* **2020**, *55*, 893–898.
23. Chhikara, D.; Singh, V.; Bhagol, A.; Dahiya, A. Mental nerve shielding from possible injury during mandibular surgical procedures: Technical note. *Int. J. Oral Maxillofac. Surg.* **2023**. [CrossRef]
24. Ruan, J.; Yang, X.; Zhao, J.G.; Tao, L.; Ning, X.J.; He, F.; Zhou, C.Y.; Zhou, C.; Karcz, W.K. Axillary channel-assisted TOETVA: An effective way to prevent mental nerve from iatrogenic injury? *J. Minim. Access. Surg.* **2022**, *18*, 450–458.
25. Kajjari, S.; Gowtham, A.; Meharwade, P.; Uppin, C.; Hugar, S.M.; Badakar, C. Infected Radicular Cyst of Deciduous Second Molar Mimicking Dentigerous Cyst of Second Premolar in a Young Child: A Rare Entity. *Int. J. Clin. Pediatr. Dent.* **2021**, *14*, 434–437. [PubMed]
26. Hyomoto, M.; Kawakami, M.; Inoue, M.; Kirita, T. Clinical conditions for eruption of maxillary canines and mandibular premolars associated with dentigerous cysts. *Am. J. Orthod. Dentofac. Orthop.* **2003**, *124*, 515–520. [CrossRef]
27. Vinereanu, A.; Bratu, A.; Didilescu, A.; Munteanu, A. Management of large inflammatory dentigerous cysts adapted to the general condition of the patient: Two case reports. *Exp. Ther. Med.* **2021**, *22*, 750. [CrossRef] [PubMed]
28. Hasegawa, T.; Yamada, S.I.; Ueda, N.; Soutome, S.; Funahara, M.; Akashi, M.; Furuno, S.; Miyamoto, H.; Hayashida, S.; Amano, R.; et al. Treatment modalities and risk factors associated with refractory neurosensory disturbances of the inferior alveolar nerve following oral surgery: A multicentre retrospective study. *Int. J. Oral Maxillofac. Surg.* **2018**, *47*, 794–801. [CrossRef]
29. Traina, G. The neurobiology of acetyl-L-carnitine. *Front. Biosci.* **2016**, *21*, 1314–1329. [CrossRef]
30. Ali, A.S.; Benton, J.A.; Yates, J.M. Risk of inferior alveolar nerve injury with coronectomy vs surgical extraction of mandibular third molars-A comparison of two techniques and review of the literature. *J. Oral Rehabil.* **2018**, *45*, 250–257. [CrossRef] [PubMed]

31. Mohajerani, S.H.; Tabeie, F.; Bemanali, M.; Tabrizi, R. Effect of Low-Level Laser and Light-Emitting Diode on Inferior Alveolar Nerve Recovery After Sagittal Split Osteotomy of the Mandible: A Randomized Clinical Trial Study. *J. Craniofac. Surg.* **2017**, *28*, 408–411. [CrossRef] [PubMed]
32. Mensink, G.; Gooris, P.J.; Bergsma, J.E.; van Hooft, E.; van Merkesteyn, J.P. Influence of BSSO surgical technique on postoperative inferior alveolar nerve hypoesthesia: A systematic review of the literature. *J. Cranio-Maxillofac. Surg.* **2014**, *42*, 976–982. [CrossRef]
33. Degerliyurt, K.; Akar, V.; Denizci, S.; Yucel, E. Bone lid technique with piezosurgery to preserve inferior alveolar nerve. *Oral Surg. Oral Med. Oral Pathol. Oral Radiol. Endod.* **2009**, *108*, 1–5. [CrossRef] [PubMed]

MDPI AG
Grosspeteranlage 5
4052 Basel
Switzerland
Tel.: +41 61 683 77 34

Medicina Editorial Office
E-mail: medicina@mdpi.com
www.mdpi.com/journal/medicina

www.ingramcontent.com/pod-product-compliance
Lightning Source LLC
Chambersburg PA
CBHW062042220926
51850CB00010B/2642
* 9 7 8 3 7 2 5 8 6 5 2 0 8 *